D1129834

Parasitology
for
Veterinarians

FOURTH EDITION

JAY R. GEORGI, D.V.M., Ph.D.

Professor of Parasitology
New York State College of Veterinary Medicine
Cornell University
Ithaca, New York

With a chapter on Antiparasitic Drugs *by*

Vassilios J. Theodorides, D.V.M., Ph.D.

Manager, Parasitology and Toxicology
SmithKline Animal Health Products
West Chester, Pennsylvania

And a chapter on Histopathological Diagnosis *by*

Marion E. Georgi, D.V.M.

Director of the Laboratory of Parasitology
New York State College of Veterinary Medicine
Cornell University
Ithaca, New York

W. B. SAUNDERS COMPANY

PHILADELPHIA   LONDON   TORONTO   MEXICO CITY   RIO DE JANEIRO   SYDNEY   TOKYO

W. B. Saunders Company: West Washington Square
Philadelphia, PA   19105

1 St. Anne's Road
Eastbourne, East Sussex BN21 3UN, England

1 Goldthorne Avenue
Toronto, Ontario M8Z 5T9, Canada

Apartado 26370—Cedro 512
Mexico 4, D.F., Mexico

Rua Coronel Cabrita, 8
Sao Cristovao Caixa Postal 21176
Rio de Janeiro, Brazil

9 Waltham Street
Artarmon, N.S.W. 2064, Australia

Ichibancho, Central Bldg., 22-1 Ichibancho
Chiyoda-Ku, Tokyo 102, Japan

Library of Congress Cataloging in Publication Data

Georgi, Jay R., 1928-
    Parasitology for veterinarians.

    1. Veterinary parasitology.   I. Title.
    SF810.A3G4   1985   636.089′696   84-10531
    ISBN 0–7216–1176–1

Cover photograph: Scanning electron micrograph of *Ctenocephalides* by
            Dr. Marguerite Frongillo.

Parasitology for Veterinarians   ISBN   0–7216–1176–1

Last digit is the print number: 9   8   7   6   5   4   3   2

PREFACE

My objectives in preparing a fourth edition of *Parasitology for Veterinarians* are first, to introduce veterinary students to those aspects of parasitology that they will find useful in their careers, and second, to provide them, as veterinarians, with a practical reference.

The text is divided into three parts. Chapters One through Six present a systematic introduction to the identification, life history, and pathogenesis of parasitic arthropods, protozoans, and helminths; the relationships of these parasites to animal and human health are emphasized. Chapters Seven through Ten are devoted to treatment and control of parasitisms of domestic carnivorans, ruminants, horses, and swine, taking into consideration the influences of parasite life history and epidemiology, behavior of domestic animals, and contemporary animal management practices. In Chapter Eleven, Dr. Vassilios J. Theodorides has characterized almost all of the insecticidal, antiprotozoal, and anthelmintic chemicals in current use with respect to their physical and chemical properties, posology, and indications and contraindications. Chapters Twelve through Fourteen are devoted to techniques of antemortem, postmortem, and histopathological diagnosis that ease the task of the non-specialist by exploiting host and site specificity as adjuncts to parasite morphology. Dr. Marion E. Georgi's chapter on histopathological diagnosis is new with this edition and is intended to assist the laboratory diagnostician and pathologist in identifying protozoan and metazoan parasites in tissue sections and to provide the general reader with information on their structural organization. This reorganization of text has eliminated much duplication in the presentation of information and illustrations. I hope that it will also make the book more interesting and easier to read.

Line drawings are the standard form of taxonomic illustration but students seem to have greater success in identifying specimens when they have photomicrographs to refer to instead. Therefore, I have replaced almost all of the many fine drawings, borrowed from other sources for previous editions, with photomicrographs. This effort kept me in the darkroom for a very long time and I am greatly indebted to Diane Moorman and Kay Georgi for taking those labors out of my hands for an entire summer.

I am preparing a set of videotapes that instructors may find helpful in orienting students for practical laboratory exercises in diagnostic parasitology. At present, the following titles are available:

1. Two Sheep Killers: Flystrike and Haemonchosis (27:00)
2. Identification of Ticks and Mites (18:55)
3. Identification of Nematodes (18:00)

4. Identification of Trematodes (9:40)
5. Parasitic Protozoans I: Flagellates, Ciliates, and Amebas (9:27)
6. Coprological Techniques (16:16)
7. Qualitative Coprology of the Dog and Cat (14:00)
8. Diagnosis of Canine Heartworm Infection (7:27)
9. Identification of Flies of Domestic Animals (18:00)
10. Life Histories of Parasitic Flies (18:00)
11. Identification of Lice and Fleas (11:55)

This whole set of videotapes is available for review by educational institutions. For information, write to:

Biomedical Communications
New York State College of Veterinary Medicine
Cornell University
Ithaca, New York 14853

JAY R. GEORGI

CONTENTS

ONE

PARASITIC ARTHROPODS, PROTOZOANS, AND HELMINTHS

A *parasite* is a smaller organism that lives on or in and at the expense of a larger organism called the *host*. A louse is a parasite and so is a virus. The host's expenses in supporting its parasites may be trivial or they may be substantial or even unbearable. This will depend on the number of parasites, the kind and degree of injury they inflict, and the vigor and nourishment of the host. A series of terms (e.g., mutualism, commensalism, parasitism) have been defined to express the degree of unilateral or mutual injury or benefit that is characteristic of particular symbiotic relationships. As a matter of convention, however, if the smaller organism is found in association with man or with animals or plants that man esteems, it is called a parasite, whether its presence is detrimental, indifferent, or beneficial. This convention is harmless enough provided we remember that parasites vary in pathogenicity.

A *species* of animal is an interbreeding natural population that is reproductively isolated from other such populations. For example, there are two species of ascarid parasites of dogs, *Toxocara canis* and *Toxascaris leonina*. These two species are sufficiently similar in size and appearance to present some difficulty in their differentiation, but though they may share the small intestine of the same dog, they never interbreed. The consequent distinctness of their genetic material is expressed in modest differences in structue and in very substantial differences in life history. On the other hand, *T. canis* and *T. leonina* share enough similarities to make their kinship obvious. We assume that this similarity stems from the evolution of both species from common ancestral stock (divergent evolution), because the number and nature of the similarities induce us to reject the alternative explanation, i.e., that they represent the adaptations of unrelated forms to the same selection pressures (convergent evolution). We recognize the kinship of *T. canis* and *T. leonina* by considering them both to be members of the same zoological order (Ascaridida); each is a leaf, if you will, on the same evolutionary branch.

Unfortunately, for those who seek perfection in the correspondence of their classification schemes to the true history of evolution, there is very little objective evidence for the kinship of worms. The progenitors of the horse (*Equus caballus*) left a clear fossil record of equine evolution, but the ancestors of our worms merely rotted and withered away, leaving only an occasional trace. The entire hierarchy of taxonomic categories above that of species (i.e., genus, subfamily, family, superfamily, suborder, order, class, phylum) is built of subjective inductions based on degrees of similarity and dissimilarity among the various groups of organisms. Fortunately, the result is nonetheless useful to us in organizing our information about parasites in an orderly and logical way. In short, any particular zoological classification scheme is no more than an opinion about how the relationships among various groups of organisms may best be expressed.

It is helpful to be acquainted with a few nomenclatorial conventions. The full zoological name of an animal is a binomen consisting of the genus name followed by the species name. The genus name is capitalized and both genus and species names are italicized in print or underlined in manuscript, e.g., *Filaroides milksi*. In taxonomic publications and in other scientific and professional journals, the zoological name is followed by the name of the person who described the species in question and the date that the description was first published, e.g., *Filaroides milksi* Whitlock, 1956. If, at a later date, another taxonomist decides for one reason or another that this particular species really ought to belong to a different genus, the original describer's name is now placed in parentheses and the name of the taxonomist that moved the species may follow outside the parentheses, e.g., *Andersonstrongylus milksi* (Whitlock, 1956) Webster, 1981. We are not forced to accept Webster's opinion and may continue to call this species by its original name, *Filaroides milksi*, if we feel that we have good reason to do so. The species *milksi* is objective in that it is based on real and tangible specimens that Whitlock studied and described in 1956. Assigning *milksi* to any particular genus is, on the other hand, largely subjective and based on *taxonomic judgement*. That is why we frequently come across the same species relegated to two or even more genera.

Certain categories have characteristic suffixes that help to identify them. For example, the genus *Strongylus* belongs to the following hierarchy of higher taxa: subfamily Strongylinae, family Strongylidae, superfamily Strongyloidea, order Strongylida. In this text, the suffixes -inae, -idae-, -oidea, and -ida are respectively applied to all subfamily, family, superfamily, and order names.

The principal objectives of zoological nomenclature are to promote stability and universality of zoological names and to ensure that each name is unique and distinct. Not every taxonomist is hard at work "changing the names to confuse the innocent," as students are prone to suspect.

1

INSECTS

PHYLUM ARTHROPODA

Well over three quarters of the million or so species of animals that inhabit the earth belong to the phylum Arthropoda, to which the insects belong. Fortunately, the arthropod parasites and disease vectors of domestic animals and man compose only a small fraction of this overwhelming horde. The body of a typical arthropod is composed of a series of segments, some of which bear jointed legs. Not all arthropods display these characteristics. Thus, body segmentation has all but disappeared with the evolution of the mites and ticks, and many insect larvae have no legs. Adaptation to parasitism has led to extreme deviation in body form in certain cases. For example, mites of the genus *Demodex* have evolved into tiny cigar-shaped organisms that fit comfortably into the hair follicles and sebaceous glands of the skin. An even more extreme example is provided by *Sacculina*, a relative of barnacles that grows like a plant's root system in the body of its crab host. However, most parasitic arthropods resemble their free-living relatives morphologically but differ from them in quite remarkable physiological and behavioral adaptations to the parasitic mode of life. Thus, the bloodsucking stable fly, horn fly, and tsetse fly much resemble their scavenging cousin, the common house fly, and there is no obvious morphological difference between the many species of maggots that thrive in decaying plant and animal matter and the "screwworm" that completes its larval development in living flesh. The resemblance of certain parasites to their free-living relatives creates a diagnostic pitfall. Even presence at the scene of the crime is not sufficient proof of guilt. Fly maggots and coprophilic beetles are frequently found in fecal specimens. In almost every such case, these insects have invaded the fecal mass after defecation and never were parasites at all.

Unfortunately, even when we restrict our consideration to unambiguously parasitic arthropods, we still have too big a chore on our hands. Medical entomology is a formidable subject and the selection of appropriate information is not always an easy task because certain topics that at first appear to bear directly on current problems of veterinary practice actually lie within the responsibilities of very few veterinarians. For example, information on mosquitoes may occupy half of a textbook of medical entomology, and mosquitoes serve as vectors of such important diseases as equine encephalomyelitis and canine heartworm infection. However, few veterinarians invest the time and effort necessary to acquire a detailed knowledge of mosquitoes because control of these pests is usually the responsibility of the medical entomologist. Of more direct interest to veterinarians are the kinds of parasitic arthropods that live in more prolonged and intimate association with domestic animals. In this book, considerably more attention is therefore devoted to lice, fleas, ticks, and mites than to mosquitoes.

The arthropods of veterinary importance belong to the classes Insecta, Arachnida, Pentastomida, Crustacea, and Diplopoda. Insects are considered in this chapter and arachnids in the next. The class Pentastomida, or "tongue worms," comprises a small group of parasites of the respiratory passages of predacious reptiles, birds, and mammals. Although they are highly specialized arthropods, the pentastomids are briefly considered under "Miscellaneous Wormlike Taxa" at the end of Chapter 6 because they look and behave very much like parasitic worms; they even undergo nymphal development in intermediate hosts. The class Crustacea (copepods, crabs, crayfish, and sowbugs) contains many taxa that serve as intermediate hosts (i.e., vectors) of helminth parasites. The class Diplopoda (millipedes) contains at least one genus, *Narceus*, that serves as intermediate host of *Macracanthorhynchus ingens*, a very large acanthocephalan parasite of the raccoon and domestic dog. Crustaceans and diplopods are mentioned only in passing in this book.

CLASS INSECTA

Structure. The body of adult insects consists of *head, thorax,* and *abdomen.* The head consists of a variable number of fused segments and bears two *eyes,* two *antennae,* and a complex set of *mouthparts.* The thorax consists of three segments, the *pro-, meso-,* and *metathorax,* and bears six jointed *legs* and four, two, or no *wings,* depending on the zoological order to which the insect in question belongs. Thus, roaches (Dictyoptera), beetles (Coleoptera), and certain bugs (Hemiptera) have four wings, most flies (Diptera) have two, and the lice (Mallophaga and Anoplura) and fleas (Siphonaptera) are wingless. When four wings are present, one pair arises from the mesothorax and the second pair from the metathorax. The functional wings of Diptera arise from the mesothorax. The abdomen consists of 11 or fewer segments of which the terminal ones are modified for copulation or egg laying. As typical arthropods, insects have a *chitinous cuticle* that is secreted by the *hypodermis,* a single layer of columnar epithelial cells of ectodermal origin, and cast off or *molted* at intervals to permit growth and metamorphosis. The chitinous cuticle serves as an *exoskeleton,* thus both a body covering and a place for attachment of muscles. Heavily chitinized areas or plates of cuticle are connected by thinner, lightly chitinized areas, thus permitting movement and some degree of expansion as, for example, when the abdomen of a feeding female mosquito fills with blood. Insect muscles are striated and often capable of extraordinarily rapid contraction. The cuticle is overlain by a thin lipoidal surface layer, the *epicuticle,* which is impermeable to water but freely permeable to lipids and lipid-soluble substances. Disruption of the epicuticle by silica aerogel insecticides results in death of the insect by dehydration; such insecticides are thus physically rather than chemically active.

When a developing insect has grown too large for its cuticle, the hypodermis lays down a new, thin, elastic cuticle under the old one. The old cuticle then splits and the insect emerges from it. This process, termed *molting* or *ecdysis,* divides the life of the individual insect into a series of *stages* or *instars.* All instars of cockroaches, bugs, and lice resemble their parents except for being smaller, whereas a newly hatched fly, beetle, or flea looks more like a worm than an insect. The former situation is called *simple metamorphosis* and the series of juvenile instars are called *nymphs,* whereas the latter situation is called *complex metamorphosis* and the juvenile instars are called *larvae.* In complex metamorphosis, the complete restructuring necessary for the transformation of the wormlike larva into the adult insect takes place during the *pupal* stage and all related events are referred to as *pupation.*

Order Diptera, Flies

All adult flies, except certain specialized parasites of the family Hippoboscidae, have one pair of functional mesothoracic wings. The metathoracic pair are represented by club-shaped balancing organs called *halteres* (Fig. 1-1), which are present even in the wingless hippoboscids. Metamorphosis is complex. Most flies are oviparous but a few deposit larvae that have already hatched. Hippoboscids and tsetse flies retain their larvae within their abdomens through the third larval instar and these pupate almost immediately upon being born. There are three main groups of flies: the gnats and mosquitoes of the suborder Nematocera, the horse flies and deer flies of the suborder Brachycera, and the more highly evolved flies of the suborder Cyclorrhapha. All three contain bloodsucking species, many of which serve as disease vectors. Larvae of calliphorid and oestrid cyclorrhaphans invade living tissues to produce a pathological condition called *myiasis.*

SUBORDER NEMATOCERA

Nematocerans are typically small and relatively delicate. The antennae are long and many-segmented and the individual segments resemble one another like beads on a string. Nematocerans generally breed in aquatic or semiaquatic habitats and their larvae are suitably endowed with appendages for swimming, breathing, and gathering food

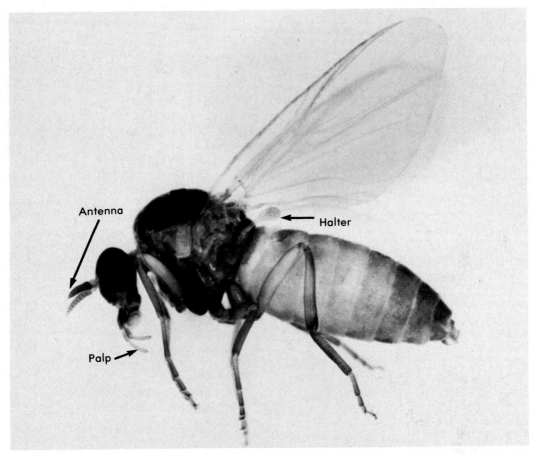

Figure 1–1. *Simulium* (Nematocera: Simuliidae), a black fly (x24). The halteres (sing., halter) are balancing organs that have evolved in Diptera in place of the metathoracic wings. The maxillary palpi are sensory structures associated with the mouthparts. The antennae of black flies consist of 11 similar segments.

in water. Only female nematocerans suck blood; the males never do and subsist instead on nectar.

FAMILY CULICIDAE, MOSQUITOES

Identification. Mosquitoes have long, 14- or 15-segmented antennae, an elongated proboscis consisting of a bundle of stylets loosely encased in a sheath formed by the labium, and fringes of scales on the wings (Fig. 1-2). These anatomical details are sufficient *taxonomic characters* to reliably distinguish the *taxon* that we recognize as mosquitoes from other insects with which they might be confused. Students occasionally make the mistake of developing their own criteria for identifying various taxa. This seems laudable in that it reflects a degree of creativity but it is a poor policy from the standpoint of diagnostic accuracy. Avoid the attractive pitfall of reinventing taxonomy; you don't have a century in which to do it. Instead, learn the

characters that experienced taxonomists have found to be reliable.

Life History. Mosquitoes lay their eggs on water or in dry places that tend to flood seasonally. Eggs laid on water hatch in less than a week. Larvae (Fig. 1-3) are air breathers and die within hours if their air supply is shut off by an oil film on the water's surface. The larvae molt four times, usually within the space of two weeks, and then pupate. As is characteristic of all nematocerans and brachycerans, the pupa emerges through a T-shaped hole in the back of the last larval skin. Culicid pupae are elaborate, free-swimming organisms with a large cephalothorax. As development proceeds, the structures of the adult mosquito become apparent (Fig. 1-4). The pupal stage ordinarily lasts from two days to a week but a few hours suffice for certain dry climate species. The adult mosquito emerges through a hole in the back of the pupal case as it floats at the water's surface. After about 24 hours, the

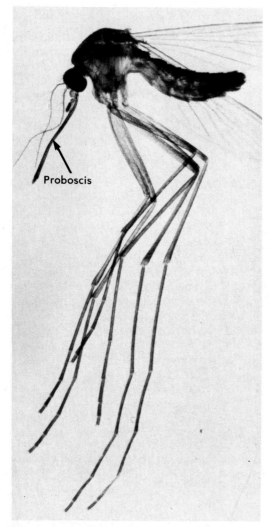

Figure 1–2. A mosquito (Nematocera: Culicidae) (x13). Note the long antennae and long mouthparts (proboscis).

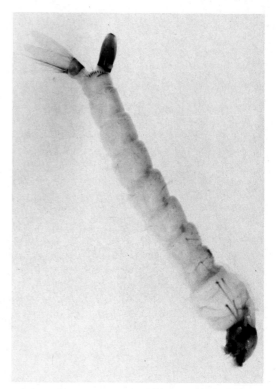

Figure 1–3. Mosquito larva (x15).

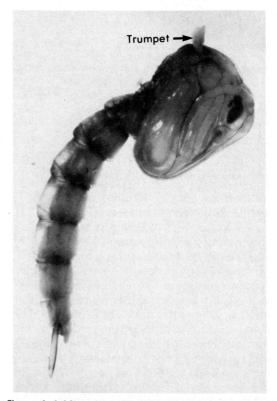

Figure 1–4. Mosquito pupa (x16). The "trumpets" on the cephalothorax are pupal respiratory structures. The eyes, legs, thorax, and abdomen of the developing adult mosquito can be seen through the pupal cuticle.

wings have expanded and hardened and the mosquito is able to fly. Only female mosquitoes suck blood, the protein of which is necessary for the maturation of the ovaries. Males and nonreproductive females get by on nectar and plant juices. In fact, there are species of mosquitoes that feed only on plants and others that normally feed on blood but in which ovarian maturation may occur without a blood meal. However, these species are of little interest as pests or disease vectors. Mammals and birds are preferred hosts (or victims) both of mosquitoes and of the various disease organisms that they transmit.

Injury. Under ordinary circumstances, the amount of blood lost to mosquito attack is entirely trivial. Sometimes, however, circumstances favor the simultaneous emergence of such enormous swarms of mosquitoes that cattle can actually be bled to death by their concerted attacks. For example, seven days after hurricane Allen (Aug. 10, 1980) brought a prolonged drought to an abrupt end and flooded 5000 acres of a Texas ranch, cattle were observed to be visibly distressed by swarms of *Aedes sollicitans* mosquitoes. The next morning, 15 cattle were found dead of exsanguination manifested by extreme pallor of the mucous membranes and postmortal evidence of severe anemia. The interval of seven days between flooding of the pastures and the sudden death of the cattle corresponded exactly to the time required for *Aedes sollicitans* to develop from egg to biting adult once their dormancy had been ended by high water. The flood led to the synchronous development of vast numbers of eggs that had accumulated during the prolonged drought and thus led to the enormous swarms of mosquitoes capable of exsanguinating mature cattle overnight. Abbitt and Abbitt, who obtained and thoughtfully analyzed the evidence in this outbreak, estimated that 3.8 million mosquito bites (5300 bites per minute for twelve hours) would be required to remove half of the total blood volume from a 366 kg. cow, assuming that a mosquito removes 0.0039 ml. per blood meal (Abbitt and Abbitt, 1981).

Disease Transmission. A *vector* is an animal, usually an arthropod, that transmits an infective organism from one host to another. A vector that transmits infective organisms directly (and necessarily, promptly) to a recipient host without development or multiplication of the organisms having occurred is called a *mechanical vector*. A *biological vector*, on the other hand, is one in which the infective organisms either undergo development or multiply or both, before being transmitted to the recipient host. Thus, a biological vector is really an *intermediate host* but, in common usage, an intermediate host that happens to be an arthropod. Mosquitoes serve as biological vectors of filariid worms such as *Dirofilaria immitis*, the canine heartworm, and *Wuchereria bancrofti*, the cause of human lymphatic filariasis, which is often manifested by a grotesque enlargement of the extremities called *elephantiasis*. These insects also transmit several viral encephalitides (e.g., equine encephalomyelitis) and the viruses of yellow fever, dengue fever, rabbit myxomatosis, and fowl pox. Mosquitoes of the genus *Anopheles* are biological vectors of the blood-inhabiting protozoon genus *Plasmodium* that causes malaria.

FAMILY SIMULIIDAE, BLACK FLIES

Identification. Black flies are small, stout-bodied, black, gray, or yellowish brown flies with relatively short antennae consisting of nine to 12 (usually 11) similar segments, and short mouthparts with prominent maxillary palps (Fig. 1-5).

Life History. Black flies breed only in running water. Mountain torrents and temporary upland streams are favored breeding sites of many species but some particularly important species breed in large rivers. Eggs are deposited on the water's surface or on partly submerged stones, twigs, or vegetation. In species that produce several broods per year (*multivoltine* species), larvae hatch from these eggs a few days later but in species that produce only one brood per year (*univoltine* species), the eggs remain in a protracted state of metabolic quiescence or *diapause* and do not hatch until the following year. Black fly larvae manage to cling to the surfaces of stones in rapidly moving, turbulent streams partly by means of little hooks on their posteriors and on a short *proleg* near the anterior end of their bodies (Fig. 1-6). By flexing their bodies, the larvae are able to move from place to place like inchworms. Black fly larvae also spin silken strands to help anchor themselves and later to form cocoons by means of which the pupae continue to cling to the rocks. Adults emerge from these pupae and are carried to the surface in a bubble of air. Blackflies attack in swarms during daylight hours and when the air is relatively still. Smoke repels them and, although various commercial repellants usually afford some degree of protection, campers, gardeners, and livestock usually find their surest relief in the lee of a smudge pot.

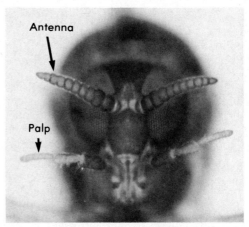

Figure 1-5. Head of a black fly (Nematocera: Simuliidae) (x27).

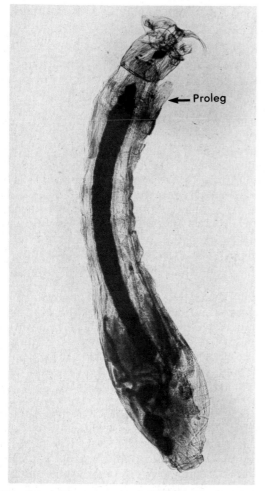

← Proleg

Figure 1–6. Black fly larva (Nematocera: Simuliidae) (x30).

Injury. The female black fly is a vicious biter. Her mouthparts consist of a bundle of flattened, serrated, bladelike stylets loosely ensheathed by the labium which itself terminates in a pair of labella. Instead of piercing a blood vessel and feeding from the lumen as a mosquito, bed bug, or sucking louse does, the female black fly lacerates tissues until a pool of blood forms and then she imbibes the blood from the pool.

Susceptibility to and severity of host reaction to the bites of many arthropods vary remarkably among individuals. With continued exposure to bites, initially susceptible individuals may become relatively immune so that they are less frequently bitten or suffer less reaction to the bites, or they may become hypersensitive so that continued attack excites a more severe and sometimes even fatal reaction. Sensitivity to the bites of black flies is a common phenomenon; the wheal may continue to itch for many days and tends to be aggravated by scratching. In a hypersensitive person, a single bite may evoke sufficient edematous reaction to force the eyelids shut. Burghardt *et al.* (1951) described a dermatitis in cattle due to *Simulium*. The lesions consisted of blisters, welts, and scabs affecting the head, thorax, and ears, and acute exudative lesions along the midabdominal line. Heavy swarms of black flies have been known to kill grazing livestock by the thousands but the exact cause of death, whether it be anemia, hypersensitivity reactions, or toxin absorbed from fly saliva injected into the bite, remains problematical.

Disease Transmission. Black flies transmit human onchocerciasis (*Onchocerca volvulus*), a form of filariasis manifested by the formation of dermal nodules and leading, at least in the African form of the disease, to blindness. Because the vectors are riverine breeders, the disease tends to be concentrated along river valleys and the ensuing blindness is called *river blindness*. *Onchocerca gutterosa*, an apparently innocuous filariid parasite of cattle, is also transmitted by black flies. These vectors of *Onchocerca* spp. serve as obligate intermediate hosts in which the worm develops from a microfilaria, the stage infective for the fly, to the third stage larva, which is infective for the definitive host.

Black flies also transmit leucocytozoonosis, a disease of poultry and wild birds caused by several species of the hemosporidian genus *Leucocytozoon*.

FAMILY HELEIDAE (CERATOPOGONIDAE), BITING MIDGES, "NO-SEE-UMS"

Identification. Heleids are tiny (less than 2 mm.), relatively glabrous flies. The antennae are long and slender and the mouthparts relatively short (Fig. 1-7).

Life History. Life histories of various species differ in detail, some requiring freshwater and others saltwater habitats. Some breed in water-filled holes in trees, others in decaying vegetation, and the like. Adults are crepuscular or nocturnal. Only females suck blood and, although they are fairly strong flyers, tend to remain close to their breeding grounds. A few may venture forth as far as a half mile when the air is still, however. Most important species belong to the genus *Culicoides*.

Injury. The bites of *Culicoides* inflict pain far out of proportion to the size of the fly. In fact, people victimized by these tiny terrors frequently don't realize that they are being

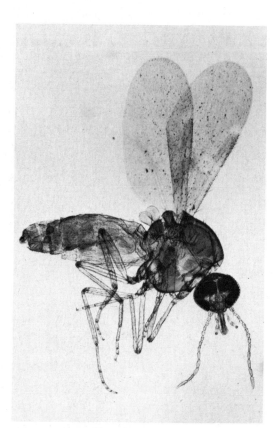

Figure 1–7. *Culicoides* (Nematocera: Heleidae), a "no-see-um" (x37). *Culicoides* differs from Culicidae in being smaller and having a shorter proboscis.

tormented by insects, sometimes mistaking them for a bit of cigarette ash because of their small size. *Culicoides* easily pass through standard window screening and make themselves obnoxious to sleepers. In sensitized individuals, the bites last longer and are more painful than mosquito bites.

"Queensland itch," demonstrated by Riek (1953a) to represent allergic dermatitis caused by the development of hypersensitivity to the bites of *Culicoides robertsi*, afflicts only certain horses. Other horses pastured with the sufferers never show any signs of disease. Initial lesions are discrete papules confined to the dorsal surfaces. Later, the hair mats and crusts form and eventually fall off, leaving hairless areas that, in severe cases, become confluent. Pruritus is intense and horses may injure themselves by scratching and rolling to relieve the itching. The attacks of *Culicoides robertsi* and associated allergic dermatitis were prevented by stabling the affected horses from four in the afternoon until seven the next morning or by weekly spraying with DDT. Antihistamine therapy accelerated regression of the lesions (Riek, 1953b).

Disease Transmission. *Culicoides* spp. transmit the viruses of bluetongue, African horse sickness and, possibly, bovine ephemeral fever. *Onchocerca cervicalis* of horses, *O. gibsoni* of cattle, and three relatively innocuous filariid parasites of man (*Dipetalonema perstans*, *D. streptocerca*, and *Mansonella ozzardi*) all develop from microfilaria to infective third stage larva in the bodies of *Culicoides*. Protozoans transmitted by *Culicoides* include *Hepatocystis* of Old World monkeys and *Haemoproteus* and *Leucocytozoon* of wild and domestic birds.

FAMILY PSYCHODIDAE, SAND FLIES

Identification. Psychodids are small, dull colored, slender flies with long antennae.

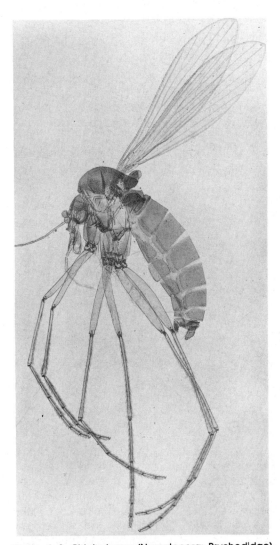

Figure 1–8. *Phlebotomus* (Nematocera: Psychodidae) (x29). The wing veins radiate in nearly straight lines from the base to the tip of the wing.

The wing veins radiate in nearly straight lines from the base to the tip of the wing (Fig. 1-8).

Life History. Psychodids lay their eggs in cracks, crevices, or burrows where there are moderate temperatures, darkness, and nearly 100% humidity. They spend at least two months as egg, larva, and pupa but are short-lived as adults. Adult psychodids are weak flyers and are nocturnal in habit. Important species belong to the genera *Phlebotomus* and *Lutzomyia*. *Phlebotomus* occurs in the Old World and *Lutzomyia* in the New World; all species are tropical or subtropical in distribution.

Disease Transmission. Psychodids transmit three-day fever virus and *Bartonella bacilliformis* infection of man, and *Leishmania* spp. hemoflagellates of man and dog.

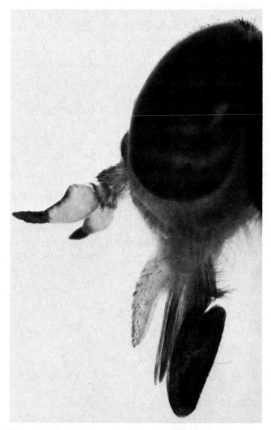

Figure 1–10. *Tabanus* (Brachycera: Tabanidae), a horse fly (x20).

SUBORDER BRACHYCERA

FAMILY TABANIDAE, HORSE FLIES AND DEER FLIES

Identification. Tabanids are stout-bodied flies varying from about the size of a house fly to as large as a hummingbird. The short, stout, anteriorly projecting antennae consist of three markedly different segments (Figs. 1-9 and 1-10). The first segment is small, the second may be expanded, and the third is marked by annulations that make tabanid antennae appear to consist of many more than three units.

Life History. Tabanids breed in damp soil or decaying organic matter. Eggs are neatly glued in masses to water plants or foliage overhanging water. Larvae hatch in a week or less and drop into the water, where they feed on insect larvae, crustaceans, snails, earthworms, young frogs, plant tissues, and dead organic matter, depending on the species of tabanid and the availability of food. In temperate regions, larvae overwinter by burying themselves in soil or dead vegetation and pupate the following spring. Thus, usually only one generation is produced each year. They are strong fliers and are very difficult to discourage.

Injury. All arthropod attacks cause some annoyance to the host and exact some expenditure of energy in efforts to avoid or relieve their effects. When flies are particularly numerous, pastured livestock may be driven frantic by incessant attacks and spend so much time and energy combating the

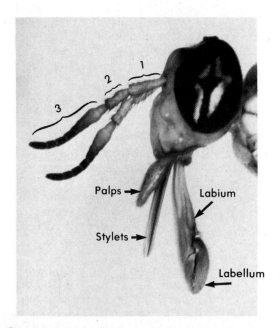

Figure 1–9. *Chrysops* (Brachycera: Tabanidae), a deer fly (x19). The distal segment of the tabanid antenna is annulated, giving the impression that the antenna consists of many segments, but there are only three.

onslaught that they cannot rest or graze adequately. The resultant exhaustion always interferes with production and sometimes proves fatal. Certain insects are particularly feared by livestock. Some horse flies are as large as hummingbirds and inflict an excruciating bite. When one of these monsters attacks, horses are likely to bolt and it behooves the rider or driver to come promptly to their aid. Vicious daylight bloodsuckers, tabanids do not usually attack indoors but, if already feeding when the host enters a building, will continue to feed until replete. Repeated attacks in the skin folds about a cow's udder and in the groove between the udder halves lead to extensive weeping eczematous lesions that may become secondarily infected with bacteria. The most efficient solution to tabanid attack is to stable the animals during the hours of peak fly activity. In biting, the mandibles and maxillae of tabanids lacerate the blood vessels and the labella lap up the blood that flows freely from the wound. After a tabanid has finished feeding, the bite wound tends to bleed for many minutes and thus attract opportunists such as *Musca*. In fact, *Musca* and other flies can often be seen clustered about a feeding tabanid, exploiting the bounty afforded by its sloppy manner of taking a meal.

Disease Transmission. The pain that a tabanid inflicts when it bites tends to increase its efficiency as a mechanical vector of disease organisms. The fly, driven away by its victim's defenses before it has had time to feed to repletion, soon alights on a second host to finish its meal and perhaps to contaminate the wound with fresh, mechanically borne bacteria (e.g., anthrax), viruses (e.g., equine infectious anemia), and the like. The large volume of blood imbibed by each tabanid also contributes to its efficiency as a mechanical vector by helping to compensate for the low concentration of microorganisms usually found in blood, and for their failure to multiply in the body of the intermediate host.

Tabanids have been incriminated in the mechanical transmission of anaplasmosis (*Anaplasma* spp.), anthrax (*Bacillus anthracis*), tularemia (*Francisella tularensis*), equine infectious anemia virus, and *Besnoitia besnoiti*, an unusual coccidian protozoan of cattle. Mammalian trypanosomes (hemoflagellate protozoans) may be transmitted mechanically or biologically by tabanids, depending on the species involved. Surra (*Trypanosoma evansi*), a fatal disease of horses, camels, elephants, and dogs in Asia, is transmitted mechanically and the flies lose their ability to transmit the infection a few hours after feeding on an animal infected with surra. *Trypanosoma theileri*, on the other hand, must multiply in the body of the tabanid because it is so scarce in the blood of cattle that one must usually resort to culture techniques to demonstrate its presence there. Otherwise, *T. theileri* would not be distributed throughout the world as a parasite of cattle and their near relatives. A vector in which such parasitic organisms multiply is sometimes referred to a *cyclopropagative host* to distinguish it from a *cyclodevelopmental host*, in which the parasite actually undergoes ontogenetic development. Examples of the latter include *Loa loa*, the African eye worm of man, and *Elaeophora schneideri*, the arterial worm of deer, elk, and domestic sheep in the southwestern United States, development from the microfilaria to the infective third stage occurring in the body of the tabanid (Hibler and Adcock, 1971).

SUBORDER CYCLORRHAPHA

The suborder Cyclorrhapha represents the apex of dipteran evolution, and the common house fly, *Musca domestica*, is a typical example. Instead of the aquatic habitats favored by nematocerans and brachycerans, cyclorrhaphans tend to breed in decaying plant and animal tissues, manure, carrion, and the like. The three larval instars are more or less conical animals with a mouth, usually armed with hooks, at the apex and a pair of prominent respiratory openings called *spiracles* or *stigmata* at the base. Slender larvae of the families Muscidae, Sarcophagidae, and Calliphoridae are usually referred to as maggots (Fig. 1-11), whereas the rather stout larvae of the family Oestridae and its relatives are called bots, grubs, or warbles (Fig. 1-12). When the third instar larva enters the pupal stage, its integument hardens to form a *puparium*, or pupal case. The adult fly emerges through a circular hole in the anterior end of the puparium. Cyclorrhaphan antennae consist of three dissimilar segments, the third, and largest of which bears a frondlike structure called an *arista* near its proximal end. The antennae are directed ventrally but the aristae project anteriorly (Fig. 1-13). Parasitic specialization has proceeded in two directions in the Cyclorrhapha. In the families Muscidae and Hippoboscidae there has been specialization from a type adapted to lapping up liquids (e.g., *Musca*, Fig. 1-13) toward a bayonetlike proboscis for piercing the skin

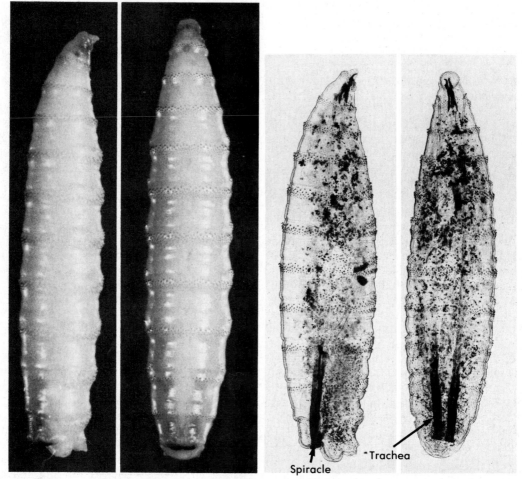

Figure 1–11. Muscoid third stage larva or *maggot* of the family Calliphoridae (x10). Note the pigmented tracheal trunks leading from the posterior spiracles. Pigmented tracheae are a specific character of *Cochliomyia hominivorax*, the American screwworm. Specimens courtesy of R. J. Gagné.

and sucking blood (e.g., *Stomoxys*, Fig. 1-14) and thus toward parasitism in the adult stage. In the families Calliphoridae and Sarcophagidae, the adult flies have retained their lapping mouthparts and remained scavengers; instead, it is in the larval stages that parasitism has evolved. The bot flies (e.g., *Hypoderma* and *Gasterophilus*) have proceeded even further in this direction. Their larvae have become highly specialized host- and site-specific parasites, whereas the mouthparts of the adult flies have become vestigial and totally nonfunctional. Parasitism by fly larvae is termed *myiasis* and is of worldwide economic importance.

FAMILY MUSCIDAE

Musca

Identification. The genus *Musca* contains 26 species of which three, *M. domestica*, the

common house fly, *M. autumnalis*, the face fly, and *M. vetustissima*, the Australian bush fly, may serve as examples. These three species resemble each other closely enough to require an expert to distinguish specimens on morphological grounds, but differ sufficiently in behavior to make their identities obvious to anyone familiar with their habits. The mouthparts of these all too familiar flies consist of a fleshy, retractable proboscis terminating in a pair of corrugated spongy organs, the *labella* (Fig. 1-13).

Life History and Disease Transmission. *Musca domestica* lays its eggs on animal manure or almost any kind of decaying organic material. A tiny, white, first stage larva (maggot) hatches from this egg in a day or less. This larva grows, molts twice, and in a few days becomes a fully developed third stage larva. When ready to pupate, the third stage larva migrates into a dryer medium, shortens, thickens, and becomes darker in color

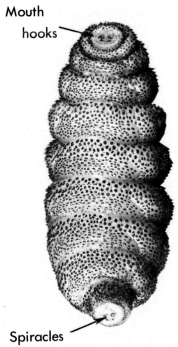

Mouth
hooks

Spiracles

Figure 1–12. A *Cuterebra jellisoni* (Cyclorrhapha: Cuterebridae) bot, or third stage bot fly larva (x2, from Baird, 1971: J. Med. Entomol., *8* (6), 616). The bot flies belong to the families Cuterebridae, Oestridae, Hypodermatidae, and Gasterophilidae.

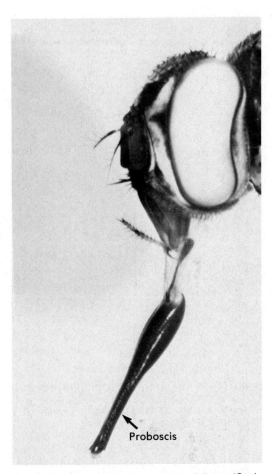

Proboscis

Figure 1–14. Head of *Stomoxys calcitrans* (Cyclorrhapha: Muscidae), the stable fly (x24). In feeding, the entire proboscis is thrust into the skin of the host.

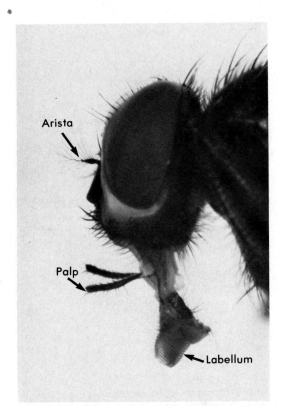

Arista

Palp

Labellum

Figure 1–13. Head of *Musca domestica* (Cyclorrhapha: Muscidae), the common house fly (x29). The proboscis is retractable into the head.

as a result of hardening and tanning of the third stage cuticle in forming the puparium. The adult fly emerges in two or three weeks by forcing off the end of the puparium with its *ptilinum*, a bladderlike structure that is inflated with hemolymph (Fig. 1-15). The ptilinum projects from the *frontal suture* and is withdrawn into the head after the fly has emerged from the puparium. Like the umbilicus of mammals, it is of no further service to the animal. The adult fly then makes its way to the surface of the medium in which the pupa lay buried, expands its wings by pumping hemolymph into the wing veins, and flies away in search of food. The housefly feeds on feces, syrup, milk, decaying fruit, and other dissolved and soluble materials. Bacteria, protozoan cysts, helminth eggs, and other disease organisms may be transported from filth to food, body openings, and wounds by way of the feces, vomit spots, sticky feet, and body hairs of houseflies. The housefly also serves as a biological vector of

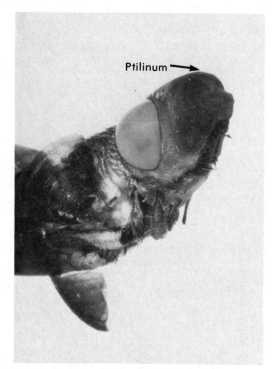

Figure 1–15. *Musca domestica* adult emerging from the puparium (x15). The baglike ptilinum is inflated with hemolymph to pop off the end of the puparium; after emergence, it is retracted into the head.

Draschia megastoma and *Habronema muscae*, nematode parasites of the stomach of the horse. A female *Musca domestica* may deposit 2000 eggs in an average lifetime of six to eight weeks.

Musca autumnalis (face fly) was introduced into North America from Europe, Asia, or Africa in the early nineteen fifties. These flies crawl about the faces of horses and cattle, feeding on the ocular and nasal discharges induced by their presence, and are extremely annoying to pastured animals. Eggs are deposited in fresh cattle dung and the larvae pupate in the dried dung or nearby soil. The adult flies overwinter in buildings. These hibernating adults, like those of *Pollenia rudis,* the cluster fly, cause considerable annoyance to the human occupants when, aroused by a spell of warmish weather, they go buzzing and blundering about the house, falling into drinks and making themselves generally disagreeable. Curiously, the active adult face fly of summer appears loath to enter buildings and may be observed to swarm off dairy cows as they enter the stable to be milked. They wait outside during milking and swarm back on as the cows emerge from the stable. This, of course, contrasts with the behavior of *M. domestica,* so appropriately called the

house fly. Face flies serve as biological vector of *Thelazia* spp. (eyeworm), a genus of nematode worms that infect the conjunctival sacs of horses and cattle (Chitwood and Stoffolano, 1971).

Musca vetustissima, the Australian bush fly, resembles *M. autumnalis* in preferring to remain out of doors, in breeding in livestock manures, and in crawling about on the faces of livestock. However, *M. vetustissima* differs in displaying an exasperating affinity for the faces of human beings as well as livestock, by involvement of its larvae in wound myiasis, and by an inability to hibernate. Instead of hibernating, *M. vetustissima* reinvades southeastern Australia each spring from the more tropical regions to the north.

These three species thus display distinct differences in behavior in spite of their morphological similarity.

Stomoxys

Identification. The stable fly, *Stomoxys calcitrans,* resembles *Musca* spp. but has a long, pointed proboscis with which it inflicts painful bites instead of the vacuum cleaner affair with which *Musca* sucks up liquids from little puddles. The palpi of *Stomoxys* are shorter than the proboscis (see Fig. 1-14; compare with *Haematobia,* Fig. 1-16). The third stage

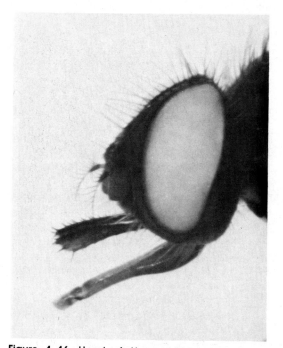

Figure 1–16. Head of *Haematobia irritans* (Cyclorrhapha: Muscidae), the horn fly (x65). *Haematobia* somewhat resembles *Stomoxys* but is only half as large and has palps almost as long as its proboscis (compare with Figure 1–14).

larvae resemble those of *Musca* and have posterior spiracles with sinuous slits but the spiracles are set farther apart than those of *Musca* (see Fig. 1-20).

Life History. Stable flies have a life history similar to that of face flies but differ in preferring decaying organic materials such as piles of lawn clippings or damp hay or grain to animal manure for egg laying. Stable flies of both sexes feed on blood once or twice a day, depending on the ambient temperature, and suspend operations entirely during cold spells.

Injury and Disease Transmission. The bite of the stable fly is painful and results in the interrupted feeding patterns observed with tabanids. The stable fly serves as biological vector of *Habronema microstoma*, a nematode parasite of the stomach of the horse.

Haematobia

Identification. The horn fly, *Haematobia irritans*, found on the backs of cattle, is about half the size of *Stomoxys* and has a relatively shorter proboscis. The palps are nearly long enough to reach the tip of the proboscis, in contrast to *Stomoxys* (compare Figs. 1-14 and 1-16).

Life History. Horn flies remain on the backs of cattle, periodically biting their hosts and sucking blood. When a cow defecates, a number of her horn flies swarm to the dropping to lay their eggs and then return to the cow. Larvae hatch in less than a day and crawl into the dropping to feed. Pupation occurs in four days and emergence of the adult follows in six more days. The entire cycle from egg to egg requires two weeks or slightly less. Because they remain on the host most of the time, horn flies are vulnerable to insecticide applications, stock oilers, and the like.

Injury and Disease Transmission. When sufficiently numerous, horn flies can impair milk production and weight gains. Cattle protected from horn fly attack by ear tags impregnated with fenvalerate achieved 18% greater live weight gains than did untreated controls (Haufe, 1982). *Haematobia irritans* serves as biological vector of *Stephanofilaria stilesi*, a filarioid nematode parasite of North American cattle and etiological agent of stephanofilariasis, a dermatitis usually confined to the midventral region of the abdomen.

Glossina

Identification. Tsetse flies (*Glossina* spp.) are limited to Africa but are included here

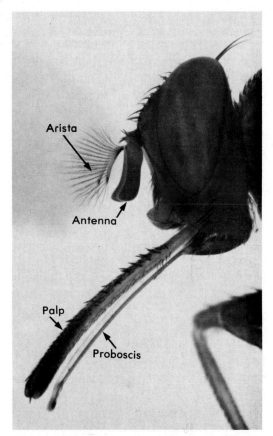

Figure 1–17. Head of *Glossina* (Cyclorrhapha: Muscidae), a tsetse fly (x22).

because of their great importance to human and animal health, to the preservation of African wildlife, and to the economy of Africa and the world at large. Each antenna of *Glossina* has a long arista that is "feathered" along one edge. The palps and long, slender proboscis are equal in length, the palps forming a sheath for the proboscis at rest (Fig. 1-17).

Life History. The female tsetse bears only one larva at a time. Larval development is completed in the abdomen of the mother, all three stages feeding on fluids from special uterine glands. It is interesting that milk secretion has evolved independently among both the highest vertebrates and the highest invertebrates! Several blood meals at regular intervals are required to support the larva during its developmental period of roughly one to four weeks. When extruded by the female tsetse, the fully developed third stage larva almost immediately burrows into the soil and prepares to enter the pupal stage. A fourth larval stage occurs within the puparium before metamorphosis to the adult stage at last takes place.

Disease Transmission. The great importance of the tsetse is its role as biological vector of various trypanosomiases of man and his domestic animals. African sleeping sickness of man and "nagana" and related diseases of domestic animals are briefly considered in Chapter 3.

FAMILY HIPPOBOSCIDAE

Identification. Hippoboscids are dorsoventrally flattened, sometimes wingless flies with piercing mouthparts. The antennae are embedded in pits in the sides of the head. *Melophagus ovinus,* the sheep ked; *Hippobosca equina,* the horse louse fly; and *Lipoptena cervi,* the deer ked, are examples (Fig. 1-18). *Melophagus* is wingless, the wings of *Hippobosca* remain well developed and functional throughout life, and *Lipoptena* have wings when they emerge from the pupal case but lose them once they have located a host. *Lipoptena* may attack horses and other domestic animals in addition to deer.

Life History. Like tsetses, hippoboscids retain their larvae in their abdomens until they are ready to pupate, nourishing them during development with uterine gland secretions. In the case of *Melophagus ovinus,* larval development requires about a week and the extruded larva pupates within a few hours. The chestnut brown pupal cases remain glued to the wool of the host sheep throughout metamorphosis of the adult fly, which

emerges in three to six weeks, depending on the ambient temperature. The entire life of the sheep ked is thus spent on the host. Shearing and organophosphorus insecticides make life very uncertain for these parasites.

Disease Transmission. *Melophagus ovinus* is host to *Trypanosoma melophagium,* which it transmits to sheep. If all keds are removed, the trypanosomes rapidly disappear from the sheep's blood, so it is the ked and not the sheep that represents the true reservoir of infection. Like *T. theileri* of cattle, *T. melophagium* appears to be totally nonpathogenic to its vertebrate host.

FAMILY SARCOPHAGIDAE

Identification. An adult sarcophagid is about twice as large as a house fly. The thorax is gray with dark, longitudinal stripes and the abdomen is checkered gray and black (Fig. 1-19). Third stage sarcophagid larvae resemble house fly maggots but are larger. The posterior spiracles are deeply sunken in a rounded concavity; the inner slit of each spiracle is directed down and away from the median line (Fig. 1-20, *3*). Differentiation of *Sarcophaga* and *Wohlfahrtia* larvae requires that adult flies be reared from them. Place the larvae in question and a piece of liver on 3 to 5 cm. of sand or loamy soil in a canning jar. When, after a day or so, the larvae have entered the substrate to pupate, remove the liver to avoid obnoxious odors and cover the

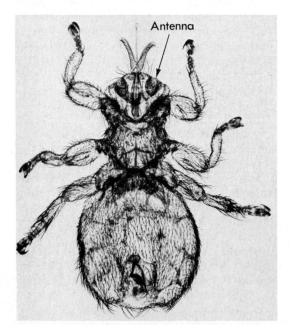
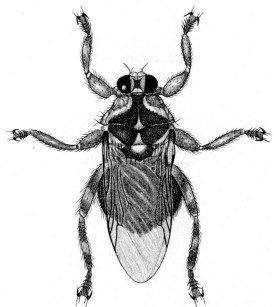

Figure 1–18. Examples of family Hippoboscidae: left, *Melophagus ovinus,* the sheep ked (x12); right, *Hippobosca equina,* the horse louse fly. (*Hippobosca* redrawn from Edwards, Oldroyd, and Smart, 1939.)

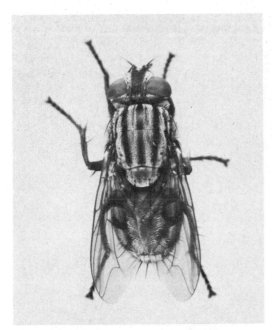

Figure 1–19. *Sarcophaga* (Cyclorrhapha: Sarcophagidae), a flesh fly (x5). About twice as large as a house fly, *Sarcophaga* is gray with longitudinal dark stripes on the thorax and checkered gray and black abdomen.

mouth of the jar with a layer of cheesecloth secured with a rubber band to provide air yet prevent the escape of flies after they have emerged from the pupal cases. The arista of *Wohlfahrtia* bears only very short hairs, whereas the arista of *Sarcophaga* is covered nearly to its tip with long hairs. The above rearing instructions serve equally well for calliphorids but best results are obtained with larvae that are almost ready to pupate, especially when obligate parasitic species are involved.

FAMILY CALLIPHORIDAE

Identification. Adult calliphorids (Gr. *kallos* beauty, plus *phoros* bearing) are usually intermediate in size between *Musca* and *Sarcophaga* and display brilliant metallic blue, green, copper, or black hues. The common names "bluebottle" and "greenbottle" fly refer to the coloration of these flies, which are also called "blowflies" because they "blow," i.e., deposit, their eggs or larvae in meat. Particular species differ in their preferences with regard to the degree of freshness of the meat, from living flesh to carrion in an advanced state of decomposition. Most calliphorids are scavengers or facultative parasites, but a few (e.g., *Cochliomyia hominivorax*, the American screwworm) are obligate parasites. Third stage larvae of Calliphoridae are muscoid maggots differing from those of Sarcophagidae in that their posterior spiracles lie flush with the posterior face of the larva (or, less commonly, are sunken in a shallow slitlike concavity) and the inner slits of the spiracles are directed obliquely downward and toward the median line (Fig. 1-20, 2). Larvae of the very important species *Cochliomyia hominivorax* may be identified by the dark pigmentation of their tracheal trunks through the last three or four segments (see Fig. 1-11).

Life History and Injury (Myiasis). Females of the American screwworm fly *Cochliomyia hominivorax* lay their eggs on fresh, uninfected wounds of all kinds. About 200 eggs are deposited in tidy rows. The eggs hatch within a day and the obligate parasitic maggots commence feeding on living flesh and, in so doing, produce a foul-smelling, brownish red discharge. The larvae leave to pupate in five to seven days, and the adults emerge from the pupal cases one to several weeks later. Wherever it occurs, *Cochliomyia hominivorax* is a serious menace to man and beast alike. Unconscious victims of accidents or alcohol intoxication lying helplessly exposed have been fatally infected or have had their facial bones completely eaten away by screwworm maggots. Docking and castrating wounds, wire cuts, the navels of newborn animals, tick bite wounds, shear cuts, needle grass wounds, and even fresh brands may attract the attentions of *C. hominivorax*. A nationwide control program based on treating wounds of all infected animals with insecticidal smears and releasing billions of sterilized flies has almost succeeded in eliminating screwworm myiasis from the United States. The adult flies are sterilized by gamma radiation, which induces dominant lethal mutations in the sperm. Because the female screwworm mates only once and because the wild population of the fly is relatively small, the addition of hordes of sexually competent but sterile males reduces the probability of successful fertilization to nil. Unfortunately, after almost a decade of excellent control, the incidence of screwworm myiasis began to increase in the southwestern United States. This was believed to be related to a loss of competitive ability of factory-reared flies resulting from selection for survival under conditions of domestication and rapid development at constant high temperatures (Bush *et al.*, 1976).

Facultatively parasitic calliphorids are drawn to such attractions as suppurating wounds, skin soiled with urine, vomitus, or

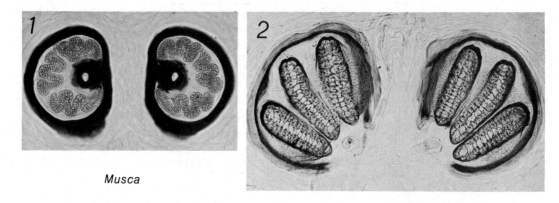

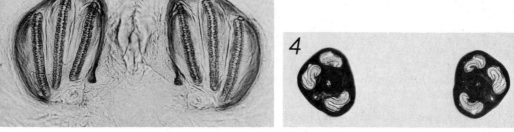

Figure 1–20. Muscoid spiracles (1, 2, and 4 x108; 3 x70).

feces, and bacterial decomposition products that tend to accumulate in the fleece of a wet sheep. Once established in exudate or necrotic tissue, some kinds of these facultative parasites may later invade living tissue, whereas others do not. For example, the "surgical maggots" of *Phaenicia sericata* and *Phormia regina* are still occasionally used in the treatment of osteomyelitis and other refractory suppurative lesions to clear away necrotic debris and promote healing. Ideally, the surgical maggots do not invade healthy tissue but strains vary and some of them don't know where to stop. A brave and resourceful gentleman of my acquaintance applied this technique in treating his own wounds when a prisoner of war in Vietnam; once the maggots had done their work to his satisfaction, he flushed them away with his urine.

Wool strike is a common and serious problem in many sheep raising regions of the world. Adult calliphorids are attracted to areas of fleece that have become soiled by feces or urine or kept damp long enough for bacterial growth to occur and generate odors that lure flies to feed and lay their eggs. The

areas involved in wool strike thus include the perineum, prepuce and, during periods of considerable rainfall, water-soaked wool of the flanks, withers, and ventral neck region. Several genera of calliphorid flies are commonly involved and each geographical region has its particular scourge among the general assemblage of facultative parasites and scavengers. In Australia, one species, *Lucilia cuprina*, stands out as a specialist in wool strike. This fly, although still a facultative parasite in that it is able to develop in carrion, has become so adept at locating suitable sheep on which to deposit its eggs that it has become the culprit responsible for initiating most cases of wool strike in Australia. The maggots feed on scales and exudate at the surface of the skin and may occasionally penetrate into the underlying tissues. When ready to pupate, the larvae of *L. cuprina* wait until night to leave the carcass (Smith *et al.*, 1981). In this way, the pupae and emerging adults of this highly specialized parasite tend to become concentrated about the preferred resting sites or *camps* of their host species. Once *L. cuprina* has initiated a strike, other species of flies are attracted to feed and lay their eggs in the developing lesions. As the morbid process advances, these less specialized newcomers tend to replace *L. cuprina*. Toxins absorbed from the myiasis lesion rapidly incapacitate the sheep and lead to its death in a matter of days. Eventually, scavenger species take over the carcass and reduce it to hair and bone. Financial loss caused by wool strike is reckoned in terms of outright death losses, loss of wool, decreased quality of wool, loss of weight, and costs of treatment and preventive measures.

A condition analogous to wool strike occurs in old, weakened or paretic dogs with urine-soaked haircoats. As such an unfortunate animal lies in the "healing rays of the sun," the blowflies are busy laying eggs in its haircoat and, in a few days, maggots will be skinning it alive. Frequently, owners that present long-haired dogs suffering from advanced cases of cutaneous myiasis are totally unaware of the mayhem taking place underneath the haircoat.

Weakened or defective calves born at pasture are also fair game for members of the family Calliphoridae. It is amazing how quickly the shiny flies appear out of nowhere and how rapidly their egg masses accumulate about the umbilicus of a newborn calf with cerebellar hypoplasia or muscle contracture. The possibility of myiasis must always be considered in the case of animals incapacitated during warm weather, especially if they are forced to remain outdoors.

FAMILIES OESTRIDAE, HYPODERMATIDAE, GASTEROPHILIDAE, AND CUTEREBRIDAE; THE BOT FLIES

The bot flies are highly host-specific and site-specific parasites in the larval (i.e., bot) stage and total slaves to reproduction in the adult stage. The adults have vestigial mouthparts and must carry on their courtship rituals and egg laying on energy stored away when they were larvae. Fully developed bots are larger and stouter than are muscid, sarcophagid, and calliphorid maggots, from which they can readily be distinguished by their posterior spiracles (Figs. 1-20 and 1-21). In fact, when found in their accustomed locations in their normal hosts, bots present very little in the way of a diagnostic challenge; a bot in a sheep's nasal passages is an *Oestrus*, a bot in a cow's dorsal subcutis is a *Hypoderma*, a bot in a horse's stomach is a

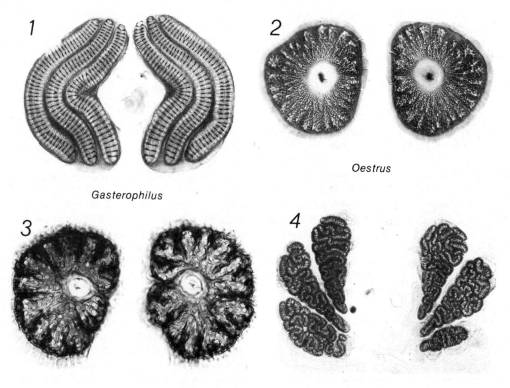

1 Gasterophilus

2 Oestrus

3 Hypoderma

4 Cuterebra

Figure 1–21. Bot spiracles (*1* and *2* x27; *3* x55, and *4* x65).

Gasterophilus, and there's hardly any sense in making more of an exercise of it than that. However, the earlier stages of bots are more difficult to distinguish from maggots and, if found migrating in other than its normal host, will require the services of an expert entomologist for identification. First stage *Hypoderma* larvae have been found migrating aberrantly through the brain of horses, and *Cuterebra* larvae, normally parasites of rodents and lagomorphs, have been found in the brains of cats and dogs. *Hypoderma* also occasionally invades man, in which it tends to migrate subcutaneously, and *Oestrus ovis* may larviposit in the eyes of shepherds and thus cause a temporary but painful ocular myiasis.

Oestrus ovis

Oestrus ovis, the "sheep nasal bot fly," somewhat resembles a honeybee. It is a stout, grayish-brown fly, about one cm. long and covered with short hairs; the mouthparts are vestigial. The flies are most active during the warmer hours of the day and especially during intervals of bright sunshine. In early morning and late afternoon, they are more likely to be found resting on buildings, tree trunks, water tanks, and the like. It is interesting to watch a mob of Australian Merino sheep on a warm, sunny day with a bit of scattered cloud. While in the shadow of a cloud, the sheep tend to distribute themselves more or less at random over the paddock, but as the sun emerges from behind the cloud, the sheep immediately huddle together and continue to graze with their heads toward the center of the huddle, only to disperse again with the arrival of the next cloud. This behavior may represent a defensive adaptation to the "attack" of the larvipositing female *Oestrus ovis;* it seems plausible, anyway,. While *Oe. ovis* females are actively depositing their larvae in sheep's nostrils, the sheep hold their noses close to the ground or in each other's fleeces, stamp their feet as if annoyed, and occasionally bolt away. The tiny first stage larvae may be demonstrated on postmortem by sawing the skull in half longitudinally, rinsing the nasoturbinates and nasal sinuses with water, and examining the collected rinsings with a hand lens or stereoscopic microscope. The fully developed third stage bots can hardly escape notice in the frontal sinuses.

Life History. Upon being deposited in the nostril of a sheep, the larva crawls onto the mucous membrane of the nasal passage, where it will remain for at least two weeks anchored to the mucous membrane by its mouth hooks. Larvae arriving late in the season remain arrested in the first stage throughout the winter and development proceeds only with the return of warm weather. After a sojourn in the nasal cavity, the larvae proceed to the frontal sinuses, where development to the third stage is completed. On reaching full development, the third stage larvae crawl down into the nasal passages and are expelled by the sheep's sneezing and enter the soil to pupate. Adults may emerge in about four weeks in summer but require considerably longer in cool weather. When pupation occurs in autumn, adult flies do not emerge until the following spring. Thus, both arrested first stage larvae in the nasal cavities of sheep and pupae in soil represent overwintering forms.

Pathologic Significance. Moderate numbers of *Oe. ovis* larvae in the nasal and paranasal sinuses do no apparent harm but heavy infections cause sneezing, nasal discharge, and partial blockage of the nasal passages.

Other Nasal Bots

Rhinooestrus purpureus infects horses in parts of Europe, Asia, and Africa, *Cephalopsis titillator* infects camels and dromedaries in Africa, and *Cephenemyia* spp. infect deer, elk, caribou, and other cervids in the Northern Hemisphere. Their life histories resemble that of *Oe. ovis.*

Hypoderma

Identification. *Hypoderma bovis* and *Hypoderma lineatum* or "heel flies" occur in cattle raising areas of the Northern Hemisphere between 25 and 60 degrees North latitude. The adult fly is about 15 mm. long and looks rather like a bumble bee. Although these flies have no functional mouthparts to bite with and the process of oviposition on the hairs is presumably painless, cattle tend to become apprehensive and excited at their approach and gallop off aimlessly with their tails held high over their backs. Such behavior, termed "gadding about" tends to involve the whole herd simultaneously in needless, hysterical exertion and distract it from the more profitable business of grazing. Agricultural research administrators, practiced in the art of extracting financial support for their institutions from legislative bodies, can tell you exactly how much this form of bovine entomophobia costs the American stockman each year. The fully developed third stage *Hypoderma* larva or "cattle grub" is found in walnut-sized lumps or "warbles" on the backs of cattle in spring. Each warble has a small hole at its summit to which the posterior spiracles of the larva are pressed to obtain air. When it emerges or is extracted from the warble, the larva (sometimes also called a warble) is about 25 mm. long and whitish to light brown in color.

Life History and Pathogenesis. Hypoderma lineatum and *H. bovis* females glue their eggs to the hairs on the legs of cattle. *Hypoderma lineatum* appears with the advent of warm weather and remains active for about two months. Then, *H. bovis* takes over and persists into summer. The eggs hatch spontaneously in less than a week, and the larvae burrow through the skin and set off on prolonged migrations through the connective tissues of their host. Larvae of *H. lineatum* accumulate in the tissues of the esophagus five months later and remain there for about three months. Finally, they migrate to the subcutaneous tissues of the back, cut breathing holes in the skin to which they appose their spiracles, and, molting twice, grow larger. When fully developed, the larvae enlarge their breathing holes, emerge through them, and fall to the ground to pupate. Adult flies emerge from pupal cases about one month later and immediately set about their reproductive duties. *Hypoderma bovis* larvae tend to accumulate in the spinal canal instead of the esophagus and appear in the subcutaneous tissues of the back about two months later than *H. lineatum*. Migrating *Hypoderma* larvae can be killed and development of "grubby backs" prevented by application of organophosphorus insecticides.

Hypoderma larvae occasionally invade horses and render them useless for equitation by warble formation in the saddle area or even cause fatal neurological disease by migrating in the brain (Olander, 1967). In man, *Hypoderma* tends to produce bouts of creeping subcutaneous myiasis ("migrating lumps") as the confused larvae try to find the top of the cow they "think" they're migrating in. Local paralysis may result from invasion of the spinal cord and blindness may result from invasion of the eye. These are fortunately rare accidents.

Related Species. Hypoderma diana occurs in deer and occasionally in man in Europe. Other species of *Hypoderma* parasitize sheep, goats, and deer in Mediterranean countries and India. *Oedemagena tarandi* is a serious enough pest of reindeer, musk-oxen, and caribou in the subarctic regions to require prophylactic organophosphorus medication, which may be administered by injection to these wild or semi-wild hosts. In one study, 70% of untreated reindeer harbored more than 100 *Oe. tarandi* larvae (Washburn *et al.*, 1980).

Gasterophilus

Identification. The adult fly superficially resembles a honeybee, with a long, curved ovipositor carried beneath the abdomen. The females may be observed on warm, sunny days hovering near horses and darting very rapidly to attach an egg to a hair. *Gasterophilus nasalis* females deposit their eggs on the hairs of the intermandibular space, *G. hemorrhoidalis* on the short hairs that adjoin the lips, and *G. intestinalis* on the hairs of the forelegs and shoulders (Fig. 1-22). First stage

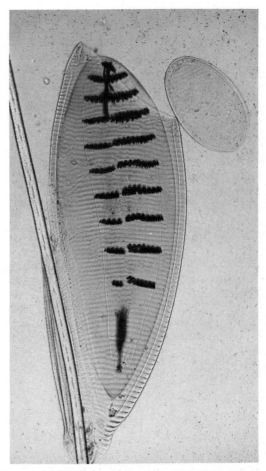

Figure 1-22. Egg of *Gasterophilus intestinalis* (Cyclorrhapha: Gasterophilidae) on a horse hair (x63). The egg shell contains a first stage larva and the operculum has become dislodged.

larvae of *G. intestinalis* can be found in tunnels in the epithelium covering the dorsal surface of the rostral two-thirds of the tongue and in pockets between the molar teeth where the first molt occurs. Second stage larvae are found in interdental pockets, attached to the root of the tongue, and attached to the wall of the stomach (Cogley, Anderson, and Cogley, 1982). Less is known regarding the initial migrations of other species of *Gasterophilus*. First and second stage larvae of *G. nasalis* are usually completely hidden well below the gum line in interdental pus pockets extending into the root sockets of molar teeth (Schroeder, 1940). The third stage larva of *G. nasalis* is yellowish and has one row of spines on each segment (Fig. 1-23); it is usually found in the pylorus and duodenum. All of the following species of *Gasterophilus* have two rows of spines per segment. The *G. intestinalis* third stage larva is red, has coarse spines that are blunted at their tips, and is usually found in the part of the stomach that is lined by stratified squamous epithelium. The following species have small spines that taper to a fine point: *G. hemorrhoidalis*, which is reddish; *G. inermis*, which is light yellow.

Life History. *Gasterophilus nasalis* females deposit their eggs on the hairs of the intermandibular space. These eggs hatch spontaneously in five or six days and the larvae crawl downward toward the chin until they arrive at a point opposite the commisures of the lips, whereupon they proceed directly toward the mouth and pass between the lips. The black eggs of *G. hemorrhoidalis* on the hairs adjoining the lips hatch after two to four days' incubation on contact with moisture, penetrate the epidermis of the lips, and burrow into the mucous membrane of the mouth. The eggs of *G. intestinalis* on the hairs of the front legs are far removed from their destination and depend on direct assistance from the horse to find their way into the mouth. After an incubation period of five days, these eggs contain first stage larvae that are prepared to hatch rapidly in response to the sudden rise in ambient temperature that occurs when the horse brings its warm muzzle and breath in contact with them; they do not respond to gradual warming. The larvae then enter the horse's mouth and burrow into the stratified squamous epithelium on the dorsal surface of the tongue. The first and second stage larvae of *Gasterophilus* spp. spend about one month in the oral cavity, after which they proceed to the stomach and duodenum, where, as second and third stage larvae, they will remain for nine or ten months. At last, they release their grip and pass out with the feces to pupate in the soil. Adult bot flies emerge from the pupal cases in three to nine weeks, depending on the ambient temperature. Bot fly activity continues through summer and fall but ceases completely when cold weather sets in.

Cuterebra

Identification. The rarely seen (or noticed) adult fly somewhat resembles a bumble bee and has vestigial mouthparts (Fig. 1-24). The fully developed third stage larva is large (up to 45 mm.) and dark brown to black, the color being due to the stout, black spines that cover the body (see Fig. 1-12). The posterior spiracles consist of groups of elegantly curved openings (see Fig. 1-21, 4). Earlier stages are much paler or even white and the posterior spiracles are quite different from

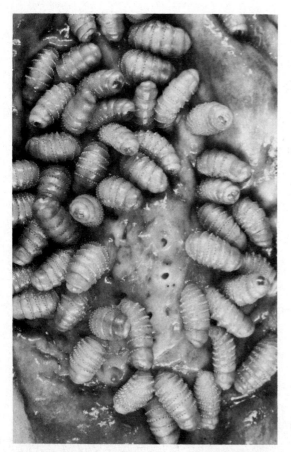

Figure 1–23. *Gasterophilus nasalis* (Cyclorrhapha: Gasterophilidae) third stage larvae attached to the gastric mucosa of a horse. Former attachment sites are visible as shallow, round ulcers in the lower center (approximate natural size).

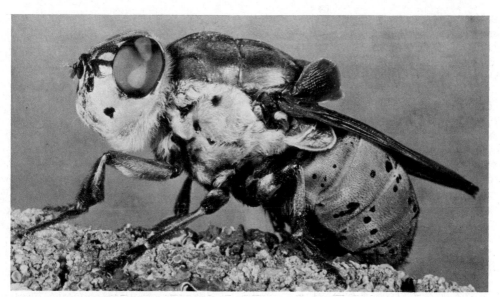

Figure 1–24. *Cuterebra jellisoni* (Cyclorrapha: Cuterebridae), a bot fly (approx. x8). From Baird, 1971: J. Med. Entomol., *8* (6), 616. The mouthparts of bot flies are vestigial.

those of the third stage, but the dark spines covering the body furnish evidence of the larva's identity as *Cuterebra*.

Life History and Pathogenesis. *Cuterebra* spp. infect rabbits, squirrels, chipmunks, mice, cats, dogs, and, occasionally, man (Baird *et al.*, 1982). Female *Cuterebra* flies lay their eggs along rabbit runs and near rodent burrows. As the host brushes past, the first stage larvae hatch instantaneously and crawl immediately into the host's fur. Once thought to burrow directly into the skin, these larvae are now known to enter the host through its natural body openings (Baird, 1971, 1972; Timm and Lee, 1981). *Cuterebra* larvae are usually found in the cervical subcutaneous connective tissue of cats and dogs during August, September, and October. The breathing hole should be judiciously enlarged with surgical scissors and the larva extracted with tissue forceps. The wound may heal slowly. *Cuterebra* larvae may also locate in the nasal and oral regions and sometimes migrate through the brains of cats and dogs with fatal results. At the present state of knowledge, it is impossible to differentiate species of even fully developed third stage larvae of *Cuterebra* except in the few cases in which their life histories have been worked out in detail.

Dermatobia

Identification. The adult of *Dermatobia hominis*, another member of the family Cutere-

bridae, somewhat resembles a brilliant blue calliphorid fly but, like all bot flies, has vestigial mouthparts. The fully developed third stage larva is pear-shaped and has posterior spiracles with straight slits deeply sunken in a concavity.

Life History and Pathogenesis. The *Dermatobia hominis* female uses a slave to carry her eggs to a prospective host. She captures another fly, usually a bloodsucker such as a mosquito or a stable fly, and glues her eggs to its abdomen. The eggs develop in a week or two and the larvae inside them stand ready to disembark when the slave fly alights upon the skin of a warm-blooded animal to feed. Each *D. hominis* larva that succeeds in penetrating the skin develops at or near the site of penetration in a separate warble. The larva emerges through the breathing hole to pupate about six weeks later. The *D. hominis* larva is a serious pest of man, cattle, sheep, dogs, and other mammals in Central and South America. The adult fly tends to concentrate at the edges of large forests.

EXPERT IDENTIFICATION OF MYIASIS LARVAE

The major taxa of fully developed myiasis larvae can be identified by means of the criteria set forth above. More detailed information will be found in James, M. J. (1947): *The Flies That Cause Myiasis In Man*. U.S.D.A. Misc. Publication 631. However, identification of all three larval stages of even the more common species is a chore for a taxonomic specialist. If your preliminary findings are inconclusive, intriguing, or of great practical importance, clean some larvae by shaking them vigorously in water, fix them in 70 per cent ethyl alcohol or 10 per cent formalin, and submit these specimens for expert identification. Precise identification in certain cases requires rearing the adult fly; instructions are provided under Sarcophagidae, above. Living larvae may also be submitted for expert identification in addition to but not in lieu of fixed specimens; include these in a separate jar loosely packed in moist cotton.

Orders Anoplura, Bloodsucking Lice, and Mallophaga, Chewing Lice

There are two main kinds of lice, represented by the orders Anoplura, or bloodsucking lice, and Mallophaga, or chewing lice. Anoplurans have piercing mouthparts

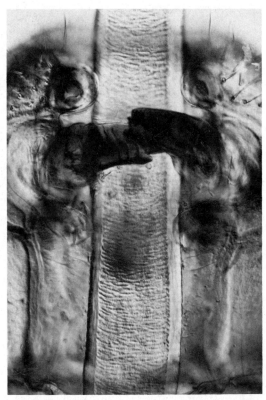

Figure 1–26. Mandibles of a mallophagan louse grasping a goat hair (x210).

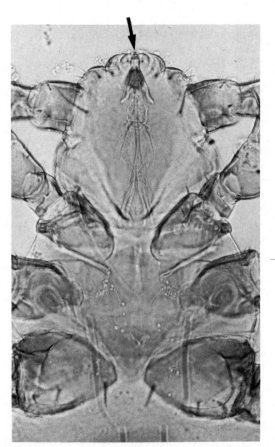

Figure 1–25. Head and thorax of an anopluran louse (x312). The bloodsucking stylets occupy the median plane of the head; mouth at arrow.

consisting of three stylets that, in fixed specimens, are usually concealed within the relatively narrow head (Fig. 1-25). Anoplurans are parasites of placental animals only. Mallophagans have stout mandibles on the ventral side of their relatively broad heads (Fig. 1-26), and these lice feed on epidermal scales, feathers, and sebaceous secretions of birds and mammals. Both anoplurans and mallophagans spend their entire lives among the hairs or feathers of their hosts and display a high order of host specificity. Even the eggs are securely attached to the hairs or feathers of the host (Fig. 1-27). The lice that hatch from these eggs are tiny replicas of the adults; they molt several times but undergo only minor changes in appearance (i.e., simple metamorphosis). The cycle from egg to egg requires several weeks, and only one or two eggs may be found developing within the abdomen of a female louse at any one time, but enormous populations may develop notwithstanding. The hatching process itself is of passing interest. The young louse swallows air and ejects it through its anus to form a cushion of compressed air that forces the animal against the operculum (i.e., lid) of the eggshell until it pops open. Thus it may be said (with due application of etymology and low humor) that *every louse is hoist by its own petard.*

Because of the sedentary habits of lice, one searches for them by carefully examining the hair coat or plumage of the host. The one exception to this generalization, the human body louse *Pediculus h. humanus*, clings to the fibers of the clothing instead of to body hairs while it feeds upon its host.

With a little practice, bloodsucking lice and chewing lice can be distinguished by inspection. This plus high host specificity simplifies identification, especially for hosts that have only one species of louse (e.g., *Haematopinus suis* on *Sus scrofa* and *Felicola subrostratus* on *Felis catus*). The next simplest case involves one anopluran and one mallophagan species per host species (e.g., *Haematopinus asini* plus *Damalinia equi* on *Equus caballus* and *Linognathus setosus* plus *Trichodectes canis* on *Canis familiaris*). Cattle (*Bos taurus*) present a more complex case; they are infested by three anoplurans and one mallophagan and attention to generic morphological characteristics is required for their diffentiation. Occasionally, a few lice are collected from other than their normal host. For example, *Pthirus pubis*, the human crab louse, has been reported now and again from dogs. In such cases, it is necessary to note the obvious morphological differences displayed by *Linognathus setosus*, the anopluran normally found on dogs, and *Pthirus pubis*, denizen of the human pubic hairs, in order to avoid misdiagnosis.

ORDER ANOPLURA

Anoplurans have pincerlike tarsal claws for clinging to the hairs of their hosts. The size of these claws is related to the diameter of the hair shaft and is probably an important factor in establishing host specificity and site specificity. Without hair, these lice are helpless; they pass from host to host most efficiently when a "bridge" of hair exists between host individuals. This is why *Pthirus pubis* is frequently transmitted during sexual intercourse. According to Chandler and Read (1961), the French call this parasite "papillon d'amour."

Pthirus

The large tarsal claws of *Pthirus pubis* (Fig. 1-27) are adapted to the coarse hairs of the pubic and perianal regions, armpits, mus-

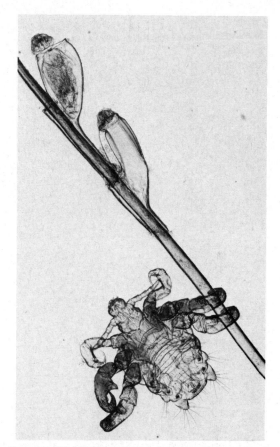

Figure 1–27. *Pthirus pubis* (Anoplura), the human crab louse, and two of its eggs on a pubic hair (x25). Dogs occasionally acquire *Pthirus pubis* by contact with infested human beings or their clothing.

tache, beard, and, particularly in young children, the eyebrows and eyelashes; these latter two furnishing the nearest approximation to a pubic hair that a child has to offer. Pruritus is intense and a papular dermatitis with discoloration of the skin develops. Once feeding, these lice display a marked disinclination to move and tend to remain fixed at one point for days while their feces accumulate about them. The life cycle requires about one month from egg to egg, so that considerable time may elapse between aquisition and awareness of infestation. Although sexual contact is the principal means of transmission between individuals, towels, clothing, and bedding used by an infested person are to be avoided. Entire families, children and family dog included, may become infested through fomites such as these. During crises of this sort, the dog may be presented to the veterinarian for euthanasia in the mistaken belief that the dog is the culprit and reservoir of pestilence. Dealing with a family

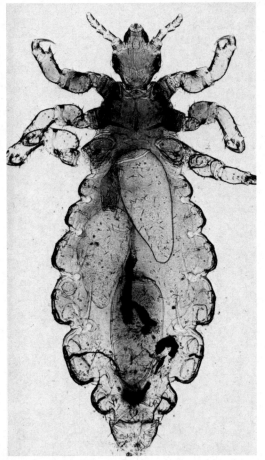

Figure 1–28. *Pediculus humanus capitis* (Anoplura), the human head louse (x34).

outbreak of crab lice and falsely incriminated dog requires considerable tact.

Another species in this genus is *Pthirus gorillae* of *Gorilla gorilla*.

Pediculus

The human head louse, *Pediculus humanus capitis* (Fig. 1-28), stays mainly on the human head, especially about the ears and nape of the neck. Dogs are rarely infested. Eggs are attached firmly to the hairs and hatch within a week. Infestation spreads rapidly because of the ease with which hairs are shed and wafted about. Outbreaks of head lice may occur under the best conditions of sanitation and personal deportment. The human body louse, *Pediculus h. humanus*, does not cling to hair. Instead, this louse clings to the fibers and deposits its eggs in the seams of clothing. Except in very heavy infestations, all one need do to be rid of body lice is to remove his or her clothing. When people are unable to bathe and change clothing for extended periods, as, for example, during wars and natural disasters, body louse populations are likely to expand rapidly. Under such circumstances, epidemic typhus (*Rickettsia prowazekii*), which is transmitted by the body louse, is likely to break out, and it is not for mere comfort's sake that vigorous delousing measures must be adopted.

Haematopinus

Identification. All tarsal claws are of equal size and the lateral margins of the abdomen are heavily sclerotized (Fig. 1-29). The two other anopluran genera found on cattle, i.e., *Linognathus* and *Solenopotes* differ in having smaller claws on their first pair of legs. Species of *Haematopinus* infesting domestic animals include *H. asini* of horses (see Fig. 9-1), *H. suis* of swine, and *H. eurysternus*, *H. quadripertussus*, and *H. tuberculatus* of cattle. *Haematopinus eurysternus* is a common parasite of domestic cattle (*Bos taurus*) in North America and tends to concentrate on the

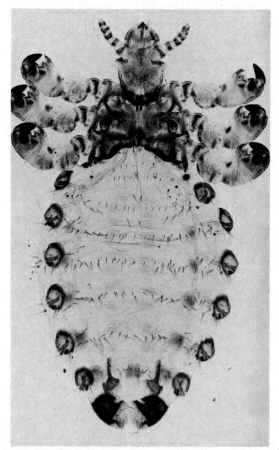

Figure 1–29. *Haematopinus eurysternus* (Anoplura) of cattle (x31). All tarsal claws are of equal size.

bers of the same herd support only light infestations. These "louse breeders," as they are called, are likely to perish during winter storms, weakened as they are by their louse burdens. Such animals may be saved by insecticide applications. The rate of increase in hematocrit is, however, considerably slower than one would expect in a simple blood loss anemia.

Linognathus

Identification. Unlike *Haematopinus*, the first pair of tarsal claws of *Linognathus* is smaller than the second and third pairs and the lateral margins of the abdomen are not heavily sclerotized (Fig, 1-30). *Linognathus* differs from *Solenopotes* in having more than one row of setae per abdominal segment and in lacking a sternal plate and protuberant abdominal spiracles. Species of *Linognathus* infesting domestic animals include: *Linognathus vituli* of cattle, *L. ovillus*, *L. pedalis*, and *L. oviformes* of sheep, *L. stenopsis* of goats, and *L. setosus* of dogs and foxes (see Fig. 7-1).

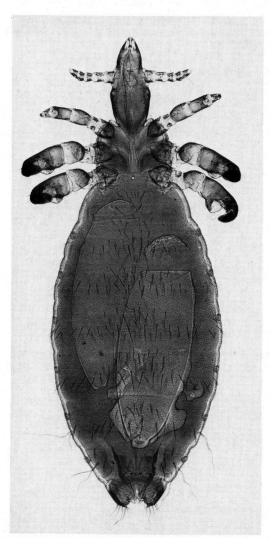

Figure 1–30. *Linognathus vituli* (Anoplura) of cattle (x45). The first pair of tarsal claws is smaller than the second and third pairs. Spiracles are flush with the surface of the abdomen, and there are more than one row of setae per abdominal segment.

neck, poll, brisket, and tail but in heavy infestation may be generally distributed over the body. *H. quadripertussus,* normally a tropical and subtropical parasite of *Bos indicus* and indicus-taurus hybrids, lays its eggs in the tail switch but may be found around the eyes and long hairs of the ears (Roberts, 1952). *H. tuberculatus* is an Old World parasite of water buffalo (*Bubalus bubalus*) and of domestic cattle associated with them (Meleney and Kim, 1974).

Heavy infestations of *H. eurysternus* are capable of causing severe anemia in adult range cattle (Peterson *et al.,* 1953). Certain individuals are predisposed to the growth of large populations of lice, while other mem-

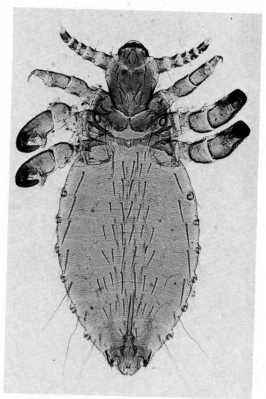

Figure 1–31. *Solenopotes capillatus* (Anoplura) of cattle (x60). The first pair of tarsal claws is smaller than the second and third pairs. Spiracles protrude above the surface of the abdomen, and there is only one row of setae per abdominal segment.

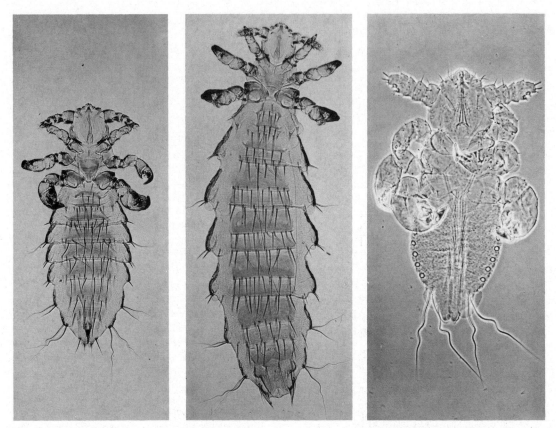

Figure 1–32. *Polyplax serrata* (Anoplura) of the mouse: male (left, x70), female (center, x70), and nymph (right, x168).

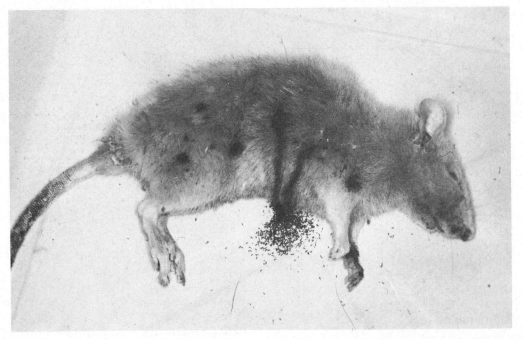

Figure 1–33. *Polyplax spinulosa* leaving a rat that died of the effects of its louse population. Urged on by the heat of an incandescent bulb, these lice are emulating their host's legendary tendency to flee from unpromising situations. This is a general phenomenon among the more mobile ectoparasites and can be exploited to advantage in diagnosis. However, if it is necessary to euthanize the host, do not use chloroform, ether, or other agents that will as surely kill the parasites as their hosts.

Solenopotes

Identification. *Solenopotes capillatus*, the "little blue louse" of cattle, is distinguished from *Linognathus* in having only one row of setae per abdominal segment, a sternal plate at least half as wide as it is long, and protuberant abdominal spiracles (Fig. 1-31).

Polyplax

Polyplax spinulosa is a parasite of the rat and *P. serrata* is a parasite of the mouse (Fig. 1-32). Both of these anoplurans may develop into serious nuisances in laboratory animal colonies and, when sufficiently abundant, may even bleed animals to death (Fig. 1-33).

ORDER MALLOPHAGA

Mallophagans, or chewing lice, are parasites of birds and mammals. All bird lice are biting lice and there is a rich variety of them,

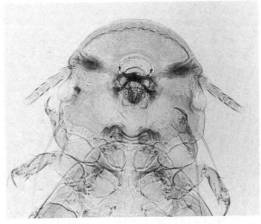

Figure 1–35. *Goniocotes* sp. (Mallophaga: Ischnocera) of the chicken (x79). Typical of ischnocerans parasitizing birds, *Goniocotes* has five-segmented antennae.

more than 40 species. Because their hosts are insectivorous and very fastidious, bird lice are in constant hazard of being eaten by their host instead of *vice versa.* However, they tend to be far less sluggish than their relatives that parasitize mammals; they have long legs to help them keep "one step ahead" and frequently develop enormous populations. Mallophagans may cause their hosts considerable irritation when present in large numbers and especially in situations where it is difficult for the animals to groom themselves, as in the case of stanchioned cattle. There are three suborders of chewing lice: Ischnocera, Amblycera, and Rhynchophthirina.

Suborder Ischnocera

Ischnocerans have salient antennae that are three-jointed in species infesting mammals (Fig. 1-34) and five-jointed in species infesting birds; all lack maxillary palps (Fig. 1-35).

Damalinia (*Bovicola*). Species infesting domestic mammals include: *D. bovis* on cattle, *D. equi* on horses, *D. ovis* on sheep, and *D. caprae*, *D. limbata*, and *D. (Holokartikos) crassipes* on goats.

Trichodectes. *Trichodectes canis*, the canine chewing louse (Figs. 1-36 and 1-37), may serve as intermediate host (cyclodevelopmental vector) of the tapeworm *Dipylidium caninum*, although the flea *Ctenocephalides* is more important in this respect. *Trichodectes canis* must be differentiated from the anopluran *Linognathus setosus* and from the warm climate amblyceran, *Heterodoxus spiniger.*

Felicola. *Felicola subrostratus* is the only louse found on cat (see Fig. 7-2).

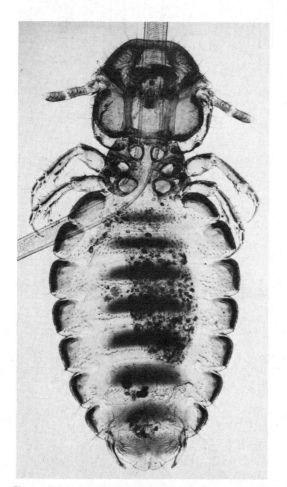

Figure 1–34. *Damalinia (Holokartikos) crassipes* (Mallophaga: Ischnocera) of the goat (x33). Typical of ischnocerans parasitizing mammals, *D. crassipes* has three-segmented antennae.

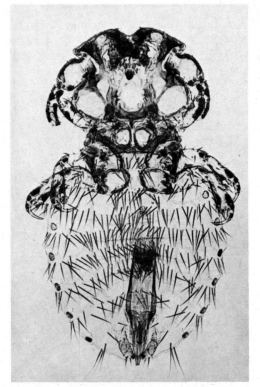

Figure 1–36. *Trichodectes canis* (Mallophaga: Ischnocera), male, of the dog (x51).

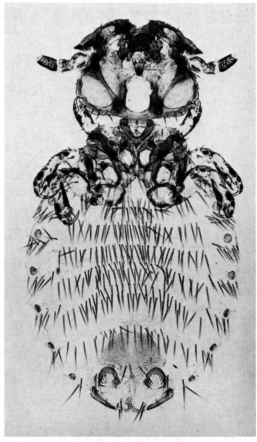

Figure 1–37. *Trichodectes canis* (Mallophaga: Ischnocera), female, of the dog (x51).

Suborder Amblycera

Amblycerans have club-shaped antennae that lie in grooves in the head and four-segmented maxillary palpi (Fig. 1-38). Many amblycerans are parasites of birds but one species, *Heterodoxus spiniger*, is a parasite of dogs in warm climates, and three species, *Gliricola porcelli*, *Gyropus ovalis*, and *Trimenopon hispidum*, are parasites of the guinea pig (Fig. 1-39).

Suborder Rhynchophtherina

Haematomyzus spp. are parasites of elephants and wart hogs (Fig. 1-40).

Order Siphonaptera, Fleas

Fleas are principally parasites of dogs, cats, pigs, people, rodents, and birds. The adults are obligate bloodsucking parasites and are extremely annoying because of their bites. Most species of fleas show limited host specificity and when hungry enough will attack any source of blood, even a fresh steak. Unfed *Ctenocephalides* adults can survive for about two months waiting for a host to hap-

pen by. People returning home after an absence of several weeks may be greeted by hordes of bloodthirsty *Ctenocephalides* fleas that, although preferring to feed on dogs, are quite willing to make do with humans when no dog is available. One of our learned mentors used to deal with this situation as

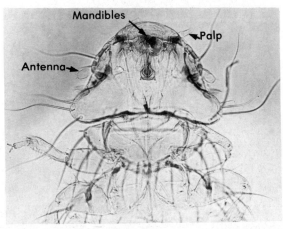

Figure 1–38. *Menopon* sp. (Mallophaga: Amblycera) of the chicken (x75).

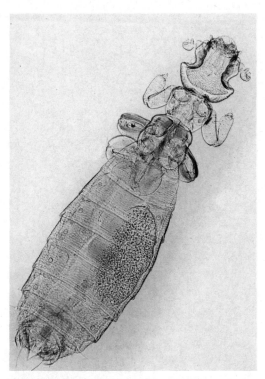

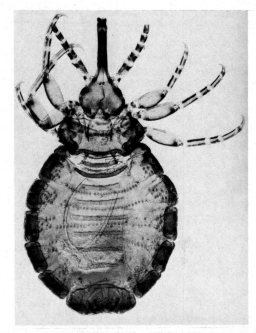

Figure 1–40. *Haematomyzus elephantis* (Mallophaga: Rhynchophthirina) of the elephant (x34).

Figure 1–39. *Gliricola porcelli* (Mallophaga: Amblycera) of the guinea pig (x90).

follows. On arriving back in town, he would go directly to the kennel where his dog had been housed during his absence and take the dog home to collect the hungry fleas that were sure to be lying there in wait. After a brief tour of the house the dog was immediately taken back to the kennel for a flea bath.

Ctenocephalides

Identification. *Ctenocephalides* spp. are parasites of cats and dogs but frequently attack other domestic animals and man. *Ctenocephalides* have both genal and pronotal *combs* (Fig. 1-41), easily distinguishing them from *Echidnophaga* (Fig. 1-42), *Xenopsylla* (Fig. 1-43), and *Pulex* (Fig. 1-44), which have neither genal nor pronotal combs, and from certain rodent fleas that have only pronotal combs. *Cediopsylla* (Fig. 1-45), a rabbit flea, resembles *Ctenocephalides* in having both genal and pronotal combs but can be distinguished as follows. If a line drawn along the bases of the genal teeth runs parallel to the long axis of the head, the specimen is *Ctenocephalides*, whereas if it runs at an angle it is *Cediopsylla*.

Diagnosis of dog and cat flea infestation is sometimes difficult partly because only a few fleas are required to cause great misery, especially in a sensitized individual. Many fail

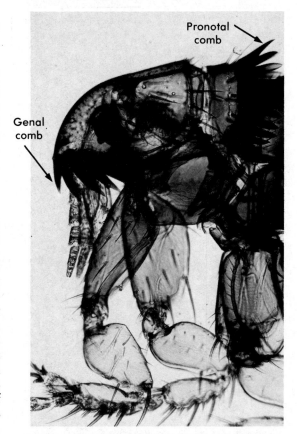

Figure 1–41. *Ctenocephalides* (Siphonaptera) of the cat and dog (x88). The bases of the genal teeth of *Ctenocephalides* lie on a line running parallel to the long axis of the head, thus serving to distinguish this genus from certain rodent and leporid fleas that have both genal and pronotal combs.

to recognize the eggs and larvae of fleas (Figs. 1-46 and 1-47) and wonder what the "tiny caterpillars" are that accumulate below a cat as it stands on the examining table. *Ctenocephalides*, more than most other fleas, tend to lay their eggs on the host instead of in the nest. Many of these 0.5-mm.-long, glistening, white eggs remain on the host long enough to hatch, and so we find not only adults but eggs and larvae of *Ctenocephalides* in the haircoat of infested dogs and cats. Adult fleas are bloodsuckers and their feces consist of only partly digested blood. The larval fleas eat their parents' dried feces as well as other organic debris. The accumulation of flea feces in the haircoat may be detected by a sort of paper chromatography. Detritus suspected of being flea feces may be placed on filter paper or other absorbent material that has been dampened with dilute soap or detergent solution. Hemoglobin will diffuse out of flea feces in a few minutes and form a red halo about the speck of suspect detritus. Or, a similarly dampened pledget of absorbent cotton may be rubbed over the haircoat and skin to pick up particles of flea feces yielding a like result.

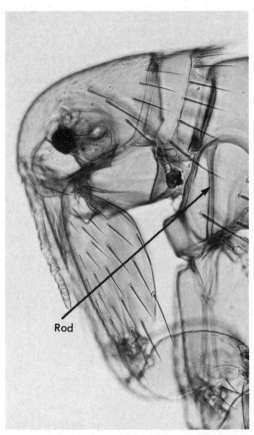

Figure 1–43. *Xenopsylla* (Siphonaptera), a rat flea and biological vector of plague (*Yersinia pestis*) and endemic typhus (*Rickettsia typhi*) (x82). The vertical rod on the mesothorax distinguishes this genus from *Pulex*.

Life History. As with all fleas, metamorphosis is complex, with egg, larval, pupal, and adult instars. Development of *Ctenocephalides felis* from egg to adult occurs within the ranges 13 to 32°C and 50 to 92 per cent relative humidity and requires from 14 to 140 days at the extremes of temperature. Temperatures above 35°C are lethal to larvae and pupae. Unfed adults may survive for many weeks under cool, humid conditions but probably cannot long withstand the low relative humidities associated with subfreezing conditions (Silverman *et al.*, 1981).

Disease Transmission. *Ctenocephalides canis* and *C. felis* are true intermediate hosts (biological vectors) of the tapeworm *Dipylidium caninum* and the filariid nematode *Dipetalonema reconditum*. Fleas acquire *D. caninum* infection as larvae, as this is the only stage with chewing mouthparts suitable for ingesting solid material such as the eggs of this tapeworm. The cysticercoid that develops from the egg is passed along through metamorphosis to the adult flea and infects the

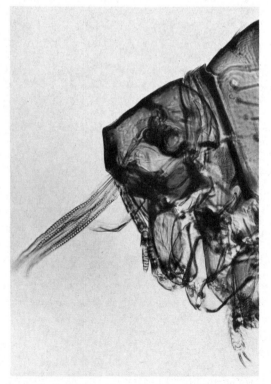

Figure 1–42. *Echidnophaga* (Siphonaptera) (x87). *Echidnophaga gallinacea*, the poultry sticktight flea, may be found firmly attached in clusters on chickens' heads and on the eyelids or in the ear canals of dogs, cats, and other animals.

dog or cat that chances to ingest that particular flea. Microfilariae of *Dipetalonema reconditum,* on the other hand, are ingested by the blood-feeding adult flea and develop into third stage larvae capable of infecting a dog at a subsequent feeding.

Echidnophaga

Echidnophaga gallinacea, the "sticktight flea" of poultry, attacks all kinds of domestic birds as well as dogs, cats, rabbits, horses, and man in subtropical America. I once found several embedded in the eyelids of a cat recently arrived in New York from Alabama. On birds, *E. gallinacea* embeds itself in the skin around the eyes and cloaca and on the combs, wattles, and other glabrous areas. These are small fleas with angular heads and are devoid of genal and pronotal combs; the thoracic tergites (dorsal sclerites of the thorax) are very narrow (Fig. 1-42).

Tunga

Tunga penetrans, the "jigger" or "chigoe," is a small (1 mm.) flea of tropical America and Africa that somewhat resembles *Echid-*

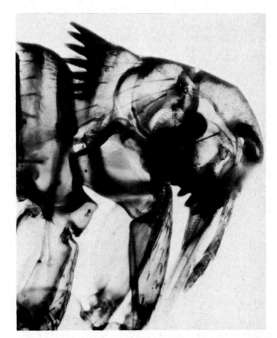

Figure 1–45. *Cediopsylla* (Siphonaptera) of the rabbit (x71). The bases of the genal teeth lie on a line running at an angle to the long axis of the head, thus serving to distinguish this genus from *Ctenocephalides.*

nophaga in having an angular head and narrow thoracic segments and in lacking combs. The impregnated *Tunga* female embeds in the host's skin with only the last few abdominal segments protruding. Eggs are retained in the abdomen and the flea swells to the size of a pea. Lesions caused by this flea are painful and subject to secondary infection and are supposedly the inspiration for the sailor's oath, "I'll be jiggered" (Chandler and Read, 1955).

Xenopsylla

Xenopsylla is a widely distributed genus of rat fleas that also attack man and are an important vector of plague (*Yersinia pestis*) and murine (endemic) typhus (*Rickettsia typhi*). Combs are absent and the head is smoothly rounded, thus distinguishing *Xenopsylla* from the foregoing genera; it differs from *Pulex* in having a vertical rod on the mesothorax (Fig. 1-43).

Pulex

Identification. *Pulex irritans,* the human flea, is widely distributed and attacks a wide range of hosts including man, swine, and dogs. *Pulex* resembles *Xenopsylla* but lacks the mesothoracic rod (Fig. 1-44).

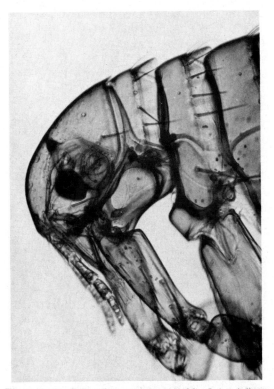

Figure 1–44. *Pulex* (Siphonaptera) (x81). *Pulex irritans,* the human flea, attacks a wide range of hosts.

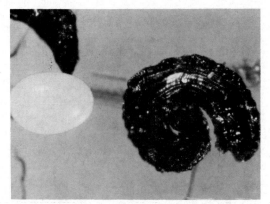

Figure 1–46. Egg of *Ctenocephalides* and two masses of flea feces (x50). Flea feces consists essentially of dried host's blood and serves as food for the flea larvae, which have chewing mouthparts.

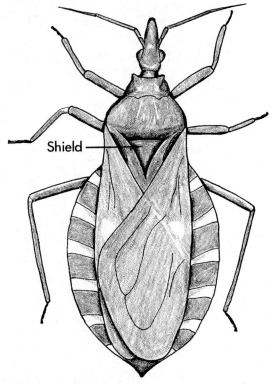

Figure 1–48. *Triatoma sanguisuga* (Hemiptera: Reduviidae), an assassin bug. Redrawn from Kitselman and Grundman, 1940.

Order Hemiptera, Bugs

Hemipterans have two pairs of wings (which may be vestigial), a triangular shield between the wing bases, four-segmented antennae, and a three-segmented beak that is directed caudally beneath the head when not in use (Figs. 1-48 and 1-49).

Metamorphosis is simple. Some hemipterans feed on plants, some kill insects and suck

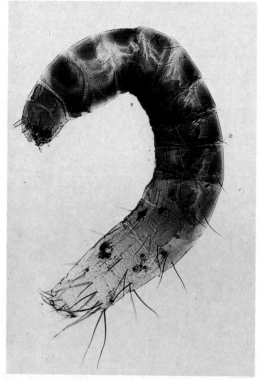

Figure 1–47. Larva of *Ctenocephalides* (x67). Flea larvae are frequently overlooked or misidentified.

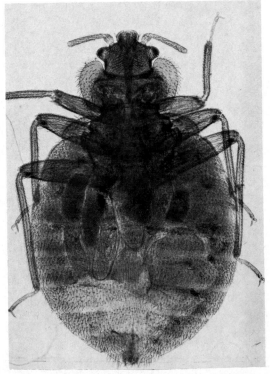

Figure 1–49. *Cimex lectularius* (Hemiptera: Cimicidae), the bed bug (x15).

their juices, and some are bloodsuckers and pests of rodents and man and occasionally attack other animals. Predacious reduviids (assassin bugs) inflict painful bites, and many such species have been reported to attack man, but the bites of the more specialized parasitic reduviids (conenoses) and cimicids (bed bugs) are painless.

FAMILY REDUVIIDAE, ASSASSIN BUGS AND KISSING OR CONENOSE BUGS

The reduviids (Fig. 1-48) have wings and a characteristic three-segmented beak. The parasitic species of the subfamily Triatominae, which feed exclusively on the blood of vertebrates, have a more slender beak than the predatory species and are able to feed sufficiently painlessly as not to awaken a sleeping host. They hide in crevices by day and attack their sleeping hosts by night in the manner of bed bugs, argasid ticks, and various mesostigmatid mites. Triatomins of the genera *Triatoma, Rhodnius,* and *Panstrongylus* transmit American trypanosomiasis or Chagas' disease (*Trypanosoma cruzi*). *Triatoma sanguisuga* may play a minor role in the transmission of equine encephalomyelitis.

FAMILY CIMICIDAE, BED BUGS

Bed bugs (Fig. 1-49) have oval, dorsoventrally flattened bodies, vestigial wings, three-segmented beaks, and a disagreeable odor. They are nocturnal and secretive bloodsucking parasites of man, chickens, bats, and nesting birds. Like triatomins, bed bugs hide in crevices by day and attack their sleeping host at night. They lay their eggs in their hiding places and molt five times at approximately weekly intervals, taking one blood meal between each molt and another before egg laying. Bed bugs can endure starvation for several months. Although such a blood-feeding pattern as this would seem ideally suited to the transmission of disease organisms, bed bugs, though frequently indicted, have yet to be convicted on any such counts.

Order Dictyophora, Cockroaches

Cockroaches are important as intermediate hosts of certain parasitic worms such as the spirurid nematodes *Spirura, Oxyspirura,* and *Gongylonema,* the acanthocephalans *Moniliformis, Prosthenorchis,* and *Homorhynchus,* and

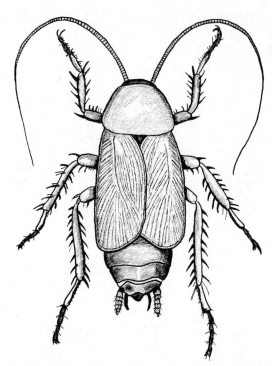

Figure 1–50. A cockroach, *Blatella orientalis* (Dictyophora). (Redrawn from Belding, 1942).

the pentastomid *Raillietiella*. They also serve as mechanical vectors of filth-borne diseases of man. Inspection of premises where food is prepared is often a veterinary function. Presence or absence of cockroaches is an important criterion of the adequacy of food sanitation (Fig. 1-50).

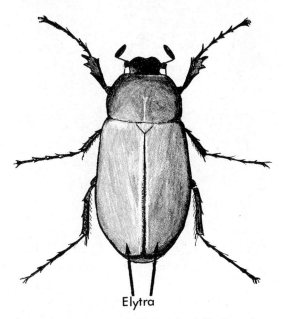

Elytra

Figure 1–51. A May beetle (Coleoptera). (Redrawn from Matheson, 1944).

Order Coleoptera, Beetles

Beetles have hard, shell-like outer wing covers called *elytra* that lack venation (Fig. 1-51). Metamorphosis is complete; the larvae are grubs.

Beetles, like cockroaches, are important as intermediate hosts of parasitic worms that infect domestic animals and man. The spirurid nematodes *Gongylonema* and *Physocephalus*, the acanthocephalans *Macracanthorhynchus* and *Moniliformis*, and the cestodes *Hymenolepis* and *Raillietina* (not to be confused with the pentastomid *Raillietiella* or, for that matter, with the mesostigmatid *Raillietia*) all develop in beetles to the stage infective for the vertebrate host.

Some species of beetles are also extremely toxic. For example, blister beetles (*Epicauta* spp.; Fig. 1-52) release an irritant and vesicant chemical (*cantharidin*) when crushed during single operation mowing-crimping of alfalfa hay. Hay containing these crushed beetles is lethal for horses and may remain so even after years of storage. Clinical signs of cantharidin toxicosis include abdominal

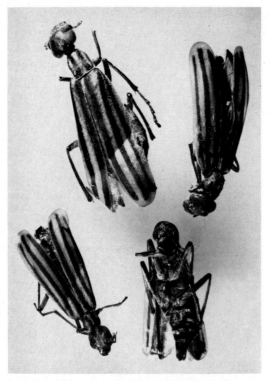

Figure 1–52. *Epicauta* sp. striped blister beetles (approx. x2). Consumption of alfalfa hay containing dead striped blister beetles causes acute cantharidin toxicosis in horses. Specimens kindly provided by Dr. R. J. Panciera.

pain, fever, depression, frequent urination, shock, and, occasionally, synchronous diaphragmatic flutter; mortality may exceed 70 per cent of affected individuals. Hematologic findings included hemoconcentration, neutrophilic leukocytosis, and hypocalcemia. As in all clinical poisonings, locating the source of the toxic agent is essential both to reaching a definitive diagnosis and to preventing further losses; the beetles should be sought in hay fed to the affected horses (Schoeb and Panciera, 1978; 1979). The lethal dose of cantharidin for the horse is probably less than 1 mg./kg. of body weight (Beasley *et al.*, 1983).

REFERENCES

Abbitt, B., and Abbitt, L. G. (1981): Fatal exsanguination of cattle attributed to an attack of salt marsh mosquitoes (*Aedes sollicitans*). J. Am. Vet. Med. Assn., *179* (12), 1397-1400.

Baird, C. R. (1971): Development of *Cuterebra jellisoni* (Diptera: Cuterebridae) in six species of rabbits and rodents. J. Med. Entomol., *8* (6), 615-622.

Baird, C. R. (1972): Development of *Cuterebra ruficrus* (Diptera: Cuterebridae) in six species of rabbits and rodents with a comparison of *C. ruficrus* and *C. jellisoni* third instars. J. Med. Entomol., *9* (1), 81-85.

Baird, C. R., Podgore, J. K., and Sabrosky, C. W. (1982): *Cuterebra* myiasis in humans: six new case reports from the United States with a summary of known cases (Diptera: Cuterebridae). J. Med. Entomol., *19* (3), 263-267.

Beasley, V. R., Wolf, G. A., Fischer, D. C., Ray, A. C., and Edwards, W. C. (1983): Cantharidin toxicosis in horses. J. Am. Vet. Med. Assoc. *182* (3), 283-284.

Belding, D. L. (1942): Textbook of Clinical Parasitology. New York, Appleton-Century Co., 888 pages.

Burghardt, H. F., Whitlock, J. H., and McEnerney, P. J. (1951): Dermatitis due to *Simulium* (black flies). Cornell Vet., *41* (3), 311-313.

Bush, G. L., Neck, R. W., and Kitto, G. Barrie (1976): Screwworm eradication: Inadvertent selection for noncompetitive ecotypes during mass rearing. Science, *193*, 491-493.

Chandler, A. C., and Read, C. P. (1961): Introduction to Parasitology. 10th ed. New York, Wiley, 822 pages.

Chitwood, M. B., and Stoffolano, J. G. (1971): First report of *Thelazia* sp. (Nematoda) in the face fly, *Musca autumnalis*, in North America. J. Parasitol., *57* (6), 1363-1364.

Cogley, T. P., Anderson, J. R., and Cogley, L. J. (1982): Migration of *Gasterophilus intestinalis* larvae (Diptera: Gasterophilidae) in the equine oral cavity. Int. J. Parasitol., *12* (5), 473-480.

Edwards, F. W., Oldroyd, H., and Smart, J. (1939): British Blood-Sucking Flies. London, British Museum (Natural History), 156 pages.

Haufe, W. O. (1982): Growth of range cattle protected from horn flies (*Haematobia irritans*) by ear tags impregnated with fenvalerate. Canadian J. Anim. Sci., *62* (2), 567-573.

Hibler, C. P., and Adcock, J. L. (1971): Elaeophorosis.

In Davis, J. W., and Anderson, R. C., editors, Parasitic Diseases of Wild Mammals. Iowa State University Press, Ames.

James, M. T. (1948): The Flies That Cause Myiasis In Man. U.S.D.A. Misc. Publication No. 631.

Kitselman, C. H., and Grundman, A. W. (1940): Equine encephalomyelitis virus isolated from naturally infected *Triatoma sanguisuga* Le Conte. Kansas State College Agricultural Experiment Station, Technical Bulletin 50.

Matheson, R. (1944): Entomology for Introductory Courses. Ithaca, N.Y., Comstock Publishing Co.

Olander, H. J. (1967): The migration of *Hypoderma lineatum* in the brain of a horse. A case report and review. Path. Vet., *4*, 477-483.

Peterson, H. O., Roberts, I. H., Becklund, W. W., and Kemper, H. E. (1953): Anemia in cattle caused by heavy infestation of the bloodsucking louse *Haematopinus eurysternus*. J. Am. Vet. Med. Assoc., *122*, 373-376.

Riek, R. F. (1953a): Studies on allergic dermatitis ("Queensland itch") of the horse. I. Description, distribution, symptoms, and pathology. Australian Vet. J., *29*, 177-184.

Riek, R. F. (1953b): Studies on allergic dermatitis of the horse. II. Treatment and control. Australian Vet. J., *29*, 185-187.

Roberts, F. H. S. (1952): Insects Affecting Livestock. Sydney, Angus and Robertson Ltd., 267 pages.

Schoeb, T. R., and Panciera, R. J. (1978): Blister beetle poisoning in horses. J. Am. Vet. Med. Assoc., *173*, 75-77.

Schoeb, T. R., and Panciera, R. J. (1979): Pathology of blister beetle poisoning in horses. Vet. Pathol., *16*, 18-31.

Schroeder, H. O. (1940): Habits of the larvae of *Gasterophilus nasalis* (L.) in the mouth of the horse. J. Econ. Entomol., *33* (2), 382-384.

Silverman, J., Rust, M. K., and Reierson, D. A. (1981): Influence of temperature and humidity on survival and development of the cat flea, *Ctenocephalides felis* (Siphonaptera: Pulicidae). J. Med. Entomol. *18* (1), 78-83.

Smith, P. H., Dallwitz, R., Wardhaugh, K. G., Vogt, W. G., and Woodburn, T. L. (1981): Timing of larval exodus from sheep and carrion in the sheep blow fly, *Lucilia cuprina*. Entomologica Experimentalis et Applicata, *30* (2), 157-162.

Timm, R. M., and Lee, R. E., Jr. (1981): Do bot flies, *Cuterebra* (Diptera; Cuterebridae), emasculate their hosts? J. Med, Entomol., *18* (4), 333-336.

Washburn, R. H., Klebsadel, L. J., Palmer, J. S., Luick, J. R., and Bleicher, D. P. (1980): The warble fly problem in Alaska reindeer. Agroborealis, *12*, 23-28.

2

ARACHNIDS

Although the class Arachnida includes spiders, scorpions, whip scorpions, and other forms that are of occasional interest to veterinarians, the following exposition is restricted to the ticks and mites. Larval stages of both ticks and mites normally have three pairs of legs and the nymphs and adults have four pairs. The head, thorax, and abdomen are fused; antennae and mandibles are absent. The mouthparts (*palps, chelicerae,* and *hypostome*) together with the *basis capituli* form a false head or *capitulum* (Fig. 2-1).

SUBORDER METASTIGMATA, TICKS

All ticks are bloodsucking parasites. The hypostome is armed with backward-projecting teeth and the chelicerae are armed with movable denticles (Fig. 2-1). The lateral stigmata are caudodorsal to the fourth coxae (Fig. 2-2) and lack the sinuous peritremes characteristic of the somewhat similar suborder Mesostigmata. Important morphological and biological characteristics help to distinguish the two main families, Argasidae and Ixodidae.

Family Argasidae

The family Argasidae, or *soft ticks,* is a small family of 140 species belonging to four genera, *Argas, Ornithodorus, Otobius,* and *Antricola. Antricola* spp. are limited to bats and will not be considered further here. Argasids live in nests, burrows, buildings, and sleeping places of their host animals and are distributed mostly in arid regions or in drier habitats in moist regions. The life stages consist of the egg (laid in several batches of

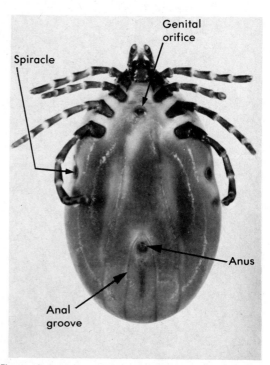

Figure 2–2. Ventral aspect of *Ixodes* (x11). The anal groove of *Ixodes* curves anteriorly around the anus.

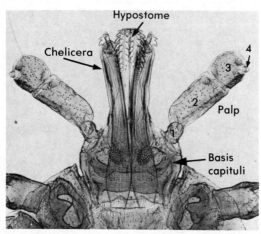

Figure 2–1. Capitulum of *Amblyomma* (x40).

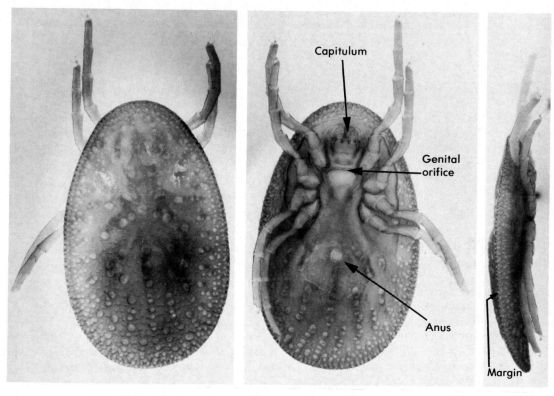

Figure 2–3. *Argas*, dorsal (left), ventral (center), and lateral (right) aspects (x10).

hundreds), larva, two or more nymphal stages, and adult male and female. Unlike ixodid nymphs and adults, which require several days to complete engorgement and feed only once during each stage, argasid nymphs and adults feed to repletion on their sleeping hosts in minutes or hours and feed repeatedly. Females lay a clutch of eggs after each blood meal. Argasid larvae, on the other hand, feed for several days and nymphs of *Otobius* may remain in the external ear canal of cattle for several weeks.

Argas

Identification. *Argas* spp. are 5–10 mm., flattened, ovoid, and yellow to reddish-brown ticks with leathery, mamillated and wrinkled dorsal and ventral surfaces meeting at a sharp lateral margin. The mouthparts are on the ventral surface and are hidden when the tick is viewed from above (Fig. 2-3). *Argas* is rarely found on the host. Search cracks and crannies in the hen house for this parasite. In the United States, *Argas* is distributed along the Gulf of Mexico and Mexican border.

Life History. Female *Argas* ticks deposit their eggs in clutches of 25 to 100 in the crevices that serve as hiding places during the day. Several clutches are laid, each preceded by a blood meal lasting 45 minutes or less. The six-legged larva hatches in one to four weeks, attaches to a host, and feeds for about five days; the larva is thus active day and night. When replete, the larva leaves the host and finds a hiding place in which to spend a week or so molting into a nymph. The eight-legged nymph feeds at night and undergoes a second molt to a second nymphal stage, which again feeds and undergoes a third molt into an adult male or female. Development from egg to adult may be completed in as little as 30 days but lack of suitable hosts may prolong the process. Larvae and nymphs may survive for months and adults for more than two years without a blood meal. It doesn't pay to try to "starve them out."

Disease Transmission. In South America, *Argas* spp. transmit fowl spirochetosis (*Borrelia anserina*), via tick fecal contamination, to domestic poultry, grouse, canaries, guinea fowl, and pigeons. Ticks may remain infective for six months or more and transmit the spirochetes to their offspring via the ovaries (transovarial transmission). *Argas* spp. also transmit a rickettsial agent, *Aegyptianella pul-*

lorum, to chickens and geese in the tropics and subtropics of the Old World.

Ornithodorus

Identification. *Ornithodorus* differs from *Argas* in being more globular, in lacking a sharp lateral margin, and in not being distinctly ovoid when viewed from above. The body is flattened in unfed specimens but strongly convex dorsally when distended with blood. These ticks (Fig. 2-4) are found in cracks and crannies of avian roosts and nests, rodent burrows, and the resting places of large mammals.

Life History. Species of *Ornithodorus* differ as to whether the larvae feed, in the number of larval instars (three to five), and in host and lair preferences. *Ornithodorus hermsi* is a rodent parasite in the Rocky Mountain and Pacific Coast states, breeding in rodent burrows and rodent-infested buildings, whereas *O. coriaceus* of California and Oregon attacks deer and cattle from the soil of their bedding areas. As typical argasids, *Ornithodorus* spp. can survive unfed for months or even years.

Disease Transmission. *Ornithodorus* spp. are most important as vectors and reservoirs of relapsing fever spirochetes (*Borrelia recurrentis*) of man. Infection may be maintained in tick populations for many years by transovarial transmission of the spirochetes from female ticks to their offspring and tends to remain endemic in wild rodent populations. Tick-borne relapsing fever typically involves an individual or small group of campers who have slept in a tick-infested cabin out in the wilderness. Because the *Ornithodorus* ticks involved in transmission are nocturnal and surreptitious, relapsing fever victims are frequently unaware of recent tick exposure.

Otobius

Identification. Larvae and two nymphal stages of *Otobius megnini*, the spinose ear tick, parasitize the ear canals of cattle, remaining in a particular host for as long as four months. Other domestic animals and man also sometimes serve as hosts. One of my former students reported that he had suffered several painful attacks by *Otobius*. As implied by the common name, the cuticle of *Otobius* is covered by spines. The second nymphal stage is particularly distinctive (Fig. 2-5).

Life History. Larvae feed in the ear canal and molt into the first nymphal stage, which in turn feeds in the same host's ear canal and molts into the second nymphal stage, which again feeds but leaves the ear canal and drops to the ground to molt to the adult stage. Adult *Otobius* have vestigial hypostomes and do not feed; they copulate within a day or two after emergence and the females oviposit in the soil. Larvae survive unfed for as long as two months. Thus, *Otobius* differs from *Argas* and *Ornithodorus* in being a one-host tick and in laying only one clutch of eggs.

Family Ixodidae

Members of the family Ixodidae, or *hard ticks,* have a shield or *scutum* that covers the entire dorsal surface of the male but only part of the dorsal surface of the female (Fig. 2-6). The size of the scutum remains constant during engorgement of a female and consequently covers a progressively smaller proportion of her dorsum. Eggs are laid in a single clutch of thousands. The larvae, the single nymphal stage, and the adults of Ixodidae feed only once each, several days being required for engorgement. Ixodids usually live outdoors and attach to passing host animals. There are two molts: the first from

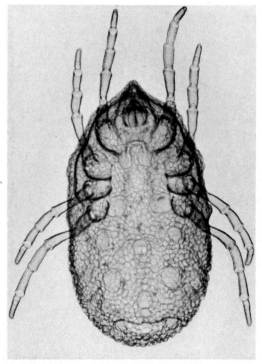

Figure 2–4. *Ornithodorus* (x14).

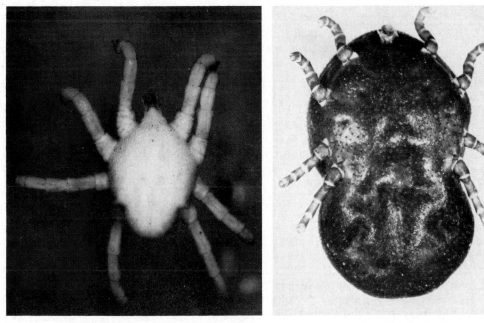

Figure 2–5. *Otobius megnini*, first nymph (left, x12) and second nymph (right, x8).

larva to nymph and the second from nymph to adult. Species that complete both molts without leaving the host are called *one-host ticks*, species whose engorged nymphs drop off to molt are called *two-host ticks*, and those whose nymphs and larvae drop off to molt are called *three-host ticks*. *Dermacentor variabilis* is a three-host tick whose larvae and nymphs engorge on small mammals and whose adults engorge on dogs. *Rhipicephalus sanguinius* is a three-host tick whose larvae, nymphs, and adults all engorge on dogs. The individual or

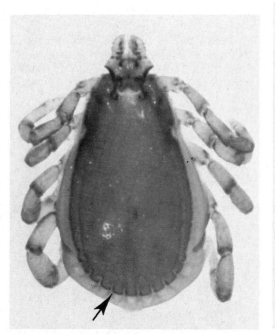
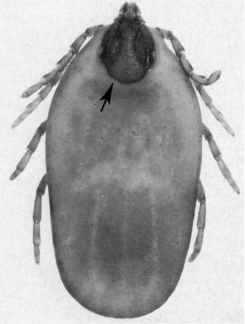

Figure 2–6. *Rhipicephalus* male (left, x23) and female (right, x 12). The scutum (arrows) covers the entire dorsal surface of male ixodid ticks but only a portion of the dorsal surface of females. As the female engorges, the scutum remains constant in size and, at last, covers only a small proportion of the fully engorged female (see Fig. 2–16).

species identity of the host has no bearing on the use of these terms.

Two- and three-host ticks can transmit disease organisms *interstadially*, that is, infection acquired by a larval tick is carried through the molt to the nymphal stage and then conveyed to the host that the nymph feeds upon, or infection acquired by a nymph is carried through the molt and conveyed to the host that the adult tick feeds upon. Thus, three-host ticks can transmit disease organisms interstadially through both larva to nymph and nymph to adult transitions, whereas two-host ticks are limited to the latter. In *transovarial* transmission, the disease organisms are passed from the adult female tick to her larvae through infection of her ovaries. *Babesia bigemina* is transmitted from the adult female *Boophilus* tick to her progeny by way of her ovaries. *Transovarial transmission* of disease organisms is the only mechanism that allows one-host ticks, such as *Boophilus*, to serve as vectors.

Ixodid ticks found attached to domestic animals may be removed individually by cautious traction with thumb forceps. The long hypostomes of *Ixodes, Amblyomma,* and *Hyalomma* are effective anchors. *Dermacentor, Rhipicephalus, Boophilus,* and *Haemaphysalis* compensate for their shorter hypostomes by secreting a cement in which the mouthparts are embedded and which attaches them securely to the skin (Moorehouse and Tatchell, 1966; Moorehouse, 1973). Therefore, unless reasonable care is exercised, the capitulum may be torn away and remain embedded as a foreign body in the skin of the host. Outdoor areas suspected as sources of ixodid tick infestation may be surveyed with a drag made by attaching one edge of a square yard of flannel to a stick and drawing it slowly over the vegetation. Hungry ticks will climb aboard the passing drag and can then be removed at intervals and placed in specimen bottles.

Identification of ticks presents some complex problems, especially below the genus level. Only expert acarologists can be relied upon to identify ticks accurately on the basis of morphological features alone. Yet identification arrived at without assuming geographical restrictions in species distribution is exactly what is required to meet one of the principal hazards posed by ticks, i.e., the introduction of exotic infectious diseases with exotic tick species. Veterinarians should carefully examine the ticks they encounter in practice. If a specimen is found that looks

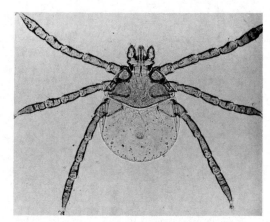

Figure 2–7. Six-legged *Rhipicephalus* larva (× 40).

different from the run of the mill, it should be sent to a diagnostic laboratory for expert identification. However, many practical problems can be solved by generic identification of adult ixodid ticks, and criteria for accomplishing that goal are presented here. No attempt will be made here to identify larvae and nymphs beyond the family level; larvae have six legs (Fig. 2-7), nymphs have eight legs and a scutum of the female type but the genital aperture is absent (Fig. 2-8).

Identification of Ixodid Ticks

In the following outline, the *italicized character* is either sufficient or nearly sufficient to represent the genus alone, provided, of course, that the corresponding morphological feature of the specimen is seen and correctly interpreted. Any ixodid tick must have one or another of these *italicized characters*

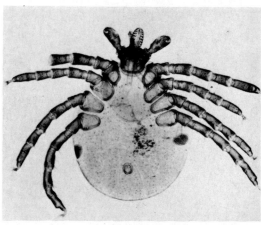

Figure 2–8. Eight-legged *Ixodes* nymph (x20).

and they serve as convenient starting points for identifying specimens but, to be on the safe side, check each subsidiary character as well. Further details may be found in *Ticks Of Veterinary Importance*, APHIS, USDA, Agriculture Handbook No. 485.

GENERA FOUND IN NORTH AMERICA

Ixodes. The anal groove forms an arch anterior to the anus; this can be seen with oblique illumination of uncleared specimens (see Fig. 2-2). Other genera have a groove posterior to the anus or no groove at all. *Ixodes* spp. have no eyes, festoons, or scutal ornamentation; their palpi are broadest at the junction of segments two and three (Fig. 2-9). A tick's eye, by the way, is a mere roundish lucent area at the margin of the scutum about opposite the second coxa.

Haemaphysalis. The palpi have laterally flared second segments (Fig. 2-10). Avoid confusing these structures with the hexagonal basis capituli of *Rhipicephalus* and *Boophilus*. Like *Ixodes*, these ticks have neither eyes nor scutal ornamentation, but they differ in having festoons and a posterior anal groove.

Rhipicephalus. The basis capituli is hexagonal (Fig. 2-11); eyes and festoons are present but the scutum is unornamented; males have salient adanal and accessory shields (Fig. 2-12).

Boophilus. The palps are ridged dorsally and laterally (Fig. 2-13). Like *Rhipicephalus*, these ticks have a hexagonal basis capituli, eyes, and an unornamented scutum and the males have adanal and accessory shields. However, *Boophilus* differs from *Rhipicephalus* in having ridged palpi and in lacking festoons. *Boophilus* specimens encountered in the field should be immediately reported to state or federal

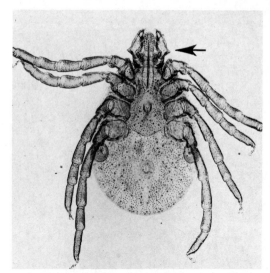

Figure 2–10. *Haemaphysalis* (x20). The second palpal segment (arrow) is flared laterally.

authorities because *Boophilus* transmits bovine piroplasmosis.

Dermacentor. The basis capituli is rectangular as viewed from above (Fig. 2-14). Coxae of males progress in size from the first to the fourth (Fig. 2-12). *Dermacentor* resembles *Rhipicephalus* in having eyes and 11 festoons, but the basis capituli is rectangular, the scutum is ornamented (Figs. 2-15 and 2-16), and the males lack adanal shields. *Dermacentor (Anocentor) nitens*, the tropical horse tick, has only seven festoons.

Amblyomma. The mouthparts are much longer than the basis capituli; the second palpal segment is at least twice as long as the third (see Fig. 2-

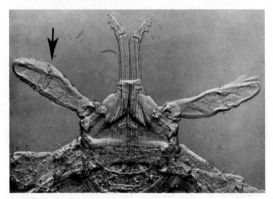

Figure 2–9. Capitulum of *Ixodes* (x40). The palps of *Ixodes* are broadest at the junction of the second and third segments (arrow).

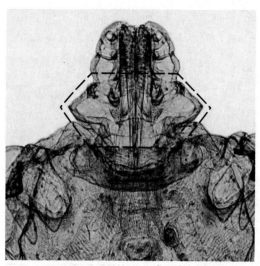

Figure 2–11. Capitulum of *Rhipicephalus* (x40). The basis capituli is hexagonal.

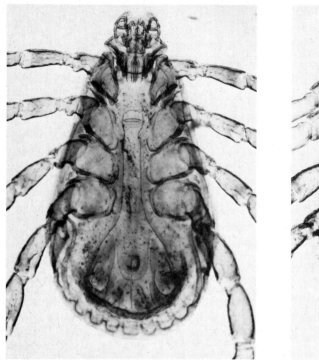 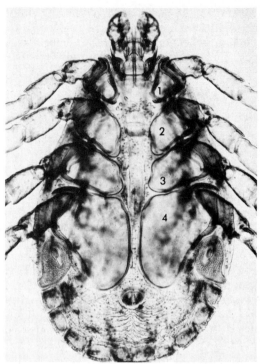

Figure 2–12. Ventral aspects of a male *Rhipicephalus* (left) and a male *Dermacentor* (right) (x21). Coxae of male *Dermacentor* progress in size from the first to fourth.

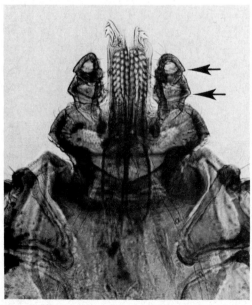 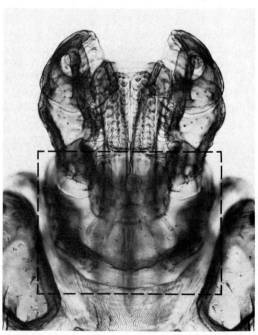

Figure 2–13. Capitulum of *Boophilus* (x60). The basis capituli is hexagonal and the palpi are ridged dorsally and laterally (arrows).

Figure 2–14. Capitulum of *Dermacentor* (x55). The basis capituli is rectangular.

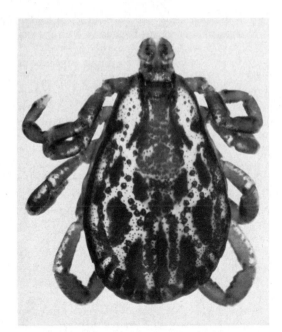

Figure 2–15. *Dermacentor* male (x14). Notice the ornamented scutum.

1). Eyes and festoons present, scutum ornamented, adanal shields absent. *Aponomma elaphensis* resembles *Amblyomma* but is smaller and lacks eyes; it is a parasite of a rat snake in Texas.

GENERA NOT FOUND IN NORTH AMERICA

Hyalomma. Resembles *Amblyomma* in having mouthparts much longer than the basis capituli but differs in that the second and third palpal segments are approximately the same length (Fig. 2-17). Eyes present, festoons irregularly coalesced; male with adanal and accessory shields.

Margaropus. Resembles *Boophilus* but the palps are not ridged and the legs of the male progress in size from the first to the fourth.

Rhipicentor. Resembles *Rhipicephalus* dorsally, *Dermacentor* ventrally; eyes and festoons present, adanal and accesory shields absent, fourth coxae greatly enlarged.

Life Histories and Disease Transmission

Ixodes spp. In Europe, species of *Ixodes* are vectors of bovine piroplasmosis and various viral diseases, including louping ill. *Ixodes holocyclus* of Australia is the most virulent tick paralysis producer known. In North America, *Ixodes scapularis* and *Ixodes pacificus* attack livestock but are not known to transmit livestock diseases. Nymphs of *Ixodes dammini*, a three-host tick that normally feeds on mice and voles as larva and nymph and on deer as adult, is held responsible for trans-

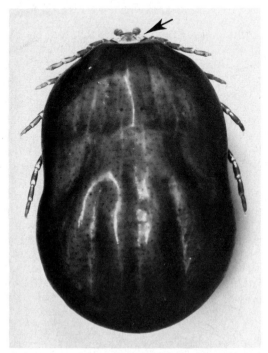

Figure 2–16. *Dermacentor* female, fully engorged (x6). The scutum (arrow) covers only a small fraction of the dorsum of a fully engorged female ixodid tick.

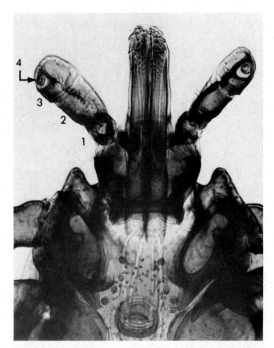

Figure 2–17. Capitulum of *Hyalomma* (x70). Palpal segments two and three of *Hyalomma* are approximately the same length, whereas the second palpal segment of *Amblyomma* is about twice as long as the third.

mission of microtine piroplasmosis (*Babesia microti*) to man (Spielman, 1976).

Haemaphysalis leporispalustris. Larvae and nymphs of *Haemaphysalis leporispalustris,* the rabbit tick, feed on ground nesting birds and small mammals, and the adults attach to rabbits, especially to the ears and around the eyes. Occasional specimens are collected from cats.

Rhipicephalus sanguineus. Larvae, nymphs, and adults of *R. sanguineus,* the brown dog tick, all feed on dogs and sometimes on man. Originally a tropical species, *R. sanguineus* has taken advantage of central heating to spread into the temperate zones, where it often generates enormous populations in homes, kennels, and veterinary hospitals; it cannot survive the winter outdoors in the north. Dogs living in temperate regions frequently acquire their *R. sanguineus* ticks in such infested premises but during summer, infestation may occur out of doors. Therefore, if enduring results are to be achieved, elimination of these ticks must include acaricidal treatment of both the dog and the home or kennel. The latter procedure is a job for a professional exterminator. Development from egg to egg may be completed in slightly over two months under favorable conditions; unfed adults may survive for well over a year.

Rhipicephalus sanguineus transmits canine piroplasmosis (*Babesia canis*) transovarially and tropical canine pancytopenia (*Ehrlichia canis*) interstadially.

African species of *Rhipicephalus* serve as vectors of the devastating East Coast fever (*Theileria parva*) and other forms of bovine theileriosis, bovine piroplasmosis (*Babesia bigemina*), and the virus of Nairobi sheep disease.

Boophilus annulatus. This transovarial vector of bovine piroplasmosis was eradicated from the United States through 40 long years of dipping cattle that began in 1906. Losses from piroplasmosis were estimated then at 40 to 100 million dollars per year at a time when cattle were selling at two to four cents a pound. Eradication was favored by the affinity of this species for cattle, and by its one-host life history; a substantial proportion of the tick population could be destroyed each time the cattle were dipped. Analogous efforts to eradicate species with broader host preferences, especially those feeding on wildlife, would be doomed to failure. *Boophilus microplus,* also a piroplasmosis vector, has a broader host range that includes horses, goats, sheep, and deer.

Dermacentor spp. *Dermacentor variabilis,* the American dog tick, is widely but discontinuously distributed over the eastern half and West Coast of the United States and parts of Canada and Mexico. Larvae and nymphs engorge on small rodents, adults engorge on man, dogs, horses, cattle, and wildlife. *Dermacentor variabilis* transmits Rocky Mountain spotted fever (*Rickettsia rickettsi*) and tularemia (*Francisella tularensis*) and causes tick paralysis.

Dermacentor andersoni, the Rocky Mountain wood tick, requires one to three years to complete its life history, depending on the latitude, altitude, and abundance of small mammals on which it feeds as larva and as nymph. *Dermacentor andersoni* transmits Rocky Mountain spotted fever, tularemia, Colorado tick fever, and Q fever and causes tick paralysis.

In the United States, *Dermacentor* (Anocentor) *nitens,* the tropical horse tick, is limited to the southern portions of Florida and Texas. Preferring the external ear canals of horses, but also found on other sites and other hosts such as cattle, sheep, goats, and deer, *D. nitens* is the vector of equine piroplasmosis (*Babesia caballi*). Other North American species of *Dermacentor* include *D. albipictus,* the winter tick, which causes heavy losses among deer, elk, and moose, *D. nigrolineatus,* the brown winter tick, and *D. occidentalis,* the Pacific Coast tick.

Amblyomma spp. In the United States, species of *Amblyomma* that attack man, livestock, dogs, and cats (e.g., *A. americanum, A. maculatum, A. cajennense,* and *A. imitator*) are distributed mainly in the southeastern costal states, Missouri, Oklahoma, and Texas, but specimens may occasionally be found as far north as Ithaca, New York. These species have been incriminated in the transmission of Rocky Mountain spotted fever, Q fever, and tularemia, and in the causation of tick paralysis. African species of *Amblyomma* transmit heartwater (*Cowdria ruminantium*) of cattle, sheep, and goats as well as the virus of Nairobi sheep disease. *Amblyomma dissimili,* the iguana tick, and *A. tuberculatum,* the gopher tortoise tick, are parasites of reptiles and amphibians; the latter is the largest ixodid tick, engorged females reaching a length of 25 mm.

Tick Injuries

Tick paralysis. In North America, the species most frequently involved in tick paralysis are *Dermacentor andersoni, D. variabilis, Am-*

blyomma americanum, and *A. maculatum.* Tick paralysis is an ascending paralysis caused by absorption of toxins from the saliva of engorging female ticks. The tick injects a considerable volume of saliva into the wound partly as an aid to digestion and partly as a means of disposing of surplus water extracted from the blood meal. A single female tick can produce paralysis in man, dog or cat, especially if the site of attachment is close to or on the head, but paralysis does not invariably occur even if many ticks of a suitable species are present. Usually, heavy infestations are required to produce tick paralysis in cattle. The first clinical sign is incoordination of the hindquarters that rapidly proceeds to complete paralysis and spreads to the forequarters, neck, and finally to the respiratory muscles, with fatal consequences. Removal of engorging ticks usually leads to gratifyingly rapid recovery. In Australia, *Ixodes holocyclus,* a parasite of the bandicoot and other marsupials, causes, in domestic animals, a particularly severe form of tick paralysis that requires, for its cure, administration of specific antitoxin and general supportive treatment as well as removal of all ticks from the victim. Even larvae and nymphs of *I. holocyclus* can induce paralysis when sufficiently numerous. The surest prevention of tick paralysis lies in careful daily examination of exposed animals and removal of ticks. Because clinical signs of paralysis do not begin to appear until the ticks have been engorging for at least four days, they should be large enough to be found relatively easily before clinical signs develop. In areas of heavy exposure, weekly acaricidal dipping is necessary.

The Bite Wound. *Ixodes, Amblyomma,* and other genera with long mouthparts produce deep, painful bite wounds that tend to become inflamed, secondarily infected with bacteria, and flyblown. In Great Britain, secondary infection of *Ixodes ricinus* bites with *Staphlyococcus* results in both local and metastatic abscessation (tick pyemia) in lambs. In the Gulf Coast states, *Amblyomma maculatum,* which prefers to attach to the ears of larger mammals, causes such pain and swelling that cattle are unable or at least reluctant to flick their ears and thus ward off flies. Before screwworm control, such ears were prone to invasion by larvae of *Cochliomyia hominivorax,* frequently with the loss of the external ear or death.

Blood Loss and Worry. Sir Arnold Theiler once collected *half* of the *Boophilus decoloratus* ticks from a horse that had died of acute anemia. His collection weighed 14 pounds (Theiler, 1911)! That horse's tick burden must have contained on the order of 13 liters of blood. This example may appear extreme to those of us who dwell in temperate zones and experience only an occasional mosquito or blackfly bite, but there are places in the tropics where light colored cattle are so totally covered by the dark bodies of engorging ticks that they appear from a distance to be black. Loss of blood, pain and swelling of bite wounds, secondary infection, myiasis, and absorption of toxins, in moderate and varying proportion, result in a form of ill-thrift referred to as "tick worry." Because tick worry is the most common practical consequence of tick infestation, it may be even more important than the more dramatic ones.

MITES

Suborder Mesostigmata

Mesostigmatids, as the name implies, have *stigmata* (respiratory pores) in the middle of their bodies. A stigma lies between the third and fourth coxae on each side of the body and is connected to a sinuous *peritreme,* a shallow groove of unknown function. The coxae are evenly spaced and crowded into the anterior half of the body, the tarsi are generally armed with claws, and the ventrum is armored with sclerotized plates (Fig. 2-18).

FAMILIES DERMANYSSIDAE AND MACRONYSSIDAE

Bloodsucking mesostigmatid mites that parasitize birds (e.g., *Dermanyssus gallinae, Ornithonyssus sylviarum*) and rodents (e.g., *Ornithonyssus bacoti, Liponyssoides sanguineus*) frequently turn on the human inhabitants of a building when deprived of their normal hosts, as may occur when fledglings leave their nests or after rodents have been exterminated. Generic or even familial identification of these mites is sufficient to establish the general nature of the epidemiological situation, but specific identification sometimes provides a very helpful lead in the search for nests. For example, a hospital administrator submitted a specimen of a mite that was causing great consternation by its abundance in the hospital's linens. I identified the specimen as a dermanyssid mite and advised the gentleman to hunt for bird or rodent nests. A few days later, he reported no success in finding nests of either kind.

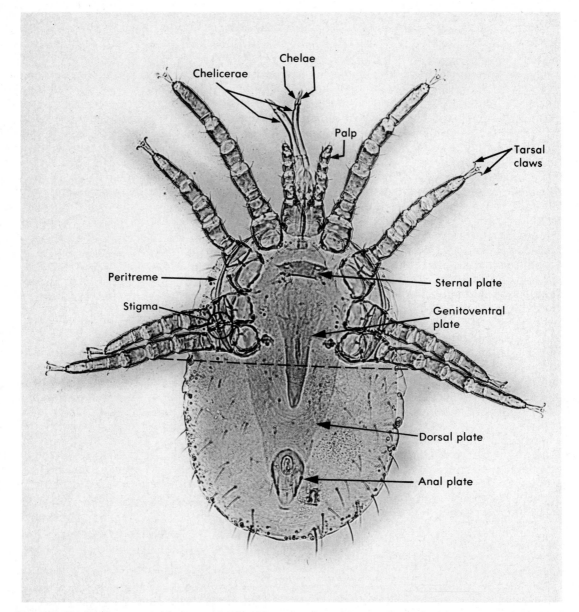

Figure 2–18. *Ornithonyssus sylviarum,* a bloodsucking mesostigmatid mite (x110). The legs are confined to the anterior half of the body of mesostigmatid mites; the stigma is located between the third and fourth coxae and has a peritreme. The chelae of *Ornithonyssus* are much larger than those of *Dermanyssus.*

However, by that time I had shown the specimen to an expert acarologist who identified it as *Dermanyssus hirundinus,* a highly host-specific parasite of swallows. Thus advised, the hospital administrator knew just where to look and the problem was quickly solved.

Dermanyssids and macronyssids all look very much alike on casual inspection, but because they vary significantly in habits and host preferences, accurate identification is a prerequisite to effective control. The *chelicerae*

(piercing mouthparts), *chelae* (scissorlike structures on the end of the chelicerae), and form and setation of various sclerotized plates provide the main taxonomic characters used in differentiating these mites.

Dermanyssus (Dermanyssidae). *The chelicerae are long and slender and the chelae minute (Fig. 2-19); there is a single dorsal plate, the sternal plate has two pairs of setae, and the anus is in the posterior half of the anal plate. Dermanyssus is infrequently found on the bird because these mites hide in nests, roosts, and*

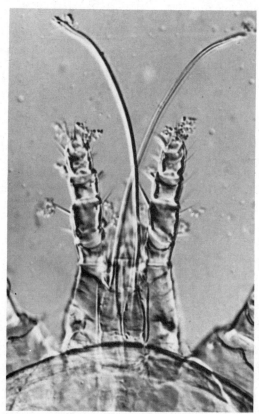

Figure 2–19. Gnathosome of *Dermanyssus gallinae* (x280). The chelicerae of *Dermanyssus* are slender and whiplike and the chelae are very small.

the like during the day and attack the sleeping bird at night. Life stages include the egg, which is deposited in the diurnal hiding places of the mites, the six-legged, non-feeding larva, and the blood-feeding protonymph, deutonymph, and adult male or female. A generation can be completed in as little as a week and large populations may build up in chicken houses or bird's nests. The adults can survive starvation for months. *Dermanyssus* mites remove enough blood to kill nestlings and reduce egg production. Their importance as disease vectors is unclear.

Liponyssoides (Allodermanyssus) sanguineus (Dermanyssidae). *The chelicerae are long and slender and the chelae minute; there are two dorsal plates, the anterior plate 10 times as large as the posterior; the sternal plate has three pairs of setae. Liponyssoides sanguineus,* a parasite of the house mouse, *Mus musculus,* and other small rodents, is the vector of rickettsial pox (*Rickettsia akari*) of man.

Ornithonyssus (Macronyssidae). *The chelicerae are much stouter than those of* Dermanyssus *and the chelae are easily visible under ordinary*

magnification; there is a single dorsal plate, and the anus is in the anterior half of the anal plate (see Fig. 2-18). Common species include O. sylviarum, the northern fowl mite, O. bursa, the tropical fowl mite, and O. bacoti, the tropical rat mite. *Ornithonyssus* spp. remain on the host much of the time and cause considerable loss of blood. Persons handling eggs from laying flocks heavily infested with *O. sylviarum* may experience serious annoyance and discomfort from the bites of these mites. *Ornithonyssus bacoti* is a serious pest in laboratory rodent stocks and serves as intermediate host for *Litomosoides carinii*, a filariid parasite of the cotton rat, *Sigmodon hispidus*. *Litomosoides carinii* is a favorite laboratory model for testing antifilarial drugs.

Ophionyssus natricis (Macronyssidae). *Ophionyssus natricis*, the snake mite, is a serious bloodsucking pest that tends to thrive on captive snakes.

FAMILY RAILLIETIDAE

Raillietia. *Raillietia auris* (Fig. 2-20), long considered a harmless parasite of the ears of cattle, has been shown to cause ulceration and blockage of the auditory canals by pus with resultant loss of hearing (Heffner and Heffner, 1983).

FAMILY HALARACHNIDAE

Pneumonyssus simicola. Groups of *P. simicola* mites may be found in the lung paren-

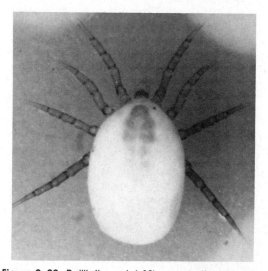

Figure 2–20. *Raillietia auris* (x30), a mesostigmatid parasite of the ear canal of cattle. In this reflected light photomacrograph, the specimen appears as it would under a stereoscopic microscope or powerful hand lens.

chyma of most if not all *Macaca mulatta* monkeys. The lesions are pinhead or larger, whitish or yellow foci that have soft or empty centers and contain mites and a black pigment. These lesions are scattered throughout the lungs and may be mistaken for those of tuberculosis. It is difficult to correlate clinical signs of pulmonary acariasis with the degree of pathological change in the lungs, and antemortem diagnosis is difficult. Monkeys can be reared free of *Pneumonyssus* infection if they are separated from their mothers at birth and reared in isolation from adult monkeys. The histopathological diagnosis of *P. simicola* infection is discussed in Chapter 14.

Pneumonyssoides caninum. A parasite of the nasal and paranasal sinuses of dogs, *P. caninum* sometimes causes chronic sneezing and epistaxis. Rhinoscopy and nasal swabbing are aids to diagnosis.

FAMILY RHINONYSSIDAE

Sternostoma tracheacolum. This mite is a bloodsucking parasite of the respiratory passages, including the abdominal air sacs, of canaries, finches, and a wide range of other wild and domestic birds. *Sternostoma tracheacolum* infection may be inapparent clinically or may cause chronic respiratory illness manifested by loss of voice, shaking of the head, and sneezing. Diagnosis in the living bird is facilitated by moistening and parting the feathers in the neck region and transilluminating the trachea with a strong light; the mites appear as shadowy spots in the trachea. On necropsy examination, these mites appear to the unaided eye as black spots in the posterior nares, trachea, air sacs, lung tissues, and abdominal cavity (Kummerfeld and Hinz, 1982).

Suborder Astigmata

In contrast to mesostigmatids, astigmatid mites lack stigmata and respiration is integumental; the first and second coxae are widely separated from the third and fourth, the ventrum is devoid of conspicuous plates, and the tarsi are equipped with suckers (sarcoptiform pretarsi). Astigmatids include the mange mites, certain hair clasping mites, two internal parasites of chickens, and the grain mites.

Mange mites (families Sarcoptidae, Knemidokoptidae, and Psoroptidae) cause mange or scabies, a dermatitis characterized by pruritus, alopecia, and epidermal hyperplasia with desquamation. Rubbing and scratching by the host frequently results in deeper wounds that ooze serum and blood. These coagulate, gluing hair, epidermal debris, and foreign matter together to form crusts and scabs. Secondary bacterial infection may complicate the situation.

The typical distribution and manner of spread of mange lesions vary with the host and parasite species and are often characteristic enough to permit accurate diagnosis by an experienced observer. However, recovery and identification of mites are necessary for positive diagnosis. Negative scrapings are inconclusive. Therefore, typical mange lesions should be subjected to persistent examination until mites are found or until further scraping would do excessive injury to the patient. For *lesions with minimal epidermal hyperplasia and lesions caused by deeply burrowing mites* (e.g., *Sarcoptes, Demodex*), dip a scalpel blade into mineral oil, pinch a fold of skin firmly between thumb and forefinger and, holding the blade at right angles to the skin, scrape until blood begins to seep from the abrasion. Much of the detritus will adhere to the layer of mineral oil on the scalpel blade and may be transferred to a microscope slide and searched for mites. For *lesions with marked epidermal hyperplasia and exfoliation and lesions caused by superficially dwelling mites* (e.g., *Chorioptes*) *and lice*, scrape the detritus into an ointment tin using the cover as a scraper. Examine the scrapings under a stereomicroscope or hand lens to find the mites crawling about. If no mites are observed directly, recourse may be had to digestion of the skin scrapings in potassium hydroxide (page 264).

Generic differentiation of mange mites likely to be encountered in routine veterinary practice requires little more than examination of their pretarsi (Figs. 2-21 and 2-22). If the pretarsus has a long, unsegmented pedicel (stalk), the specimen is most likely *Sarcoptes* or *Notoedres.* If the pretarsus has a long, three-segmented pedicel, it's bound to be *Psoroptes.* Pretarsi with short pedicels are found on *Chorioptes* from ungulates and *Otodectes* from dogs; the species identity of the host is a sufficiently reliable differential criterion in this case. *Knemidokoptes* females lack pretarsi but the males have pretarsi resembling those of *Sarcoptes.* Certain particularly destructive manges such as psoroptic mange in sheep and cattle and sarcoptic mange in cattle should be reported to state animal disease control authorities.

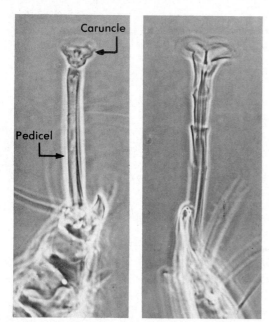
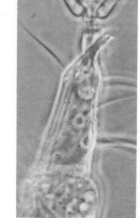

Figure 2–21. Pretarsi of *Sarcoptes* (left, x830) and *Psoroptes* (right, x870). Both have long pedicels; that of *Psoroptes* is jointed.

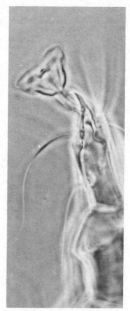

Figure 2–22. Pretarsi of *Otodectes* (left, x810) and *Chorioptes* (right, x710). Both have short pedicels. *Otodectes* is a parasite of the ear canal of carnivorans; *Chorioptes* is a parasite of the epidermis of ungulates.

FAMILY SARCOPTIDAE

Sarcoptes. *The pretarsi have long, unsegmented pedicels and the anus is at the posterior edge of the body* (Fig. 2-23). *Sarcoptes scabiei* causes sarcoptic mange or scabies of man, dogs, foxes, horses, cattle, and others. *Sarcoptic mange of cattle is reportable.* Although *S. scabiei* infests a wide range of hosts, a considerable degree of host specificity has arisen among populations of this parasite so that

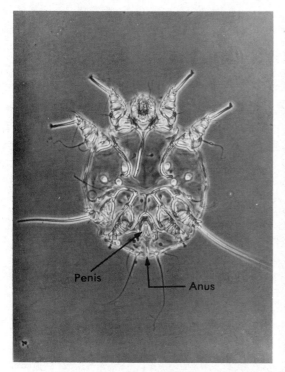
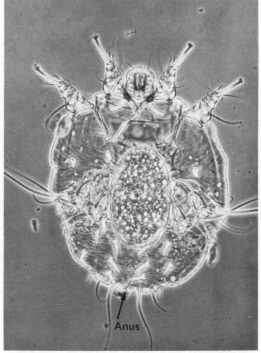

Figure 2–23. *Sarcoptes* male (left, x140) and female (right, x140).

scabies of pigs tends to spread more readily among pigs, scabies of man tends to spread more readily among man, and, when interspecific transmission does occur, the resulting dermatitis tends to be atypical and transient. In fair-skinned human subjects suffering relatively mild infestations, it is possible to see the tiny serpentine tunnels that trace the wanderings of the egg-laying female mite as she burrows through the epidermis. Along the course of the burrow, dark areas representing eggs and accumulations of feces may be observed and, at the end of the tunnel, the mite may be found and lifted out with the point of a needle. Hair obscures such lesions on domestic animals and it may be that many relatively mild cases of sarcoptic mange are overlooked. As few as 10 to 15 mites constitute a case of ordinary (but nontheless unendurable) human scabies but thousands to millions may be found on a mangy pig or fox. Curiously, however, *Sarcoptes* mites are frequently difficult to find on dogs, even those exhibiting advanced lesions.

Sarcoptic mange of domestic animals usually starts on relatively hairless areas of skin and may later generalize. In dogs, the lateral aspect of the elbow and pinna of the ear are favorite starting places; the lesions consist of follicular papules, areas of erythema, crusts of dried serum and blood, and excoriations from scratching to relieve the intense pruritus. Secondary bacterial infection is a frequent complication. In swine, sarcoptic mange usually starts around the eyes and on the nose, back, sides, and inner surface of the thighs; lesions may progress to hyperkeratosis and exfoliation of epidermal debris. The red fox, *Vulpes fulva*, suffers a lethal form of sarcoptic mange in which the epidermis may undergo a tenfold increase in thickness and contain countless hordes of mites (Fig. 14-5).

Notoedres. A parasite of cats, rats, rabbits, and occasionally and temporarily of man, *Notoedres* much resembles *Sarcoptes* but is smaller and *its anus is on the dorsal surface instead of on the posterior margin of the body* (Figs. 2-24 and 2-25). Face mange of cats caused by *Notoedres cati* starts on the medial edge of the pinna of the ears and then spreads over the ears, face, paws, and hindquarters by contiguity and contact. The lesions of notoedric mange consist principally of alopecia and marked hyperkeratosis with abundant epidermal flakes; mites are easily demonstrated. Not all cases of cat mange are caused by *Notoedres*, however, especially as regards exotic cats. For example, a half-dollar-sized area of dermatitis on the top of a pet ocelot's head was tentatively diagnosed

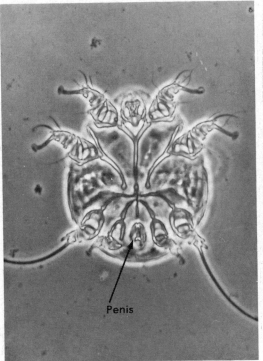
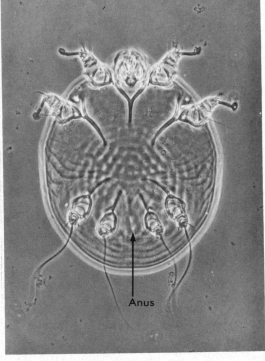

Figure 2–24. *Notoedres* male (left, x250) and female (right, x290).

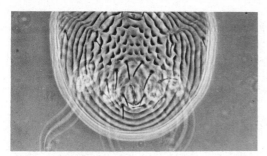

Figure 2–25. Same as Figure 2–24. right, but with dorsal anus in focus (x290).

as notoedric mange. However, a scraping revealed that the villain was *Sarcoptes* and raised the possibility of an infested human contact. And indeed, the owner had been suffering from a severe itch below her breasts, but hadn't connected her discomfort with her ocelot's skin lesion. In this particular case it wasn't at all clear who had harbored the mites first but that, after all, is an academic question. What is important is that correct generic identification of the parasite led to effective control through appropriate medication of both infested individuals.

Cosarcoptes, Prosarcoptes, Pithesarcoptes, and Kutzerocoptes. The first three genera are parasites of Old World monkeys (Cercopithecidae) and the last of New World monkeys (Cebidae). All resemble *Sarcoptes* morphologically, biologically, and pathogenetically. Mange of monkeys, at least that caused by *Cosarcoptes scanloni,* may be trasnsmissible to man (Smiley and O'Connor, 1980).

Trixacarus caviae. A parasite of the guinea pig, *T. caviae* closely resembles *Sarcoptes scabiei* but is only half as large; the anus is on the dorsal surface of the female and on the posterior margin of the body of the male. *Trixacarus* causes pruritus so intense that affected guinea pigs are subject to fits and seizures brought on by vigorous scratching or manipulation of the skin (Kummel *et al.,* 1980).

FAMILY KNEMIDOKOPTIDAE

Knemidokoptes. *Knemidokoptes mutans* causes scaly leg in chickens, turkeys, pheasants, and other gallinaceous birds. The mites burrow in the epidermis of the legs, causing the scales to lift and become loosened and the legs thickened and deformed. To demonstrate mites, simply remove a loose leg scale and examine the underside of it with a hand lens. The female *K. mutans* is about 0.5 mm. in diameter; the legs are very short and

lack pretarsi (Fig. 2-26). The males are much smaller and have longer legs equipped with pretarsi resembling those of *Sarcoptes.*

Knemidokoptes pilae and *K. jamaicensis* cause mange of the legs, base of the beak, vent area, and back of parakeets and canaries, respectively. Lesions respond well to daily applications of mineral oil to all areas where mites are likely to be found, including the vent area.

Knemidokoptes gallinae, the depluming mite of chickens, pigeons, pheasants, and geese, is found at the base of the feathers on the back, top of wing, on the vent, breast, and thighs, causing intense pruritus leading in turn to feather pulling.

FAMILY PSOROPTIDAE

Psoroptes. *The legs are long and the pretarsi have long, three-segmented pedicels* (Fig. 2-27). *Psoroptes ovis* causes a very serious and reportable form of mange (scabies or "scab") in cattle, sheep, and horses. Psoroptic mange is prevalent among cattle herds in the southwestern U.S.A., but relatively rare elsewhere in North America. *P. cuniculi* is very common and causes ear canker in rabbits, and a less severe form of otic acariasis in goats and horses.

Psoroptes ovis does not burrow in the epidermis but remains at the base of the hairs and pierces the skin with its styletlike chelicerae. This mannner of feeding results in exudation of serum, which hardens to form a scab. The mites are best demonstrated under the edges of these scabs and so it is

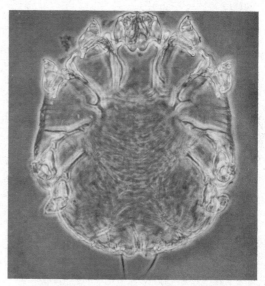

Figure 2–26. *Knemidokoptes* female (x200).

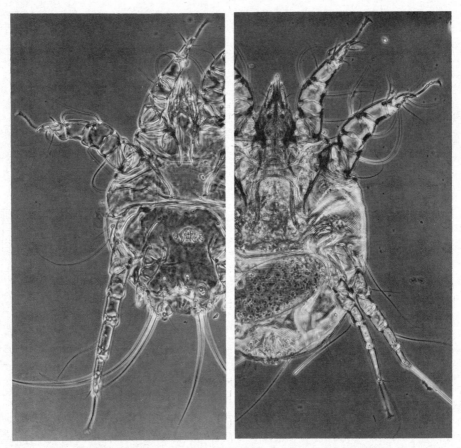

Figure 2–27. *Psoroptes* male (left, x110) and female (right, x110).

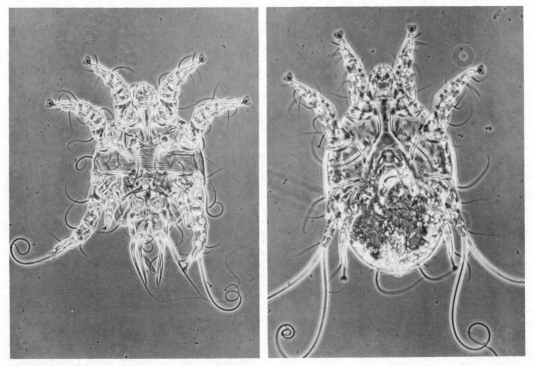

Figure 2–28. *Chorioptes* male (left, x120) and female (right, x140). The female has pretarsi on the first, second, and fourth pairs of legs; the male has pretarsi on all four pairs.

inefficient to submit great wads of wool to the laboratory, especially if the scabs are not included in the shipment. Psoroptic scab is particularly devastating in sheep, especially those maintained principally for the production of high quality wool. Pruritus is usually intense. At first, tags of wool are observed projecting from the fleece and adhered to fence posts, door jambs, trees, and other convenient objects against which an itchy sheep might obtain some measure of relief. Progressively more and more wool is shed or rubbed away by the frantic sheep, and pustules appear on the denuded, hardened, thickened, and excoriated skin. As the pustules become confluent and overlain by a scab of coagulated serum and foreign material, the area ceases to be suitable for the mites and they move on to fresh territory. In this way, the lesions tend to spread over the surface of the body. The sheep become greatly debilitated by psoroptic scab and may even die of it. *Psoroptes ovis* may survive off the host for several days or weeks. Therefore, effective control requires both acaricidal treatment of all infested livestock and either disinfection or two to four week vacation of contaminated enclosures and vehicles (Wilson *et al.*, 1977).

Psoroptes cuniculi is a ubiquitous parasite of the external ear canal and can frequently be demonstrated in apparently normal rabbits. When infested rabbits are placed under stress, as for example when a doe kindles, the population of mites tends to explode and the ear canal is laid waste as a result. A full-blown case of *ear canker* is virtually untreatable and almost surely fatal. Prevention is possible by weekly instillation of a few drops of mineral oil into the ear canal of each rabbit in the colony. *Psoroptes cuniculi* produces a less severe form of otic acariasis in goats and horses.

Chorioptes bovis. Pretarsi of C. bovis *have short, unsegmented pedicels on the first, second, and fourth pairs of legs of the female and on all legs of the male; the male has two turretlike lobes on the posterior margin of the body* (Figs. 2-28 and 2-29). *Chorioptes bovis* is a cosmopolitan, superficially dwelling parasite, displaying a distinct preference for the tail, escutcheon, and legs of cattle, where it feeds on epithelial debris. Although cattle are the principal hosts, *C. bovis* may also be found on the tail and legs of horses, sheep, and goats, and in the ear canal of rabbits. Asymptomatic infestation is far more common than obvious dermatitis.

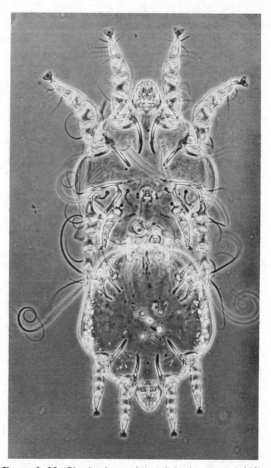

Figure 2–29. *Chorioptes* male and deutonymph (x140). The deutonymph has pretarsi on the first and second pairs of legs.

Chorioptic mange in cattle usually appears during late winter as a superficial, mildly pruritic, flaky dermatitis involving the tail, escutcheon, and hind legs of cattle. Stanchioned animals are made miserable because they are unable to take appropriate action to relieve the itching but, for unconfined cattle, chorioptic mange is probably not much more serious a burden than a crop of chewing lice and, like a suit of woolen underwear, may help keep them warm by encouraging physical activity. Chorioptic mange tends to disappear soon after the cattle are turned out to pasture in spring. *Chorioptes bovis*, like the pinworm *Oxyuris equi*, is an identifiable cause of tail rubbing in horses. Scrotal mange in rams, caused by *C. bovis*, may lead to seminal degeneration if lesions advance sufficiently to interfere with heat loss through the scrotal skin (Rhodes, 1975).

Otodectes cynotis. Pretarsi of O. cynotis *have short, unsegmented pedicels on the first and second pairs of legs of the female and on all legs*

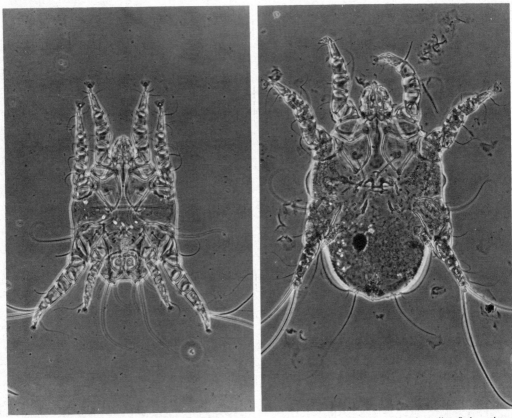

Figure 2–30. *Otodectes* male (left, x110) and female (right, x120). The female has pretarsi on the first and second pairs of legs; the male has pretarsi on all four pairs.

of the male; the body of the male is only weakly bilobed posteriorly (Fig. 2-30). *Otodectes cynotis* infests the external ear canal and adjacent skin of dogs, cats, foxes, and ferrets, causing intense irritation. Copious production of dark cerumen is characteristic of otodectic otitis. Aural pruritus sometimes causes the animal to rub and scratch its ears and shake its head violently enough to produce hematoma of the aural pinna. The mites may be demonstrated by swabbing the ear canal with a cotton applicator and then placing the applicator on a dark background under a lamp or on a sunny windowsill. The heat will drive the mites out of the debris and they will be seen as tiny white specks moving against the dark backgrounnd.

SUPERFAMILY LISTROPHOROIDEA AND OTHERS

Hair-clasping mites of the superfamily Listrophoroidea have one or more pairs of legs variously flattened, bowed, or otherwise modified for clasping a hair. Examples include *Chirodiscoides caviae*, a parasite of guinea pigs (Fig. 2-31), and *Myocoptes musculinus*, a parasite of rodents (Fig. 2-32). *Lynxacarus radovskyi* is a hair-clasping mite of domestic cats in Florida, Puerto Rico, Hawaii, Australia, and Fiji; hordes of these tiny mites clinging to the hairs impart a "scurfy" appearance (Greve and Gerrish, 1981). Not all hair-clasping mites belong to the superfamily Listrophoroidea or even to the suborder Astigmata. For examples of exceptions, see *Myobia* and *Radfordia* below.

Feather mites occur in variety and abundance. Most are members of several superfamilies of Astigmata. Feather mites are usually external, but some live within the quills. Others, such as members of the family Epidermoptidae, burrow in the skin and may cause a mangelike condition. Astigmatid feather mites may be distinguished from prostigmatid feather mites such as *Syringophilus* by their sarcoptiform pretarsi.

Figure 2–32. *Myocoptes musculinus* male (left, x230) and female (right x230), an astigmatid hair-clasping parasite of laboratory rodents. Notice how the third pair of legs of the male and third and fourth pairs of legs of the female are modified for hair clasping. The first two pairs of legs have sarcoptiform pretarsi.

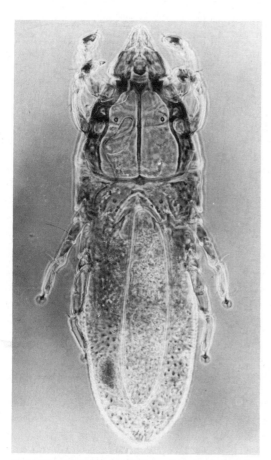

Figure 2–31. *Chirodiscoides caviae* female (x 220).

Two families of Astigmata have evolved as internal parasites of birds: *Laminosioptes* (Laminosioptidae) occur in subcutaneous nodules in chickens, and several genera of the family Cytoditidae are parasites of the air sacs and respiratory passages of chickens, canaries, and other birds.

Members of the families Acaridae and Glyciphagidae are free-living mites that feed on organic matter. They may be found in grain, cheeses, dried fruit, and other stored food products. Contact with these mites and their detritus may cause urticaria and dermatitis in human beings. "Grain mites" are frequently found as pseudoparasites in fecal smears. They may be distinguished from parasitic astigmatids by the shape of the female genital opening, which is a transverse or U-shaped slit in the parasites but a more or less longitudinal slit in grain mites.

Suborder Cryptostigmata

The Cryptostigmata, or oribatid mites, are free-living inhabitants of humus, some of which serve as intermediate hosts to tapeworms of the family Anoplocephalidae. When ingested by an oribatid mite, the egg of the tapeworm *Moniezia* develops into a

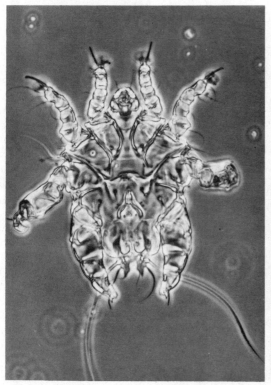

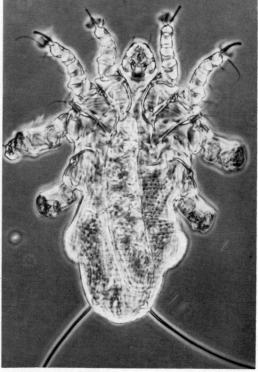

Figure 2–32. *See legend on opposite page*

cysticercoid, the larval stage infective for the ruminant definitive host.

Suborder Prostigmata

The Prostigmata is a polyphyletic amalgamation including both free-living species and such diverse obligate parasites as pilosebaceous mites (*Demodex*), hair-clasping mites (*Myobia*), and "chiggers" (Trombiculidae).

FAMILY DEMODICIDAE

Demodex spp. *are tiny, wormlike mites with short, stubby legs* (Fig. 2-33) that live in the hair follicles and sebaceous glands of mammals (see Fig. 14-7). Several distinct species of *Demodex* often parasitize the same host animal but each species tends to be restricted to a particular habitat. For example, two species, *D. folliculorum* and *D. brevis*, live in

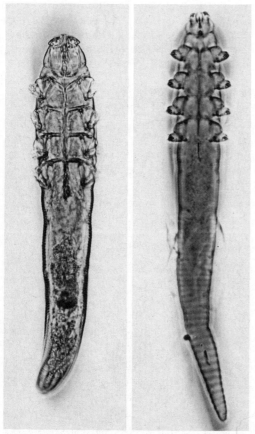

Figure 2–33. *Demodex canis* (left) and *D. cati* (right, x390).

the skin of almost every human face, *D. folliculorum* in the hair follicles and *D. brevis* in the sebaceous glands (Desch and Nutting, 1972), where they eat the epithelial cells. Some important pest species are the following:

Demodex canis is present, in small numbers, in the skin of most normal dogs. Pups acquire *D. canis* infection from their dams during the nursing period, and most cases of demodectic mange occur between three and six months of age. Affected dogs harbor much larger than normal populations of *D. canis*, apparently as a result of immunodeficiency, and display circumscribed areas of erythema and alopecia around the eyes and mouth, and over bony projections on the extremities. There is no evidence of pruritus. If the lesions remain thus localized, the prognosis for clinical recovery is excellent; the majority of such cases are mild and recover spontaneously with the attainment of sexual maturity. However, a few cases persist and these tend to become generalized and intractable and may prove fatal. In generalized demodicosis, the hair becomes sparse over wider expanses and the skin becomes coarse, dry, and erythematous ("red mange"). Concomitant staphylococcal pyoderma is the rule in generalized cases; pustules develop, break open, and ooze. Severe cases have a disagreeable odor. Generalized canine demodicosis is difficult to ameliorate and probably impossible to cure.

Demodex bovis mites are part of the normal fauna of bovine skin but sometimes pinhead- to egg-sized nodules appear, usually on the neck and forequarters. Occasionally, only the eyelids, vulva, or scrotum are involved. If a fresh nodule is nicked with a sharp scalpel, a thick, toothpastelike pus can be expressed which contains masses of *D. bovis* mites, but older lesions consist only of scar tissue and are devoid of mites. Bovine demodectic mange is practically incurable, even though individual lesions typically regress, because new nodules form to take their place. However, an unusual case of bilateral lower palpebral demodicosis in a dairy cow, characterized by chronic eosinophilic granulomatous cellulitis but without appreciable pus formation, resolved spontaneously within three months (Gearhart *et al.*, 1981).

D. caprae. causes a nodular dermatitis in milk goats.

D. caballi is a harmless parasite of the meibomian glands of horses.

D. cati is rarely noticed. Dermatitis associ-

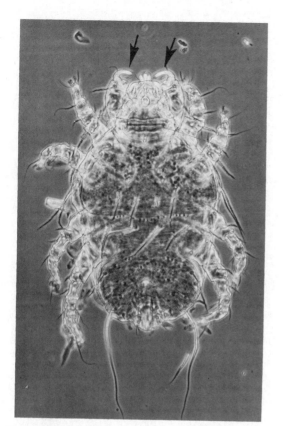

Figure 2–34. *Cheyletiella yasguri* (x130). Notice the formidable palpal claws (arrows).

ated with *D. cati* is usually localized on the head and in the ear canals.

D. cuniculi is a relatively rare parasite of the rabbit.

D. ovis is rarely noticed but probably rather common; mites are found in the skin of the eyelids and vulva.

D. phylloides is found in nodules around the eyes and on the snouts of pigs. These lesions later spread over the underside of the body.

FAMILY CHEYLETIELLIDAE

Cheyletiella spp. are easily recognized by their *big palpal claws, M-shaped gnathosomal peritremes, and comblike tarsal appendages* (Fig. 2-34). *Cheyletiella yasguri* occurs on dogs, *C. blakei* on cats, and *C. parasitivorax* on rabbits. Man may serve as an accidental or transitory host. Pups infested with *C. yasguri* develop "walking dandruff" on their backs, a dermatitis with branlike exfoliative debris that stirs with the movements of these rather large mites (see Fig. 14-6). We have observed a caged cat that passed *C. blakei* in its feces

for several weeks. Presumably, this cat was ingesting these mites while grooming itself, but there was no macroscopically visible skin lesion and we could find no mites in the fur. Other genera of the family Cheyletiellidae are parasites of birds. *Cheyletiella* spp. survive longer off the host than other mange mites and the premises may remain a source of reinfestation after treatment of affected animals.

FAMILY PSORERGATIDAE

Psorobia ovis, the sheep itch mite, sporadically causes pruritus and alopecia in sheep. The course is very chronic. Lambs under six months appear unaffected, and generalization may require three or four years. The mite is minute, almost discoidal, and has radially arranged legs. *Psorobia bos* is a non-pathogenic mite of cattle. *Psorergates simplex*, the subcutaneous mite of mice, may cause a mangelike condition. To demonstrate mites, skin an infested mouse and look for pockets of mites on the underside of the dermis.

FAMILY MYOBIIDAE

Myobiid mites cause dermatitis in stocks of laboratory rodents. In myobiids, the first pair of legs is modified for clasping hair (Fig. 2-35), whereas in *Myocoptes* spp., the third pair of legs of the male and third and fourth

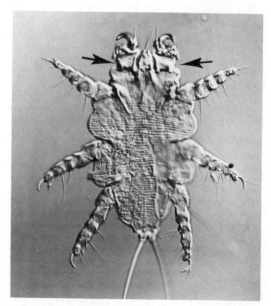

Figure 2–35. *Myobia musculi* a myobiid hair-clasping parasite of laboratory rodents. The first pair of legs (arrows) is modified for hair clasping (x170).

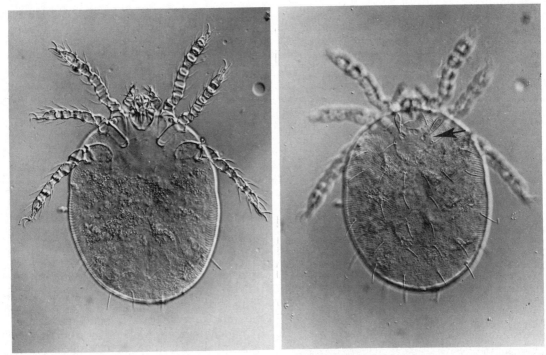

Figure 2–36. *Walchia americana*, a trombiculid mite (chigger). At left the ventral surface is in focus and at right, the dorsal surface. The scutum (arrow) with its two sensillae (large plumose setae) and four or five setae is helpful in identifying chiggers; it is on the dorsal surface near the anterior end of the body (x170).

pairs of the female are so modified (Fig. 2-32). *Myobia musculi* attacks laboratory mice and *Radfordia ensifera* attacks laboratory rats. Alopecia and erythema of the dorsal neck region is typical; severe cases are characterized by self-inflicted excoriations. Stress of overcrowding is frequently responsible for converting an asymptomatic infestation of hair-clasping mites into an outbreak of serious skin disease.

FAMILY HARPYRHYNCHIDAE

Harpyrhynchids are rounded mites, resembling psorergatids, that cause mangelike conditions in birds, Several genera include species that burrow in feather follicles or form large crusted cysts in the skin.

FAMILY SYRINGOPHILIDAE

Syringophilids are nonpathogenic inhabitants of the lumen of feather quills.

FAMILY TROMBICULIDAE

Trombiculid larvae (chiggers) are parasitic but nymphs and adults are free-living. These bright red or orange, six-legged larvae are likely to be found on the skin or in the ears of cats or dogs, on the faces or pasterns of sheep and other ungulates, and under the wings or around the vents of chickens. Infestation is usually acquired in wild or semiwild landscapes; the distribution of these nuisances is spotty but, wherever they are found, chiggers are infamous. Microscopically, the scutum is useful for recognizing a chigger as such and for generic and species identification with the help of keys. Focus on the dorsal surface (the surface opposite the one with the coxae) to see the scutum (Fig. 2-36). Chiggers remain on the skin for several days unless dislodged by the scratching host, and their saliva, injected into the skin, disintegrates host cells and the resulting material is taken into the mite as food. The surrounding skin hardens and a tube called a *stylostome* is formed in which the mouthparts remain until the chigger is replete or dislodged. The fully developed stylostome extends from the surface of the epidermis into the dermis and is lined by necrotic cells of the stratum germinativum (see Fig. 14-10). Pruritus is intense and may be protracted for many days after the chigger has been removed.

FAMILY PYEMOTIDAE

Pyemotes. "Hay itch mites" of the genus *Pyemotes* are parasites of various insect larvae that are grain-destroying pests. *Pyemotes tritici* is a tiny elongate mite that becomes enormously distended when gravid; males and females are sexually mature at birth. People and domestic animals that come into contact with infested grains, straw, hay, and the like may be attacked by these mites and develop an erythematous and intensely pruritic papular and vesicular rash. An outbreak of dermatitis in 12 horses and many persons in Florida was attributed to *Pyemotes tritici* received in a shipment of alfalfa hay (Kunkle and Greiner, 1982).

REFERENCES

Desch, C., and Nutting, W. B. (1972): *Demodex folliculorum* (Simon) and *D. brevis* Akbulatova of man: redescription and reevaluation. J. Parasitol., *58*, 169-177.

Gearhart, M. S., Crissman, J. W., and Georgi, M. E. (1981): Bilateral lower palpebral demodicosis in a dairy cow. Cornell Veterinarian, *71* (3), 305-310.

Greve, J. H., and Gerrish, B. S. (1981): Fur mites (*Lynxacarus*) from cats in Florida. Feline Practice, *11* (8), 28-30.

Heffner, R. S., and Heffner, H. E. (1983): Effect of cattle ear mite infestation on hearing in a cow. J. Am. Vet. Med. Assoc. *182* (6), 612-614.

Kummel, B. A., Estes, S. A., and Arlian, L. G. (1980): *Trixacarus caviae* infestation of guinea pigs. J. Am. Vet. Med. Assoc., *177* (9), 903-908.

Kummerfield, N., and Hinz, K. H. (1982): Diagnose und Terapie der durch die Luftsackmilbe (*Sternostoma tracheacolum*) bei Finken (Fringillidae) und Prachtfinken (Estrilididae) verursachten Acariasis. Kleintierpraxis, *27*, 95-104.

Kunkle, G. A., and Greiner, E. C. (1982): Dermatitis in horses and man caused by the straw itch mite. J. Am. Vet. Med. Assoc., *181* (5), 467-469.

Moorehouse, D. E. (1973): On the morphogenesis of the attachment cement of some ixodid ticks. Proc. 3rd. Int. Cong. Acarol., 527-529.

Moorehouse, D. E., and Tatchell, R. J. (1966): The feeding processes of the cattle tick *Boophilus microplus* (Canestrini): A study in host-parasite relations. Part I. Attachment to the host. Parasitology, *56*, 623-632.

Rhodes, A. P. (1975): Seminal degeneration associated with chorioptic mange of the scrotum of rams. Austral. Vet. J., *51*, 428-432.

Smiley, R. L., and O'Connor, B. M. (1980): Mange in *Macaca arctoides* (Primates: Cercopithecidae) caused by *Cosarcoptes scanloni* (Acari: Sarcoptidae) with possible human involvement and descriptions of the adult male and immature stages. Internat. J. Acarol. 6 (4), 283-290.

Spielman, A. (1976): Human babesiosis in Nantucket Island: transmission by nymphal *Ixodes* ticks. Am. J. Trop. Med. Hyg., *25*, 784-787.

Theiler, A. (1911): Diseases, ticks, and their eradication. Agr. J. S. Afr., *1* (4), 491-508.

Wilson, G. I., Blachut, K., and Roberts, I. H. (1977): The infectivity of scabies (mange) mites, *Psoroptes ovis* (Acarina: Psoroptidae), to sheep in naturally contaminated enclosures. Research in Vet. Sci. 22, 292-297.

PROTOZOANS

3

Most protozoans are free-living organisms and, of those that live as parasites in the bodies of mammals, only a very small proportion are associated with disease. Even then, their etiological significance is sometimes unclear. For example, certain intestinal flagellates tend to multiply when the host has diarrhea. In such cases, the presence of large numbers of flagellates in the fecal smear is the result rather than the cause of the diarrhea. On the other hand, there are protozoans that indeed behave as primary pathogens and these are responsible for some of the most important diseases of man and domestic animals. These diseases are the malarias, piroplasmoses, and coccidioses caused by apicomplexans, and the trypanosomiases caused by sarcomastigophoran hemoflagellates.

SUBPHYLUM SARCOMASTIGOPHORA

Flagellates

Flagellates bear one or more long, slender *flagella* (sing., *flagellum*) for locomotion. They multiply asexually by binary fission, and certain species form resistant cysts. The parasitic flagellates can be divided into two main groups according to their location in the host's body and type of life history. The *hemoflagellates* (e.g., *Trypanosoma, Leishmania*) live in the blood, lymph, and tissue spaces and are transmitted from host to host by blood-sucking insects. There is no collective term for the others, so we will call them *mucosoflagellates*. These live in the alimentary or genital tract, usually in intimate association with the mucous membrane, and are transmitted from host to host in the feces or genital effluvia. Certain mucosoflagellates are transmitted as trophozoites (e.g., *Trichomonas)*, others as cysts (e.g., *Giardia)*.

HEMOFLAGELLATES

Trypanosoma and Leishmania. A trypanosome is an elongated, spindle-shaped cell with a single nucleus lying near the middle of its length and a single *flagellum* that arises near a small granule of extranuclear DNA called a *kinetoplast* and passes out of the anterior end of the cell (Fig. 3-1). During development in both mammalian and arthropod hosts, trypanosomes undergo considerable morphological change. Four morphological forms are distinguished. The *amastigote* lacks a flagellum, whereas the other three all have a flagellum but differ

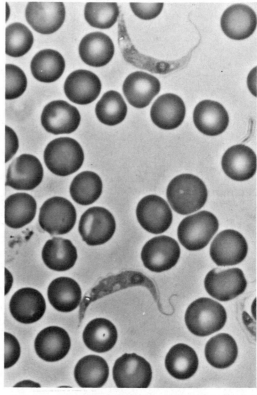

Figure 3–1. *Trypanosoma lewisi* in rat blood (x 1000).

with respect to the location of the *kinetoplast*. The kinetoplast lies posterior to the nucleus in the *trypomastigote,* immediately anterior to the nucleus in the *epimastigote,* and near the anterior end of the cell in the *promastigote.* The flagellum lies in the edge of an *undulating membrane* as it courses from kinetoplast to the anterior end of the cell body of the trypomastigote. Infection of the arthropod host occurs when it ingests the blood of an infected mammal. Infection of the mammalian host occurs by one of two mechanisms, depending on the species of trypanosome involved, i.e., either through the bite of the infected arthropod or by contamination of the host's mucous membranes or abraded skin by its feces. The former are called *salivarian,* and the latter *stercorarian* trypanosomes. Most salivarians are pathogenic and most stercorarians are nonpathogenic but the pathogenic stercorarian *Trypanosoma cruzi* forms an important exception to this generalization.

Trypanosoma cruzi, the etiological agent of American trypanosomiasis (Chagas' disease) of man and dog, is transmitted by reduviid bugs of the genera *Triatoma, Rhodnius,* and *Panstrongylus* in South and Central America and in the eastern United States as far north as Maryland. Opossums, armadillos, rats, guinea pigs, cats, raccoons, and monkeys serve as reservoirs of infection in the wild. *Trypanosoma cruzi* amastigotes multiply by binary fission in mammalian cells, including reticuloendothelial, neural, and glial cells, but most importantly, cardiac and smooth muscle cells (see Fig. 14-16). Amastigotes released by rupture of the host cell change into trypomastigotes which then appear in the circulating blood to invade other cells or to be ingested by the hemipteran as it feeds. The trypanosomes multiply and undergo metamorphosis in the bug's hindgut and are eventually passed in the feces that the bug almost invariably passes while feeding on its sleeping victim. Entry of the trypanosomes into the body is by way of the oral, nasal, and conjuctival mucosae or by rubbing the infective bug feces into abrasions in the skin. Infection can also occur transplacentally or by blood transfusion, and accidental self-injection presents a potential hazard of infection to persons handling blood samples from infected animals, even those in which trypomastigotes cannot be demonstrated in blood films. Trypomastigotes are difficult to demonstrate in the blood of chronic carriers and recourse must be had to serology or *xenodiagnosis.* In xenodiagnosis, uninfected bugs are allowed to feed upon the suspected individual and their hindguts later examined for trypanosomes, a cumbersome and inefficient procedure at best. The acute phase of Chagas' disease is characterized by prolonged fever, tachycardia, lymphadenopathy, subcutaneous edema, and hepatosplenomegaly, and the chronic phase by cardiomyopathy, megaesophagus, or megacolon. Asymptomatic carriers constitute a large proportion of the human population in endemic regions. There is no cure.

Trypanosoma equiperdum is unique among trypanosomes in not requiring an intermediate host. Transmission among hosts occurs through direct sexual contact and results in the equine venereal disease called dourine. The acute stage is characterized by swelling of the genitalia and a mucoid discharge in which *T. equiperdum* can usually be demonstrated. As the acute signs subside, circular, flattened, "silver dollar" plaques appear in the skin and then disappear within several hours or days to be replaced by others. The chronic stage of dourine is marked by emaciation, paresis, intermittent fever, and finally death. Dourine was eradicated from the United States in 1920 and again in 1949, but has since appeared at least once. Infected horses are identified by the complement fixation test and destroyed.

Trypanosoma brucei and *T. congolense* cause fatal *nagana disease* of domestic ruminants in sub-Saharan Africa but are only mildly pathogenic for the indigenous wild ruminants. The wild ruminants thus serve as reservoirs of *T. brucei* and *T. congolense,* which are conveyed through the bites of tsetse flies (*Glossina* spp.) to domestic livestock. Here is an example of well-adapted parasites actually benefiting their natural hosts. These trypanosomes and tsetses defend vast areas of African grazing lands against invasion by domestic livestock. Man has been striving to introduce his domestic animals into these areas for a long time without remarkable success and where he has succeeded he has often destroyed the grasslands by overgrazing and turned them into deserts. *Trypanosoma brucei* multiplies by longitudinal binary fission in the blood, lymph, and cerebrospinal fluid of the mammalian host. Trypomastigotes ingested by the tsetse when it feeds on the blood of an infected mammal multiply in the insect's midgut, undergo metamorphosis, and migrate to the salivary glands, where they reach the infective *metacyclic* trypomastigote stage and are then ready to be injected into the mammalian host at the next feeding. *T. gambiense* and *T. rhodesiense,* the etiological agents of African sleeping sickness in man, are closely related to *T. brucei.*

Trypanosoma evansi occurs in Asia, tropical America, and Africa north of the Sahara and causes *surra* of all species of domestic animals. Flies of the family Tabanidae and vampire bats serve as vectors. *Trypanosoma equinum* causes a disease similar to surra called *mal de Caderas* in South American horses.

Not all trypanosomes are exotic and tropical and most of them are nonpathogenic. *Trypanosoma cervi* was identified in 29 of 45 Alaskan reindeer (*Rangifer tarandus*) examined over a two year period; *T. cervi* also infects elk, mule deer, and white-tailed deer in the United States and is apparently without pathogenic effect (Kingston *et al.,* 1982). *Trypanosoma theileri* (pronounced "tyler-eye") is a harmless parasite of cattle transmitted by tabanid flies, and *T. melophagium* is an equally harmless parasite of sheep transmitted by *Melophagus ovinus;* both are worldwide in distribution. Occasionally, *T. theileri* is found contaminating culture media that have been enriched with "sterile" bovine serum, much to the surprise and confusion of the microbiologist. It is interesting that *Melophagus ovinus,* which is first cousin to a tsetse, is almost universally infected with a trypanosome, albeit fortunately a harmless one.

Leishmania donovani causes several clinical forms of visceral leishmaniasis (kala-azar), and *L. tropica* causes several clinical forms of cutaneous and mucocutaneous leishmaniasis in man, dogs, rodents, and wild mammals. These diseases are mostly confined to the tropics, where they are transmitted by psychodids of the genera *Phlebotomus* and *Lutzomyia.*

MUCOSOFLAGELLATES

Trichomonads

Trichomonads are characteristically pear-shaped and have a rodlike axostyle that protrudes from the more pointed, posterior end. There are three to five *anterior flagella* and an *undulating membrane* with a *trailing flagellum* running along its free edge. Special techniques are required for the differentiation of trichomonad genera on purely morphologic grounds. Therefore, practical diagnosis is based on host and site specificity and on the number of anterior and trailing flagella.

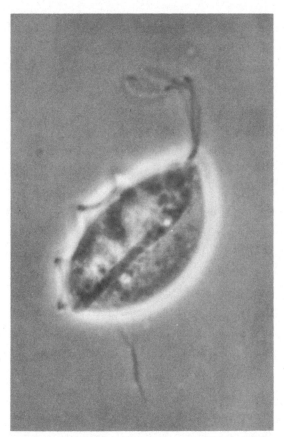

Figure 3–2. *Tritrichomonas foetus,* electronic flash, phase contrast photomicrograph of living organism from a culture provided by Dr. S. J. Shin (x5500). The three anterior flagella, undulating membrane, trailing flagellum, and axostyle are clearly visible.

Tritrichomonas foetus (Fig. 3-2) is found in the vagina, uterus, macerated fetus, prepuce, penis, epididymis, and vas deferens, and causes *genital trichomoniasis* in cattle, a disease characterized by early abortion, pyometra, and sterility. The organism displays considerable pleomorphism, varies from 10 to 25 μm in length, and has three anterior flagella and a long, trailing flagellum that extends beyond the undulating membrane. This flagellar arrangement may be abbreviated: (3+1).

Trichomonas spp. (4+0) occur as oral parasites on various hosts and tend to multiply in the presence of pyorrhea, much as their intestinal counterparts multiply in the presence of diarrhea. One species, *T. vaginalis,* causes vaginitis in women; it is transmitted by sexual intercourse, with men playing the role of asymptomatic carriers. *Trichomonas gallinae* causes necrotic ulcerations in the esophagus, crop, and proventriculus of pigeons, turkeys, and chickens.

Nonpathogenic species of *Tritrichomonas*

(3 + 1), *Trichomitus* (3 + 1), *Tetratrichomonas* (4 + 1), and *Pentatrichomonas* (5 + 0) occur in the cecum and colon of various domestic animals. These organisms tend to multiply in fluid feces, and many cases of diarrhea are mistakenly attributed to them for this reason. Their abundance in fluid feces is often the effect and not the cause of the diarrhea.

Monocercomonas spp. (3 + 1) resemble *Trichomonas* but lack an undulating membrane. *Monocercomonas* spp. are nonpathogenic; *M. ruminantium* is found in the rumen of cattle.

Histomonas meleagridis is a cosmopolitan parasite of the cecum and liver of turkeys, chickens, pheasants, guinea fowl, and the like. The cecal nematode *Heterakis gallinarum* serves as paratenic host for *Histomonas meleagridis*. When a bird ingests an infective *H. gallinarum* egg, it acquires a nonpathogenic nematode and a pathogenic protozoan parasite at one stroke. The protozoan, released from the nematode larva, spends about a week as a flagellate resident of the cecal lumen before it loses its flagella and invades the subepithelial tissues of the wall as an ameboid organism. Inflammation and necrosis of the cecal wall and the liver are particularly severe and cause high mortality in turkeys. *Histomonas meleagridis* trophozoites discharged in bird droppings perish within hours but they remain infective for years within the larvated eggs of *H. gallinae* in soil. Earthworms serve as paratenic hosts for *H. gallinae* larvae and, because birds like to eat them, actually facilitate infection with both this nematode and its protozoan guest.

The trichomonads discussed thus far do not form cysts; *Giardia* does.

Giardia

The number of species of *Giardia* is open to question. Based on differences on the shape of the *median bodies,* there appear to be at least three: *G. duodenalis* (*G. lamblia*) in mammals, *G. muris* in rats, and *G. ranae* in frogs, but there may be many more. About 7 per cent of the world's people harbor *Giardia* in their *small intestines* but very little is known about the epidemiology of this organism, especially with regard to the possible role of other mammals as sources of human infection. Beavers (*Castor canadensis*) have been incriminated as reservoirs in the wild.

Giardia trophozoites are adapted for attachment to the mucous epithelial cells of the small intestine. The *Giardia* cell is shaped like a teardrop, with one side pushed in to form a sucking disc. Within the cell are two nuclei, each with a large endosome (Feulgen-negative nucleolus) that makes the organism look like a tennis racket with eyes when viewed bottom side up under the compound microscope (see Fig. 12-35). Other subcellular structures include two slender axostyles, four pairs of flagella, and a pair of median bodies. The mature cyst containing four nuclei is the form usually found in the feces of infected hosts, although trophozoites may also be passed with diarrheal stools. Unlike all of the other intestinal flagellates, which are found in the cecum and colon, *Giardia* parasitizes the small intestine where these organisms attach to the mucosal cells by their sucking discs.

Giardia infection in man may be inapparent or cause severe enteritis. Diagnosis is usually based on finding the distinctive cysts in the feces. Sometimes, however, no evidence of infection can be found in the feces of patients suffering from severe giardial enteritis. *Giardia* is generally considered capable of causing enteritis and diarrhea in the dog, yet we have observed *Giardia* cysts in scores of well-formed canine fecal samples. The question of transmission of *Giardia* from animals to man has not been settled; feces-contaminated water supplies appear to figure in the epidemiology of human infection.

Amebas

Entamoeba histolytica causes amebic dysentery of man, an endemic disease of the tropics that occurs sporadically in the temperate regions. Man also hosts a few nonpathogenic amebas (*E. hartmanni, E. coli, Iodamoeba butschlii,* and *Endolimax nana*), some of which are shared with domestic animals. *Entamoeba histolytica* and other amebas appear to cause little if any harm to dogs.

The parasitic amebas reproduce asexually, usually by binary fission. Actively parasitic forms, called *trophozoites,* display ameboid motion when recovered from fresh feces and kept at body temperature. Most species form cysts, which in certain cases are multinuclear. Trophozoites are more likely to be found in fluid feces and cysts in formed feces.

SUBPHYLUM CILIOPHORA, CILIATES

Balantidium coli

Balantidium coli, a normal element of the intestinal fauna of the pig and rat, is very large as single cells go, measuring up to 150 μm in length. The cell surface is covered with *cilia* (sing. *cilium*) arranged in rows with a tuft of longer ones surrounding the peristome, or cell "mouth." Prominent organelles include a large *macronucleus*, a smaller *micronucleus*, two *contractile vacuoles*, and a number of *food vacuoles* in the cytoplasm. *B. coli* reproduces by transverse fission and forms cysts up to 60 μm in diameter (see Fig. 12-19).

Although harmless to the pig and usually harmless to man, *B. coli* occasionally causes ulceration of the human large intestine, manifested clinically as diarrhea and occasionally as *dysentery* (diarrhea with abdominal pain, straining, and blood and mucus in the stools) (see Fig. 14-17). Diagnosis of *B. coli* infection is based on the demonstration of motile trophozoites in direct smears of diarrheal feces or cysts in flotation preparations of formed feces. Acute enteritis characterized by watery diarrhea and lethargy involving four gorillas in the Los Angeles Zoo was attributed to *B. coli* infection (Teare and Loomis, 1982).

Symbiotic Ciliates

The forestomachs of ruminants and the cecum and colon of horses abound with large, somewhat bizarre ciliates that are neither pathogenic nor indispensable to their hosts. Sometimes, they are found in the lungs of ruminants at necropsy, the result of agonal inspiration of ruminal contents and nothing more (see Fig. 14-18).

SUBPHYLUM APICOMPLEXA

The Apicomplexa (Sporozoa) of interest to us are all intracellular parasites and cause disease by destroying those cells. The most important members are the *coccidia*, many of which develop in epithelial cells of the alimentary canal and cause a form of enteritis called coccidiosis, and the *hemosporidians*, which develop in erythrocytes and cause hemolytic anemia. Coccidians are transmitted mainly by fecal contamination and reproduce by rigid sequences of asexual and sexual phases of multiplication and development that, in an important minority of cases, require an alternation of hosts. Hemosporidians are transmitted by bloodsucking arthropods and include the *piroplasms*, which are transmitted by ixodid ticks and apparently lack sexual stages, and the *plasmodia*, which are transmitted by dipterans in which they complete the sexual phases of their life histories.

Coccidia and Coccidioses

A particular species of coccidium tends to be restricted to a very narrow range of hosts but each host species may be parasitized by a number of different species of coccidia simultaneously. Diagnosis of coccidian infection is usually based on identification of egg-like *oocysts* (o'o-sists) in the host's feces. Identification of coccidian species is usually based on oocyst morphology and host specificity but may also require micrometric measurement of the oocysts or their sporulation in culture to obtain more differential structural detail. The identification of coccidia in the feces of a host does not justify a diagnosis of the disease *coccidiosis* unless the history and clinical signs are in accord. Large numbers of oocysts may be counted in the feces of perfectly healthy hosts. On the other hand, severe and even fatal coccidiosis sometimes occurs during the early asexual stages of infection before oocysts have had time to develop. In such cases, disease is manifest, but oocysts have not yet appeared in the feces.

COCCIDIAN LIFE HISTORIES

During the past 15 years, revolutionary advances have been made in the knowledge of coccidian ontogeny and epidemiology, especially with respect to those species requiring intermediate hosts (e.g., *Toxoplasma, Sarcocystis*). The electron microscope has greatly enriched and modified previous conceptions of both structure and reproductive processes. With this progress have come innovations in taxonomic nomenclature and descriptive terminology. The terminology adopted in the following exposition is generally conservative but some of the newer synonyms are included to aid the reader in understanding the contemporary literature.

The functional unit of coccidian ontogeny is the *zoite*, a motile, banana- or cigar-shaped cell, rounded at one end and pointed at the other (apical) end. It is the zoite that migrates in the host and invades cells, the zoite that represents the beginning and end point of every coccidian life process. Relationship to a particular portion of the life history is denoted by a prefix. Thus, *sporozoites* are infective forms that are found in sporulated oocysts. Sporozoites invade hosts' cells, where they form many *merozoites* by a kind of multiple internal fission called *schizogony* (ski-zog'o-ne; synonym, *merogony*); *tachyzoites* divide rapidly, *bradyzoites* divide slowly, and so forth. The following exposition progresses from the relatively simple, highly constrained life history of an enteric coccidian genus, *Eimeria*, to the complex and varied life history of *Toxoplasma*. The genera *Eimeria*, *Isospora*, *Hammondia*, *Sarcocystis*, and *Toxoplasma* present an orderly sequence of increasing biological complexity.

Eimeria

The simplest form of coccidian life history is represented by the genus *Eimeria*, species of which are gastrointestinal parasites of a wide range of vertebrate hosts. This life history includes both asexual multiplication and sexual multiplication. Sexual multiplication culminates in the formation of cysts, which are discharged with the feces, and in the development, within each of these cysts, of eight infective organisms.

Schizogony (*Merogony*). If the infective, sporulated oocyst is ingested by a suitable host, the sporozoites emerge and each may enter an epithelial or lamina propria cell, round up as a *trophozoite* (see Fig. 14-20), grow larger, and become a first generation *schizont* (*meront*) (see Figs. 14-21 and 14-22). This schizont produces first generation *merozoites* that burst the cell and invade fresh cells to become second generation schizonts. There may be several more schizogonic generations, but two or three is the limit for many of the important species of *Eimeria*. The number of asexual generations, the type and location of the host cells parasitized, and the number of merozoites formed at each generation depend on the species of coccidium in question. The biologically significant attributes of schizogony are: (1) an exponential increase in the number of parasites arising from a single sporozoite, (2) a corresponding destruction of host cells, and (3) an automatic halting of the asexual process after a fixed number of repetitions.

Gametogony. A merozoite produced by the final schizogony (i.e., a *telomerozoite*) enters a fresh host cell and develops into either a male or a female *gamont*. The female gamont (syn., *macrogametocyte*) enlarges, stores food materials, and causes a hypertrophy of both cytoplasm and nucleus of its host cell (see Fig. 14-31). When mature, it is called a *macrogamete*. The male gamont (syn., *microgameto-*

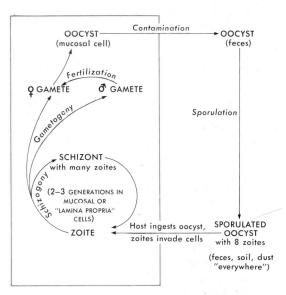

Figure 3–3. Life history of a typical *Eimeria* sp.

cyte) undergoes repeated nuclear division and becomes multinucleate (see Figs. 14-29 and 14-30). Each nucleus is finally incorporated into a biflagellate *microgamete*. Of the many microgametes formed by the male gamont, only a small fraction find and fertilize macrogametes to form *zygotes*. An *oocyst wall* forms about the zygote by the coalescence of hyaline granules at its periphery to form an *oocyst* (see Fig. 14-31). The oocyst is released by rupture of the host cell and passes out with the feces to undergo *sporulation*. Within a day or two, if provided with adequate moisture, moderate temperatures, and sufficient oxygen, the single cell (*sporont*) in the oocyst divides into four *sporoblasts*. Each sporoblast develops into a *sporocyst*, which contains two haploid *sporozoites* (see Figs. 12-28 and 12-29), thus becoming an infective, sporulated oocyst and completing the cycle of events in the life history of *Eimeria*. The details of the *Eimeria* life history are presented diagrammatically in Figure 3-3.

Isospora

The genus *Isospora* (I-sos'po-rah) until recently included species now assigned to the genera *Hammondia*, *Toxoplasma*, *Besnoitia*, and *Sarcocystis* because the sporulated oocysts of all of these genera contain two sporocysts, each of which contains four sporozoites (see Fig. 12-18A). The life history of *Isospora felis* resembles that of *Eimeria* except that its sporozoites may encyst (singly) in the tissues of a mouse. As Figure 3-4 indicates, a cat may

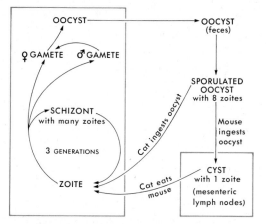

Figure 3–4. Life history of *Isospora felis*.

become infected with *I. felis* by ingesting either sporulated oocysts or sporozoite-infected mice. The mouse thus serves as a facultative, paratenic host for *I. felis*.

Hammondia

Hammondia hammondi, a rather rare parasite of the cat, goes beyond *Isospora felis* by multiplying in the tissues of an intermediate host. The zoites first multiply rapidly (tachyzoites), then form cysts in which they multiply slowly (bradyzoites). The net result is the multiplication and storage of zoites in cysts in the tissues of an animal that is likely to fall prey to a cat. As indicated in Figure 3-5, only sporulated oocysts from cat feces are

infectious for mice, and only bradyzoites from mouse tissues are infectious for cats; thus *H. hammondi* has an obligatory two-host life history. Tachyzoites are not infectious to cats and are not transmitted to the progeny of pregnant female mice via the placenta, as is true of *Toxoplasma gondi*.

Sarcocystis

Species of *Sarcocystis*, like *H. hammondi*, have an obligatory two-host life history but differ in that only sexual reproduction occurs in the definitive host and that sporogony is completed there; fully sporulated oocysts and sporocysts (see Fig. 12-22D) are discharged in the host's feces and no development occurs in the external environment. Asexual reproduction, including schizogony (see Fig. 14-23) and sarcocyst formation (see Figs. 14-25 and 14-26), occurs only in the intermediate host. The bradyzoites in *sarcocysts* differ from those in *Hammondia* cysts in that they develop into gamonts instead of schizonts when ingested by the definitive host. Bradyzoites represent a state of arrested development, or *hypobiosis*. Like sporozoites in a sporulated oocyst, bradyzoites in a sarcocyst or in a *Hammondia* cyst must enter a definitive host to develop further. The life history of *Sarcocystis* is portrayed diagrammatically in Figure 3-6.

The host relationships of several species of *Sarcocystis* are summarized in Table 3-1. In all cases, the carnivorous host becomes infected by eating the infected flesh of the herbivorous host, and the herbivorous host becomes infected by ingesting sporocysts from the feces of the carnivorous host. Schizogony and encystment occur exclusively in

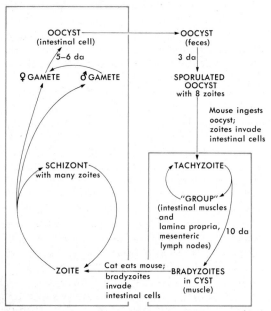

Figure 3–5. Life history of *Hammondia hammondi*.

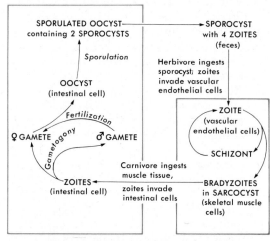

Figure 3–6. Life history of *Sarcocystis* sp.

Table 3–1. Host Relationships of Some Species of *Sarcocystis*

Intermediate Hosts	Definitive Hosts		
	Dog	Cat	Man
Cattle	S. cruzi	S. hirsuta	S. hominis
Sheep	S. ovicanis	S. tenella	—
Swine	S. miescheriana	S. porcifelis	S. suihominis
Horse	S. bertrami	—	—
	S. fayeri	—	—
	S. equicanis	—	—
Cottontail rabbit	—	S. leporum	—
Mouse	—	S. muris	—
Mule deer	S. hemionilatrantis	—	—

the herbivorous host, and gametogony, fertilization, and sporulation occur exclusively in the carnivorous host. *Sarcocystis* usually causes no illness in the carnivore but schizogony in the endothelium of herbivores may result in serious or fatal disease.

Toxoplasma

The life history of *Toxoplasma gondii* (Fig. 3-7) is like that of *Hammondia hammondi* with every conceivable constraint removed. Sporozoites, tachyzoites, merozoites, and bradyzoites of *T. gondii* are all capable of infecting both definitive and intermediate hosts; extraintestinal as well as intestinal infection occurs in the definitive host, and infection is passed transplacentally to the unborn. The definitive hosts are members of the family Felidae and the intermediate hosts are virtually all other warm-blooded animals. Infected cats shed very small unsporulated oocysts (see Fig. 12-22C) that are easily over-

looked in fecal preparations. Cats shed *Toxoplasma* oocysts in their feces 3 to 10 days after eating mice infected with encysted bradyzoites and 19 to 48 days after ingesting sporulated oocysts or mice infected with tachyzoites (Dubey and Frenkel, 1976). Apparently, the asexual reproduction preceding the formation of bradyzoites in the intermediate host satisfies a major portion of the developmental requirements preceding sexual reproduction. Cats may also serve as intermediate host inasmuch as multiplication of tachyzoites and cyst formation occur in their extraintestinal tissues (see Figs. 14-27 and 14-28).

Intermediate hosts become infected with *Toxoplasma* by ingesting sporulated oocysts from cat feces or tachyzoites or bradyzoites in the tissues of other intermediate hosts, or by transplacental migration of tachyzoites from their mothers.

Besnoitia

Large cysts (0.5 mm.) containing bradyzoites occur in the skin of cattle, where they cause scleroderma, and in various tissues of other animals. Oocysts resembling those of *Toxoplasma* are shed in the feces of cats.

Cryptosporidium

Cryptosporidium spp. are tiny coccidians that insinuate themselves under the microvillous borders of intestinal epithelial cells of mammals, birds, and reptiles (see Fig. 14-33). The oocysts are only 4 to 5 μm in diameter and therefore easily overlooked on routine fecal examination. The number of species and pathogenetic significance of *Cryptosporidium* are as yet undetermined. It appears likely that *Cryptosporidium* infection causes diarrhea in at least some species of hosts.

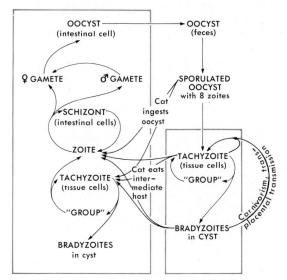

Figure 3–7. Life history of *Toxoplasma gondii*.

Equine Protozoan Myelitis (EPM) Organism

This organism causes severe neurologic disease in horses, particularly Standardbreds (Mayhew *et al.*, 1976).

Hemosporidians

PIROPLASMOSES

Babesia

Babesia spp. are apicomplexan parasites of the erythrocytes (see Fig. 3-8). *Babesia bigemina* causes bovine piroplasmosis ("Texas fever"), a disease characterized, in the acute phase, by pyrexia (up to 42° C), hemoglobinuria, anemia, icterus, and splenomegaly. The appleseedlike piroplasms are found in pairs in the erythrocytes, which they destroy, releasing hemoglobin in the process and giving rise to the characteristic clinical manifestations. Transmission of infection among cattle occurs through the bite of the one-host ticks *Boophilus annulatus* and *B. microplus;* the piroplasms multiply in the ovary of the female tick and thereby infect the larvae that hatch from her eggs. In The United King-

dom, piroplasmosis is transmitted by *Ixodes ricinus* and can be transmitted experimentally by parenteral injection of infected erythrocytes. Calves are much less susceptible than older cattle. The greater susceptibility of older hosts holds for all species of *Babesia* and is greatly increased by splenectomy.

Texas fever was once endemic south of the 35th parallel in the United States, but a cattle dipping campaign launched in 1906 to eradicate *Boophilus annulatus* virtually eliminated the disease by 1940. This prodigious effort was successful mainly because of the high degree of specificity displayed by *B. annulatus* for its bovine host. Other mammals can serve as hosts, but the majority of *B. annulatus* ticks are found on cattle. Therefore, when the cattle were rounded up for dipping, most of the feeding tick population was rounded up with them. *Boophilus microplus*, on the other hand, infests a very broad range of hosts and where *B. microplus* is involved, eradication of bovine piroplasmosis is virtually impossible with contemporary methods.

Babesia bovis, *B. divergens*, and *B. argentina* cause bovine piroplasmosis in various parts of the world. Each employs one or more different species of tick vectors. Other species

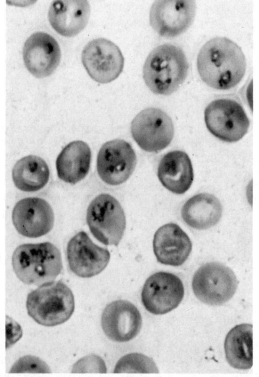
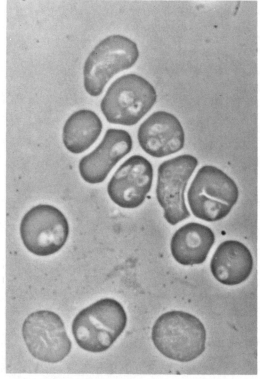

Figure 3–8. *Babesia microti* in blood film from a golden hamster *Mesocricetus auratus;* isolate provided by Dr. Jorge Benach. At left is a brightfield photomicrograph of a thin blood smear stained with Giemsa for 45 minutes, and at right is a phase contrast photomicrograph of a fresh blood film (x1000).

of *Babesia* infect sheep (*B. ovis*), horses (*B. caballi, B. equi*), swine (*B. trautmanni*), and dogs (*B. canis*). Canine piroplasmosis is cosmopolitan in distribution but relatively rare in the United States in spite of the ubiquity of its vector, *Rhipicephalus sanguineus*.

Theileria

Theileria parva, the etiological agent of East Coast fever of African cattle, occurs in the erythrocytes, lymphocytes, and endothelial cells and is transmitted interstadially by *Rhipicephalus* and *Hyalomma* spp. East Coast fever is characterized by dyspnea, emaciation, weakness, tarry feces, and exceptionally heavy mortality.

Cytauxzoon

Cytauxzoon felis. Cytauxzoonosis is a rapidly and uniformly fatal disease of cats that roam rural wooded areas of the Gulf Coast states. Clinical signs consist of pyrexia, anemia, icterus, and dehydration; death occurs within a few days. Wright's or Giemsa stained blood smears reveal 1 to 2 μm organisms with light blue cytoplasm and dark red nucleus in the erythrocytes. Late in the course of cytauxzoonosis, enormous reticuloendothelial cells packed with schizonts appear in the peripheral blood. Histologically, parasitized reticuloendothelial cells nearly occlude the lumens of small and medium sized veins in the lungs, spleen, and lymph nodes (Wightman *et al.*, 1977). The bobcat *Lynx rufus rufus* develops a parasitemia but no clinical signs of disease, and may be the natural reservoir host of *Cytauxzoon felis* (Kier *et al.*, 1982, Glenn *et al.*, 1982).

MALARIAS

Plasmodium

Plasmodium spp. are the etiological agents of malarias of man, nonhuman primates, rodents, birds, and reptiles (mainly lizards). Mammalian malarias are transmitted by anopheline mosquitoes and avian malarias by culicine mosquitoes; the vectors of reptilian malarias are unknown.

Life History. Sporozoites injected into the host by the infected mosquito during feeding enter cells such as hepatocytes, become trophozoites, and undergo schizogony. This first multiplication of plasmodia in hepatocytes is termed *pre-erythrocytic schizogony*. Merozoites released when the hepatocyte ruptures invade erythrocytes or reticulocytes of the circulating blood, pass through a trophozoite phase, and then undergo schizogony. In certain species of *Plasmodium*, some of these merozoites reinvade hepatocytes to continue *exoerythrocytic schizogony*, which is held accountable by some authorities for relapses following therapeutic elimination of erythrocytic infection by chloroquine, quinine, and the like. Merozoites released when the infected erythrocytes rupture reinvade other erythrocytes, and again undergo schizogony. Each generation of erythrocytic merozoites occupies approximately 24, 48, or 72 hours, depending on the species of *Plasmodium* involved. Synchronization of schizogony and consequent erythrocyte destruction leading to cyclic bouts of chills and fever is typical of certain malarias, pariculary those of man. The terms *quotidian, tertian,* and *quartan* refer to recurrence of fever daily, on the third day (i.e., at 48 hours), and on the fourth day (i.e., at 72 hours), the anomaly in nomenclature arising from inconsistency in the inclusion of zero in the system of natural numbers as applied to the reckoning of time. Eventually, some merozoites develop into either microgametocytes or macrogametocytes, which are the stages infective for the mosquito. When a suitable species of mosquito feeds upon a malarious host, the micro- and macrogametocytes in the blood meal mature and the microgametes fertilize the macrogametes to form zygotes. The zygotes then elongate to form motile *ookinetes*, which migrate to the hemocoel side of the mosquito's midgut where each develops into an oocyst. Thousands of sporozoites develop within each oocyst by a budding process similar to schizogony and are released into the hemocoel when the oocyst ruptures. Those sporozoites that reach the salivary glands are ready to infect another host next time the mosquito takes a blood meal and thus complete the rather involved life history of *Plasmodium*. In man, the symptoms of malaria are extremely variable and diagnosis depends on the demonstration of plasmodia in fixed, stained blood smears. Fatality can usually be attributed to cerebral involvement, renal failure, or pulmonary hemorrhage.

Identification. Differentiation of species of *Plasmodia* is based on study of Giemsa stained thin blood smears and recognition of rather subtle morphologic features of the early trophozoite ("ring form"), ameboid late trophozoite, schizont, and male and female gametocytes. The color and distribution of hematin in the cytoplasm of the parasite, as well as cytoplasmic stippling and other morphologic alterations of the infected erythrocyte, are also taken into account. The diagnosis of malaria is clearly a job for an expert.

Simian Malaria. About twenty species of *Plasmodium* have been described from non-human primates, some of which (e.g., *P. knowlsi, P. cynomolgi*) are transmissible to man through the bites of infected anopheline mosquitoes. The diagnosis of simian malaria is of particular interest to laboratories using imported primates as experimental animals (see Coatney *et al.*, 1971). Old World monkeys may also be infected with *Hepatocystis*.

Avian Malaria. Avian malaria is a complex of diseases caused by many species of *Plasmodium*. *Haemoproteus* and *Leucocytozoon*, considered below, also cause malarialike infections in birds.

Haemoproteus

Haemoproteus spp. are parasites of birds, turtles, and lizards. Schizogony occurs in vascular endothelial cells of various organs and only gametocytes appear in circulating erythrocytes. In blood films fixed with methanol and stained with Giemsa, the gametocytes appear as elongate, sometimes horseshoe-shaped cells embracing the erythrocyte nucleus; the cytoplasm of the gametocyte contains pigment granules accumulating as a result of the incomplete digestion of hemoglobin. Various species of *Haemoproteus* are transmitted by *Culicoides*, Hippoboscidae, or *Chrysops*, which become infected when they ingest erythrocytes containing gametocytes. Fertilization, development of oocysts, and salivarian transmission of sporozoites to the vertebrate host resemble the corresponding events in the life history of *Plasmodium*. *Haemoproteus* is essentially nonpathogenic.

Leucocytozoon

Leucocytozoon spp. are parasites of domestic and wild birds; *L. simondi* causes acute, fatal disease of ducks and geese, as does *L. caulleryi* in chickens, and *L. smithi* in turkeys. Schizogony occurs in hepatocytes and vascular endothelial cells of various tissues, producing merozoites which invade erythroblasts, erythrocytes, lymphocytes, and monocytes, and there develop into gametocytes. *Leucocytozoon* gametocytes differ from those of *Plasmodium* and *Haemoproteus* in not containing pigment granules and in greatly distorting the host cell. Some gametocytes are round and push the host cell nucleus to one side so that it forms a cap on the parasite. Others are oval or elliptical in cells that become elongated and quite bizarre in appearance as the parasite grows. *Simulium* spp. serve as intermediate hosts.

Hepatocystis

Hepatocystis spp. are parasites of the lower monkeys, fruit bats, and squirrels of the Old World. Schizogony occurs in hepatocytes, requires two months, and results in large schizonts called "merocysts." Merozoites released from merocysts invade erythrocytes and develop into gametocytes. *Culicoides* spp. are the probable vectors.

REFERENCES

Coatney, G. R., Collins, W. E., Warren, McW., and Contacos, P. G. (1971): The Primate Malarias. U.S. Govt. Printing Office, Washington, D.C.

Dubey, J. P., and Frenkel, J. K. (1976): Feline toxoplasmosis from acutely infected mice and the development of *Toxoplasma* cysts. J. Protozool., 23, 537–546.

Glenn, B. T., Rolley, R. E., and Kocan, A. A. (1982): *Cytauxzoon*-like piroplasms in erythrocytes of wild-trapped bobcats in Oklahoma. J. Am. Vet. Med. Assoc., *181* (11), 1251-1253.

Kier, A. B., Wagner, J. E., and Morehouse, L. G. (1982): Experimental transmission of *Cytauxzoon felis* from bobcats (*Lynx rufus*) to domestic cats (*Felis domesticus*). Am. J. Vet. Res., *43*, 97-101.

Kingston, N., Morton, J. K., and Dietrich, R. (1982): *Trypanosoma cervi* from Alaskan reindeer, *Rangifer tarandus*. J. Protozool., *29* (4), 588-591.

Teare, J. A., and Loomis, M. R. (1982): Epizootic of balantidiasis in lowland gorillas. J. Am. Vet. Med. Assoc., *181* (11), 1345-1347.

Wightman, S. R., Kier, A. B., and Wagner, J. E. (1977): Feline cytauxzoonosis: clinical features of a newly described blood parasite disease. Feline Practice 7 (3), 23-26.

4

TREMATODES

PHYLUM PLATYHELMINTHES

The phylum Platyhelminthes contains three classes, Turbellaria, Trematoda, and Cestoda. All are typically soft-bodied, flattened dorsoventrally, and hermaphroditic. The Turbellaria (planarians) are free-living, carnivorous flatworms. Aquarists finding them in fish tanks may mistake planarians for parasites, but otherwise they are of only passing interest to veterinarians. Adult cestodes (tapeworms) are parasites of the small intestine or bile ducts of vertebrates, and their larvae are parasites of alternate vertebrates or of invertebrates. The class Cestoda includes many important parasites of domestic animals and is the subject of Chapter 5.

CLASS TREMATODA

The class Trematoda contains three orders, Monogenea, Aspidogastrea, and Digenea. Monogeneans and most Aspidogastreans undergo direct development and are parasites of aquatic and amphibious animals. *Gyrodactylus* and *Dactylogyrus,* for example, are common and pathogenic monogenean parasites of the skin and gills of aquarium fishes.

Order Digenea

LIFE HISTORY

The order Digenea is so called because its members undergo indirect development with sexual and asexual generations parasitizing alternate hosts. All flukes infecting dogs, cats, ruminants, horses, and swine are digeneans. The life history of *Fasciola hepatica* is typical of the order.

Life History of Fasciola hepatica. Adult *F. hepatica* (Fig. 4-1) live in the bile ducts of ruminant and other mammalian hosts. Their

eggs are carried first to the bowel lumen with the bile and then to the exterior with the feces. When deposited, each of these eggs consists of a fertilized ovum and a cluster of vitelline cells enclosed in an operculated capsule (Fig. 4-2). Only if the egg falls into water will a ciliated larva called a *miracidium* develop inside it (Fig. 4-3). The miracidium is completely covered with cilia, has a conical papilla at its anterior end for boring into the snail intermediate host, a pair of eye spots, a brain, a rudimentary excretory system, and a cluster of germinal cells, the progenitors of the next generation of larvae (Fig. 4-4). The miracidium escapes from the egg capsule by pushing aside the operculum and swims about in search of a suitable species of snail (e.g., *Limnea truncatula).* If it fails to find such a snail within 24 hours, the miracidium exhausts its energy stores and dies.

If the miracidium is more fortunate, it bores into the snail's body, loses its ciliated covering, migrates to the gonad or digestive gland ("liver"), and forms a *sporocyst.* Each germinal cell, by growth and repeated divisions, becomes a *germinal ball,* and each germinal ball develops into a *redia* (Fig. 4-5).

The rediae grow until they burst the sporocyst wall and are thus liberated into the tissues of the snail. The redia has a mouth and digestive organs and eats its way through the snail's tissues. Like the sporocyst, the redia is packed with germinal balls, these being the progenitors of a second generation of rediae. Each germinal ball of second generation rediae develops into yet a third kind of larva, the *cercaria* (Fig. 4-6).

The cercaria is a tadpolelike larva with a discoidal body and a long tail for swimming. The cercaria displays certain adult organs (e.g., oral and ventral suckers, mouth, pharynx, forked intestine, and excretory canals with flame cells) and primordia of the reproductive organs. Special secretory cells alongside the pharynx are purely larval structures;

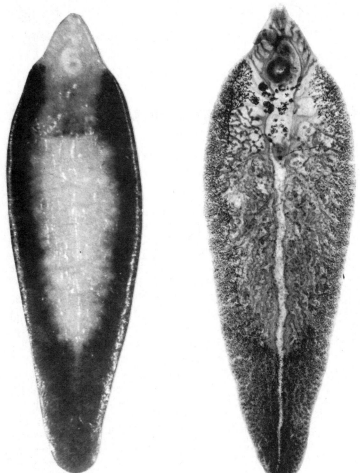

Figure 4–1. *Fasciola hepatica:* an uncleared specimen at left and a cleared, stained specimen at right (x6.5).

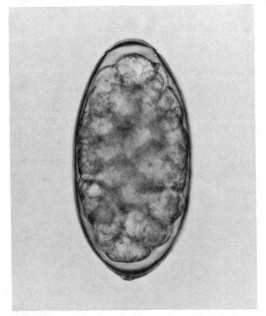

Figure 4–2. Egg of *Fasciola hepatica* from a sheep's bile duct (x 380).

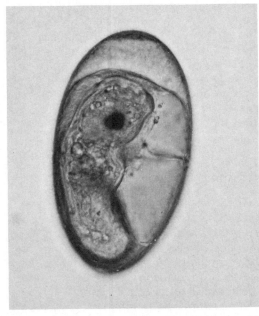

Figure 4–3. Egg of *Fasciola hepatica* containing a fully developed miracidium (x380).

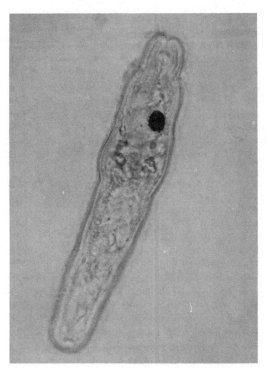

Figure 4–4. Miracidium of *Fasciola hepatica* swimming; electronic flash photomicrograph (approx. x400).

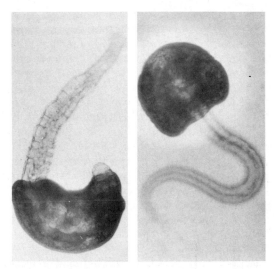

Figure 4–6. Cercariae of *Fasciola hepatica*; electronic flash photomicrograph (approx. x125).

they secrete a cyst wall within which the final larval stage will lie in wait for a grazing ruminant. When fully developed, the cercaria leaves the redia through a birth pore and makes its way out through the snail's tissues and into the surrounding water. After a brief swim, the cercaria migrates a short distance above the water level on the surface of some plant and encysts, losing its tail in the process to become a *metacercaria*, the stage that is infective to sheep and other grazing mammals (Fig. 4-7).

When ingested, the metacercarial cyst is digested in the host's small intestine. The young fluke, now called a *marita*, penetrates the wall of the intestine and crosses the

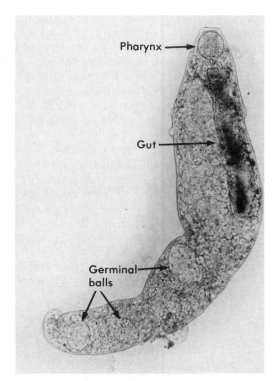

Figure 4–5. Redia of *Fasciola hepatica* from a snail's digestive gland (x90).

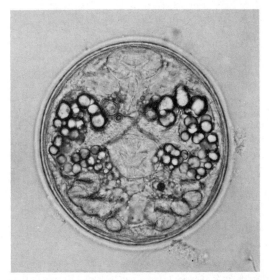

Figure 4–7. Metacercaria of *Fasciola hepatica* (x250).

peritoneal space to the liver, which it penetrates. After several weeks of boring about in the hepatic parenchyma, the maritas enter the bile ducts, mature into adult flukes, and begin laying eggs.

Digenean trematodes are very discriminating in their choice of snail hosts and the geographic distribution of trematode species is therefore largely dictated by the geographic distribution of suitable species of snails. Adult trematodes, on the other hand, seem to be able to make do with a rather broad range of definitive host species. Hosts' food preferences somewhat limit the range of possibilities; that is, fish-eating animals tend to serve as hosts for trematodes whose metacercariae encyst on fish and, as we have already seen, *Fasciola hepatica* metacercariae have a strategic advantage when it comes to getting into grazing ruminants. However, *Fasciola hepatica* has found its way into human beings (by way of water cress) and so has *Dicrocoelium dendriticum*, whose cercariae are contained in the bodies of ants.

The preceding details of early larval development, as outlined for *Fasciola hepatica*, vary considerably among species of trematodes and, though fascinating, are of less practical consequence than the ecological relationships of the snail host at one end of the cycle and of the cercariae or metacercariae at the other. In Figure 4-8, life history variations displayed by important families of trematodes parasitizing domestic animals are portrayed diagrammatically. Further details are set forth in the discussion of families of trematodes below.

IDENTIFICATION

An adult trematode is little more than a bag of reproductive organs with both sexes represented. Typically, there are two *testes* and one *ovary*, the anatomical positions of which provide diagnostic criteria. The genital pore may be identified by the convergence of male and female reproductive ducts. Usually the presence of a *cirrus*, or intromittent organ, helps to identify the male duct, and a procession of well-tanned eggs the female duct. The *oral sucker* surrounds the *mouth*, which is connected by way of the *esophagus* to a pair of blind *ceca*. The ceca are simple tubular sacs in most species but are intricately branched in the family Fasciolidae. The *ventral sucker* or *acetabulum* is often but not always near the genital pore. In the family Heterophyidae, both the ventral sucker and the genital pore are enclosed in an invagination, the *ventrogenital sac*, and an extra *genital sucker* or *gonotyl* surrounds the genital opening. The anatomical structures most used as taxonomic characters are labeled in Figure 4-9. Diagnostic criteria sufficient for identification of these families are presented in the following discussion. In general, identification of trematodes to family level combined with the host and organ listings provided in Chapter 13 will result in sufficiently precise diagnosis to serve practical needs. An excellent guide to the identification of families and genera of trematodes of North America north of Mexico is S. C. Schell's *How to Know the Trematodes*, Wm. C. Brown Company, Dubuque, Iowa. Because only a limited set of trematode species is likely to be found in domestic animals in any particular locality, a knowledge of the endemic species is valuable. Sometimes, the only way to acquire this information is to submit collections for expert identification. The specimens should be relaxed by overnight storage at 5 C and fixed in FAA or shipped fresh and packed in plenty of ice in a well-insulated container.

A FEW REPRESENTATIVE FAMILIES OF TREMATODES

Family Fasciolidae

Identification. The body is large and leaflike with suckers close together at the anterior end, the

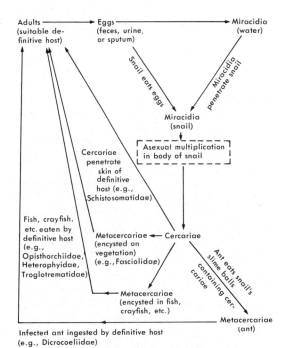

Figure 4–8. Some life history variations followed by trematode parasites of domestic animals.

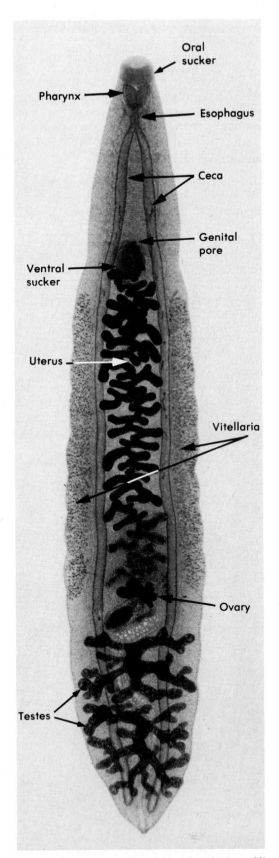

Figure 4–9. *Clonorchis sinensis* (Opisthorchiidae; x30).

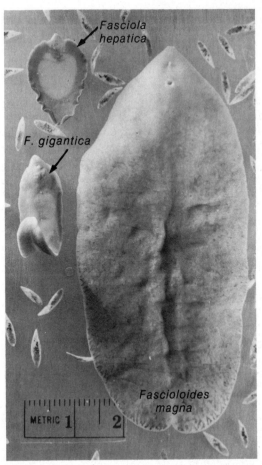

Figure 4–10. Liver flukes of ruminants. *Fasciola hepatica,* *F. gigantica,* and *Fascioloides magna* belong to the family Fasciolidae. The small flukes scattered about are *Dicrocoelium dendriticum* of the family Dicrocoeliidae.

ceca have numerous diverticula, and the ovary and testes are dendritic (Figs. 4-1 and 4-10). *Fasciola hepatica, F. gigantica,* and *Fascioloides magna* are parasites of the liver and bile ducts of herbivorous mammals and man. *Fasciolopsis buski* is a parasite of the small intestine of pigs and man in Asia; the ceca of this species do not have diverticula.

Life History. The life history of *Fasciola hepatica,* as presented above, is typical of the family. *Fascioloides magna,* one of the largest known trematodes, is widely scattered over North America. Adult *F. magna* are found in cysts that communicate with the bile ducts of its normal definitive host, the white-tailed deer *Odocoileus virginianus.* In cattle, however, these cysts usually do not communicate with the bile ducts, and in sheep and goats, *F. magna* maritas do not mature but wander extensively and destructively in the liver tissue. Therefore, *F. magna* infection is nonpatent in cattle, sheep, and goats and cannot be diagnosed by fecal examination in these hosts.

Importance. Several clinical syndromes may be associated with liver fluke infection, depending on the numbers and stage of development of the parasite and on the presence or absence of *Clostridium novyi. Acute fluke disease* occurs during invasion of the liver by recently ingested metacercariae. In heavy invasions, the trauma inflicted by the maritas tunneling about in the liver and consequent inflammatory reaction result in highly fatal clinical illness characterized by abdominal pain with a disinclination to move. Postmortem examination reveals an abdominal cavity containing blood-stained exudate and an enlarged, friable liver covered with fibrin tags; large numbers of maritas can be recovered from the cut surfaces. Heavy invasions of the sort associated with acute fluke disease may occur when lambs are turned into pastures containing marshy areas that were heavily contaminated the previous season.

In certain cases, all that is needed to precipitate rapidly fatal disease is a minor trauma that provides clostridial organisms with some damaged and poorly oxygenated tissue in which to multiply and secrete their deadly toxins. Even the minor trauma associated with the migrations of a few *F. hepatica* (or *Taenia hydatigena* larvae) is enough to provide an appropriate environment for *Clostridium novyi.* As is typical of clostridial infections, sheep die so fast that they hardly have time to be sick. Necropsy reveals focal liver necrosis and extensive subcutaneous hemorrhage; the latter is possibly responsible for the colloquial name "black disease." *Clostridium novyi* also causes a lethal condition called "big head" in young rams, but here the precipitating trauma results from contests of physical prowess instead of parasite migrations.

Chronic fluke disease is associated with the presence of adult trematodes in the bile ducts and characterized by the classical clinical signs of liver fluke infection. There is gradual loss of condition, progressive weakness, anemia, and hypoproteinemia with development of edematous subcutaneous swellings, especially in the intermandibular space and over the abdomen. Necropsy reveals distended, thickened bile ducts packed with adult trematodes. In cattle, the fibrotic ducts later calcify to produce what looks like a branching system of clay pipes. Isseroff and colleagues (1977) have demonstrated that the bile duct wall inflammation is related to the excretion of large amounts of the amino acid proline by *F. hepatica.*

Fascioloides magna causes considerable economic loss as wasted cattle livers that are condemned as unfit for human consumption, and its destructive migrations in the livers of sheep and goats virtually preclude small ruminant production in endemic areas.

Family Schistosomatidae

Identification. Sexes are separate with the slender female lying in the gynecophoric canal of the somewhat stouter male (Fig. 4-11). Adult schistosomes are parasites of veins of the digestive and urinary tracts of birds and mammals. Other trematodes are hermaphroditic and parasitize tissues other than blood vessels. Eggs lack an operculum and contain a fully developed miracidium when discharged in the feces (e.g., *Schistosoma mansoni, S. japonicum*) or urine (e.g., *S. haematobium*); eggs of some species are armed with a spine. Other trematode eggs have a polar operculum and lack a spine.

Life History of Heterobilharzia americana. The miracidium hatches very soon after the egg comes in contact with water and enters a freshwater snail, *Lymnaea cubensis,* in which

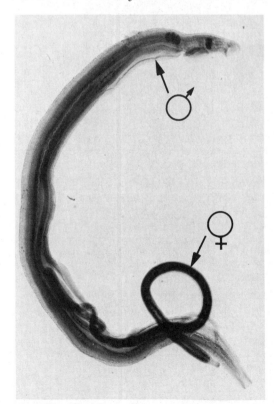

Figure 4–11. *Schistosoma* spp. (Schistosomatidae; x24). The body of the slender female can be seen protruding from the gynecophoric groove of the stouter male.

cercariae develop in daughter sporocysts. Upon emergence from the snail, the cercariae penetrate the skin of a raccoon, dog, bobcat, rabbit, or nutria, and migrate by way of the lungs to the liver. After a period of development in the liver, mature males and females make their way to the mesenteric veins and mate, the more or less cylindrical female lying in the gynecophoric groove of the male. The eggs, laid in the terminal branches of the mesenteric veins, passively work through the bowel wall to the lumen, and escape with the feces. The eggs evoke a granulomatous reaction that eventually prevents their egress and favors their carriage to other organs, with the consequent production of widely disseminated granulomas. The life histories of other schistosomes differ in detail from that of *H. americana.*

Schistosomiasis is second only to malaria as a scourge of mankind, especially in the Caribbean area, South America, Africa, and the Orient. Domestic animals in various tropical areas may be affected with *S. bovis* (cattle and sheep), *S. indicum* (horses, cattle, goats, and, in India, buffalo), *S. nasale* (cattle in India), *S. suis* (swine and dogs in India), and *S. mathiei* (sheep, southern Africa). In North America, schistosomes present only two small problems, *Heterobilharzia americana*, a parasite of Florida lynx that occasionally infects dogs, and "swimmer's itch," a dermatitis caused by cercariae of wild waterfowl schistosomes (*Trichobilharzia, Austrobilharzia, Bilharziella*) penetrating and abortively migrating in human skin. Of course, many cases of human schistosomiasis exist in North America among immigrants from endemic localities but human schistosomiasis is unlikely to become endemic because the snail intermediate hosts (*Biomphalaria, Tropicorbis, Oncomelania, Bulinus*) do not occur here.

Family Troglotrematidae

Identification. *The genital pore is immediately posterior to the ventral sucker;* the genital pore of other trematodes is located elsewhere. The location of the genital pore and the fact that the testes lie opposite one another are about all that unite the diverse assemblage of genera thrown together in the family Troglotrematidae. Troglotrematids are parasites of the lungs (*Paragonimus*, Fig. 4-12) or intestines (*Nanophyetus*, Fig. 4-13).

Life Histories. *Nanophyetus salmincola* adults parasitize the small intestine of piscivorous carnivorans of the Pacific Northwest. Eggs are undeveloped when passed in the

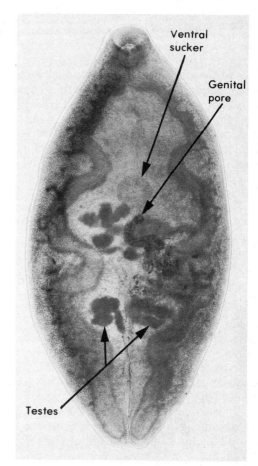

Figure 4–12. *Paragonimus kellicotti* (Troglotrematidae; x13).

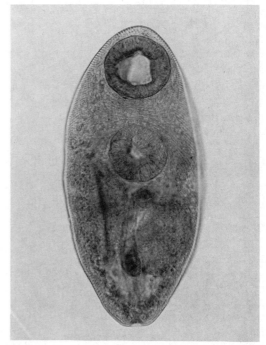

Figure 4–13. *Nanophyetus salmincola* (Troglotrematidae; X108).

host's feces. Miracidia require about three months to develop in eggs laid in water and hatch spontaneously still later. The miracidia penetrate the freshwater snail *Oxytrema silicula* in which cercariae develop in rediae. After emergence from the snail, these cercariae penetrate the skin of salmonid fishes and encyst in various tissues. The dog, cat, coyote, fox, bear, raccoon, or mink becomes infected by eating salmon or trout infected with metacercariae of this trematode. *N. salmincola* is host in turn to a rickettsial agent, *Neorickettsia helminthoeca*, the etiological agent of "salmon poisoning" in dogs. "Salmon poisoning" is characterized by hemorrhagic enteritis and lymph node enlargement, is diagnosed by the presence of trematode eggs in the patient's feces, and is usually fatal unless treated with broad spectrum antibiotics.

Paragonimus kellicotti occurs, usually in pairs, in pulmonary cysts. Cats, dogs, and many species of wild mammals may become infected by eating crayfish containing the encysted cercariae or by eating animals that have recently fed on crayfish. The large, vase-shaped eggs (see Fig. 12-17) are swept up the tracheobronchial tree, swallowed, and passed out with the feces. If the eggs arrive in water, miracidia develop and hatch in about two weeks and enter an operculate snail, *Pomatiopsis lapidaria*, in which cercariae develop through one sporocyst and two redial stages. The cercariae leave the snail and encyst as metacercariae in crayfish. Radiographically demonstrable cysts develop in the lungs of cats at 28 days, and eggs are first shed in the feces about a month after infection. Signs of respiratory disease may be associated with *P. kellicotti* infection.

Family Paramphistomatidae

Identification. *The ventral sucker is at the posterior end of the body;* the ventral sucker of other trematodes is either on the ventral surface of the body or absent (Fig. 4-14). Genera include *Paramphistomum* and *Cotylophoron* (rumen flukes), *Gastrodiscoides hominis* (a parasite of the intestine of man, monkey, and ape), and *Megalodiscus* spp. (parasites of the colon and cloaca of frogs).

Life Histories. Eggs of *Paramphistomum cervi* are undeveloped when passed in the feces of cattle, sheep, and goats. Miracidia develop in eggs deposited in water and hatch to invade snails of the genera *Physa*, *Bulinus*, *Galba*, and *Pseudosuccinea*, where cercariae develop through one sporocyst and two re-

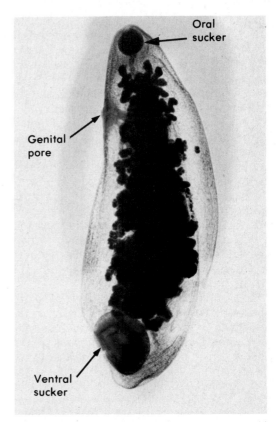

Figure 4–14. A "rumen fluke" of the family Paramphistomatidae (x16).

dial stages. Upon emergence from the snail, the cercaria swims away to encyst on aquatic vegetation. Thus, the extramammalian portion of the life history of *Paramphistomum* is very much like that of *Fasciola*. Metacercariae of *Paramphistomum* excyst in the small intestine and migrate back to the rumen. In so doing, they occasionally cause enteritis, especially when there are many of them; otherwise, rumen flukes are not at all pathogenic.

Instead of encysting on aquatic vegetation like other paramphistomatids, *Megalodiscus* cercariae encyst on the skin of frogs and tadpoles. The frogs become infected when they eat pieces of molted epidermis or tadpoles bearing metacercariae.

Family Diplostomatidae

Identification. *The body of these intestinal parasites of birds and mammals is divided into a flattened or spoon-shaped forebody containing oral and ventral suckers and a bulbous tribocytic organ, and a cylindrical hindbody containing the reproductive organs* (Fig. 4-15). Diplostomatids are most likely to be confused with members of the families Strigeidae, which have cup-

where it transforms into a metacercaria. In a few weeks, the metacercaria migrates up the trachea, is swallowed, and matures in the intestine. Eggs appear about 35 days after ingestion of mesocercariae (see Fig. 7-3).

Importance. Adult *Alaria* spp. are attached to the mucous membrane of the small intestine but apparently do their host little harm. However, because the mesocercariae migrate through the lungs and sometimes wander into other tissues, they may at times cause clinical illness. For example, a case of human infection with mesocercariae of *A. americana* terminated fatally as a result of extensive pulmonary hemorrhage. The circumstances suggested that the victim had eaten inadequately cooked frog's legs while hiking (Freeman *et al.*, 1976).

Family Heterophyidae

Identification. The ventral sucker and genital pore are withdrawn in a ventrogenital sac; one or more gonotyls (muscular suckers surrounding the genital pore) may be present (Fig. 4-16). *Metagonimus yokagawi* and *Heterophyes heterophyes*

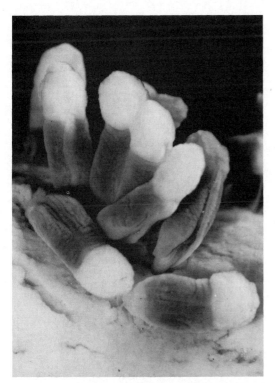

Figure 4–15. *Alaria* sp. (Diplostomatidae) attached to the mucosa of a dog's small intestine (x6.5).

shaped forebodies and leaflike tribocytic organs, and Cyathocotylidae, which have bulbous tribocytic organs but undivided bodies.

Life History of Alaria canis. The large, unembryonated egg (see Fig. 12-17A) is passed in the feces of the infected canid. If the egg is deposited in water, a miracidium develops and hatches in about two weeks to penetrate a snail of the genus *Helisoma* in which cercariae develop in daughter sporocysts. Each cercaria that succeeds in penetrating the skin of a tadpole transforms into a special larval stage called a *mesocercaria*, which is unique to the genus *Alaria*. If the tadpole is eaten by a frog, snake, or mouse, the mesocercariae take up residence and wait for their new host to fall prey to a dog or other suitable definitive host. The frog, snake, or mouse that harbors these metacercaria is called a *paratenic host* or *collector host*, which, by definition, is an intermediate host in which immature helminths may survive indefinitely but undergo no development. The paratenic host helps to distribute the parasite in space and time and often bridges the gap of food preferences or overcomes some other obstacle to the union of parasite and definitive host. When a dog eats a paratenic host, the mesocercaria migrates directly through the diaphragm to the lungs,

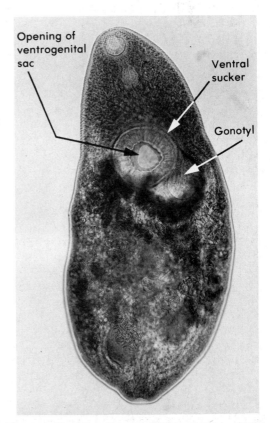

Figure 4–16. *Heterophyes* sp. (Heterophyidae; x8). This specimen was generously provided by Dr. John Pearson of the University of Queensland.

are parasites of cats, dogs, pigs, and human beings in the Orient; infection is acquired by eating insufficiently cooked fish in which metacercariae have encysted. *Cryptocotyle lingua*, a parasite of gulls and terns, produces severe enteritis in dogs, foxes, and minks a few days after eating a small North Atlantic fish, the cunner, in which metacercariae are found in the subcutaneous tissues surrounded by black host capsules. The appearance of infected fish leads to the colloquial name "black spot disease." A black host capsule is also observed surrounding various other species of trematode metacercariae and is not peculiar to *C. lingua*. Cercariae of *C. lingua* develop in the periwinkle *Littorina littorea*, a marine snail.

Family Dicrocoeliidae

Identification. *The body is translucent and the ovary is posterior to the testes of these parasites of the gall bladder and bile and pancreatic ducts of mammals, birds, and reptiles* (Figs. 4-17 and 4-18).

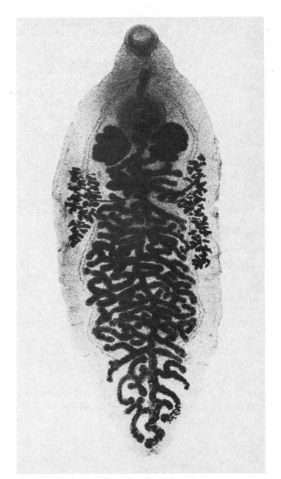

Figure 4–18. *Platynosomum fastosum* (Dicrocoeliidae; x24).

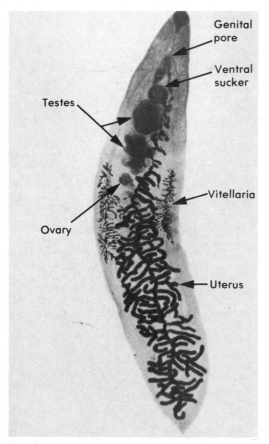

Figure 4–17. *Dicrocoelium dendriticum* (Dicrocoeliidae; x25).

Life History of Dicrocoelium dendriticum. Whereas most trematode life histories involve water, this species is adapted to a sequence of hosts that frequent dry habitats. Adult *D. dendriticum* are parasites of the bile ducts of sheep, cattle, pigs, deer, woodchuck, and cottontail rabbit. Embryonated eggs deposited in the host's droppings are ingested by the terrestrial snail *Cionella lubrica* in which long-tailed cercariae develop in daughter sporocysts. As the cercariae leave the sporocysts, the snail secretes mucus around masses of them to form so-called "slime balls" in which they are expelled from the snail. The slime balls are apparently esteemed as food by the ant *Formica fusca*, in which the cercariae encyst as metacercariae. The definitive host becomes infected by inadvertently ingesting infected ants while grazing; the metacercariae excyst in the small intestine and migrate up the common bile duct into the finer ramifications of the biliary tree.

Importance. Dicrocoelium dendriticum causes no clinical illness in cattle, lambs, or yearling sheep but these trematodes are long-lived and the pathological changes in the liver increase in severity and extent with the duration of the infection. Therefore, in older sheep, *D. dendriticum* infection causes progressive hepatic cirrhosis manifested clinically as cachexia, lowered wool production, decreased lactation, and premature aging. In short, *D. dendriticum* makes sheep husbandry unprofitable by curtailing the reproductive life of the ewe flock.

Platynosomum fastosum, a parasite of the bile and pancreatic ducts of cats, occurs in the southeastern United States and the Caribbean; infection is acquired by eating lizards containing metacercariae.

Family Opisthorchiidae

Identification. The uterus and ovary are anterior to the testes, there is no cirrus sac, and the genital pore is immediately anterior to the ventral sucker of these flat, translucent, fusiform or oval parasites of the bile and pancreatic ducts of mammals, birds, and reptiles (Figs. 4-9 and 4-19). Opisthorchiids might be confused with dicrocoeliids because they are similar in size, shape, and location in the host but, in dicrocoeliids, the ovary is posterior to the testes. Species include *Opisthorchis tenuicollis, O. felineus, Metorchis conjunctus, M. albidus, Parametorchis complexus, Clonorchis sinensis,* and others.

Life History of Opisthorchis tenuicollis. The adult trematodes are parasites of the bile and pancreatic ducts and small intestine of dog, cat, fox, pig, and man. Eggs containing miracidia when deposited in the host's feces are eaten by a snail *Bithynia tentaculata*, in which cercariae develop in rediae. The cercariae encyst as metacercariae in carp, bream, and roach. The definitive host becomes infected by eating these freshwater fish.

Importance. Opisthorchiids display a rather low order of host specificity and each species is capable of infecting many species of fish-eating mammals. Uncomplicated in-

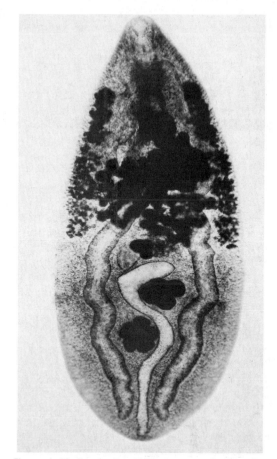

Figure 4–19. *Parametorchis* sp. (Opisthorchiidae; x50).

fection with moderate numbers of opisthorchiids is usually asymptomatic, but chronic infection with heavy worm burdens may lead to severe hepatic insufficiency.

REFERENCES

Freeman, R. S., Stuart, P. F., Cullen, J. B., Ritchie, A. C., Mildon, A., Fernandes, B. J., and Bonin, R. (1976): Fatal human infection with mesocercariae of the trematode *Alaria americana*. Am. J. Trop. Med. & Hyg., *25,* 803-807.

Isseroff, H., Sawma, J. T., and Reino, D. (1977): Fascioliasis: Role of proline in bile duct hyperplasia. Science, *198,* 1157-1159.

5

CESTODES

With few exceptions, adult cestodes (tapeworms) are parasites of the small intestine of vertebrates, and their larvae are parasites of either alternate vertebrates or invertebrates. In general, the definitive host becomes infected when it ingests an intermediate host containing metacestodes (immature tapeworms), and the intermediate host, in turn, becomes infected when it ingests tapeworm eggs discharged with the feces of the definitive host. Often, the relationship of the definitive host to the intermediate host is clearly that of predator to prey but, in certain cases involving small arthropods as intermediate hosts, these are ingested as incidental contaminants of the host's food or during self-grooming, as when a dog nips a flea that happens to be infected with cysticercoids of *Dipylidium caninum*. In a unique case, *Hymenolepis nana*, both larval and adult stages may develop and even coexist in the same mouse or man.

A recent treatise on cestode classification divides them into two main groups, the class Cotyloda, or pseudotapeworms, and the class Eucestoda, or true tapeworms (Wardle *et al.*, 1974). The class Cotyloda is represented by only one family of veterinary importance, Diphyllobothriidae, with two genera, *Diphyllobothrium* and *Spirometra*. The rest are all eucestodes. The diphyllobothriids are associated with aquatic food chains, whereas the eucestodes are associated with terrestrial food chains. It is helpful to keep this in mind when considering differences in the structure and life histories displayed by members of these two classes.

LIFE STAGES OF CESTODES

Adult Cestodes

A tapeworm is a chain (*strobila*) of progressively maturing, independent, reproductive units (*proglottids* or segments) that is anchored at one end in the wall of the host's intestine by a holdfast organ (*scolex*) (Fig. 5-1). When a metacestode is ingested, all parts except the scolex are discarded or digested away. The scolex, which has attained full development in the larval stage, attaches itself to the intestinal wall and begins to form segments by budding. At first, these segments display little in the way of internal structure but, as the chain lengthens, reproductive organs first appear, then mature, and finally "go to seed." Thus, in a fully developed tapeworm, all stages of development are displayed in a linear array starting at the scolex and terminating at the distal end. Although, from a reproductive viewpoint, a tapeworm appears to be a colony instead of an individual, all segments are served by common osmoregulatory and nervous systems, and the animal moves in a rhythmic and coordinated manner by means of the concerted activity of its two zones of muscle fibers. There are no organs of prehension or digestion; all nutrients are absorbed through the tapeworm's specialized integument.

THE SCOLEX

Compared with the rest of the mature worm, which may be several meters long, the scolex is minute, frequently measuring less than a millimeter. The eucestode scolex has four radially disposed muscular cups (*acetabulae* or *suckers*) that serve the functions of attachment and locomotion (Fig. 5-2). These suckers and the tissue immediately surrounding them are quite mobile. I have watched a severed scolex of *Taenia pisiformis* "walk" with remarkable agility across the bottom of a Petri dish. Each sucker in turn was advanced on a stalk of tissue and fixed to the bottom of the dish. Then the scolex was drawn toward the point of fixation by

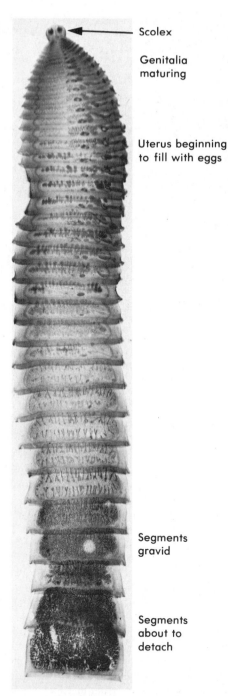

Scolex

Genitalia
maturing

Uterus beginning
to fill with eggs

Segments
gravid

Segments
about to
detach

Figure 5–1. *Paranoplocephala mamillana* (Anoplo-cephalidae), entire tapeworm (×3).

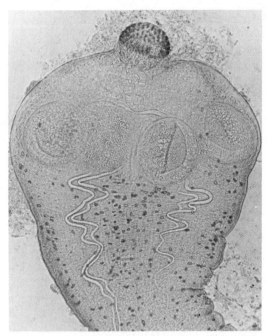

Figure 5–2. *Dipylidium caninum* (Dipylidiidae), scolex of fresh mount (x108). The scolex of *D. caninum* is less than 0.5 mm. in diameter; the rostellum is retractable and armed with small, thornlike hooks.

nonretractable rostellum is armed with two concentric rows of hooks (Fig. 5-3). Strong muscles operate these hooks in a concerted and rhythmic clawing motion; the points are projected in a manner similar to a cat baring its claws, but in a centrifugal direction. This clawing motion ceases once the scolex has found safe anchorage in the intestinal wall. Eucestode families that lack rostellar hooks (e.g., Anoplocephalidae, Mesocestidae) tend

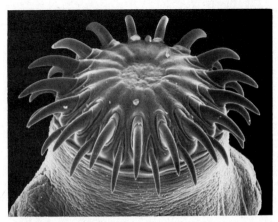

Figure 5–3. *Hydatigera taeniaeformis* (Taeniidae), scanning electron micrograph by Dr. Ronald Minor (x90). The rostellum of taeniid tapeworms is nonretractable and is armed with a row of long hooks and a concentric row of short hooks.

contraction of the stalk of tissue, another sucker advanced, and so on. At the apex of the scolex of many eucestodes there is a dome-shaped projection, the *rostellum*. The rostellum is sometimes retractable into the scolex and, if so, may be armed with small hooks (Fig. 5-2). In the family Taeniidae, a

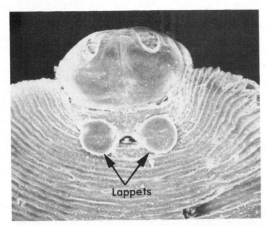

Figure 5-4. *Anoplocephala perfoliata* (Anoplocephalidae), scanning electron micrograph (x18). The scolex of *A. perfoliata* is about 2 mm. in diameter and has four large suckers and four projections called *lappets*.

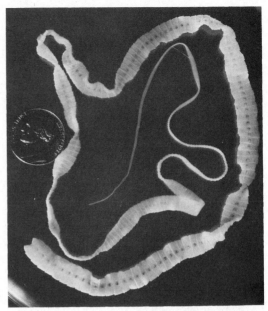

Figure 5-6. *Spirometra mansonoides* (Diphyllobothriidae), entire specimen from a cat. Notice how small the scolex is relative to the mature segments and also the central location of the genitalia throughout the length of the tapeworm.

to have more strongly developed suckers (Fig. 5-4).

The scolex of diphyllobothriids has only two shallow longitudinal grooves (*bothria*) for locomotion and attachment (Fig. 5-5). The two most important genera, *Diphyllobothrium* and *Spirometra*, have no hooks to assist the weak grip of their bothria. The considerable area of contact that exists between the long chain of broad segments and the intestinal mucosa apparently affords sufficient traction to maintain the tapeworm in place (Fig. 5-6).

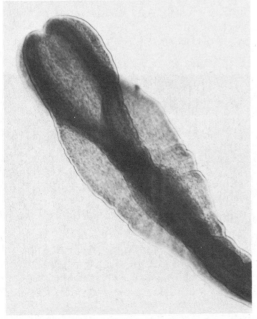

Figure 5-5. *Diphyllobothrium latum* (Diphyllobothriidae), scolex of stained, permanent mount (x50).

THE STROBILA

The body of a tapeworm is so flattened that for descriptive purposes it can be said to have two surfaces and two edges. This shape affords maximum surface area per unit volume, a distinct asset for an animal that absorbs all of its nourishment through its skin.

The anatomical details and nomenclature of the genitalia are presented in Figure 5-7. These are important in detailed taxonomic work but need not be emphasized here because a reliable identification can usually be made on the basis of host identity and somewhat more accessible morphological features as outlined below. However, differences do exist between eucestodes and diphyllobothriids that are important in diagnosis and in understanding their particular life histories.

Segments of the eucestode strobila have genital pores for fertilization but no opening to allow the eggs to escape, so that the eggs accumulate until the segment becomes packed full like a ripe seed pod. As they reach the end of the chain, these gravid segments are detached and pass out with the feces or crawl out the anus onto the perianal skin. Diphyllobothriid segments have a uterine pore that permits the escape of eggs. Segments over a considerable length of the

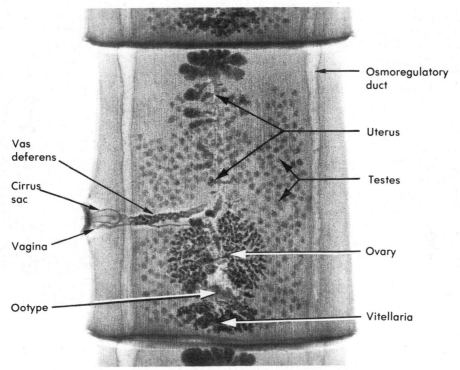

Figure 5–7. Mature *Taenia* segment (x22).

strobila discharge their eggs until their supply is exhausted. The terminal segments of diphyllobothriid tapeworms become senile rather than gravid and are usually detached in chains instead of individually. Thus, eucestode infections are usually diagnosed by identifying gravid segments on the host or in its environment, whereas diagnosis of diphyllobothriid infections depends on distinguishing the operculate eggs in fecal sediments from those of trematodes, sometimes not an easy matter (Fig. 12-15).

CESTODE EGGS

Eggs of eucestodes contain fully developed *oncospheres* (*hexacanth embryos*) when they are passed and are immediately infective for the intermediate host (Figs. 5-8, 5-9, 5-10). Diphyllobothriid eggs resemble those of trematodes in having an operculum at one pole of the shell (Fig. 5-11). The ciliated larva (*coracidium*) that develops within these eggs after they have been deposited in water is also reminiscent of the trematode miracidium (Fig. 5-12).

Cestode eggs are all of the same basic pattern but certain structures display special adaptations. At the center of a fully developed cestode egg is the *oncosphere* or *hexacanth*

embryo, the larval stage that is infective for the intermediate host. The oncosphere is immediately surrounded by an *embryophore*. In diphyllobothriids the embryophore is ciliated and propels the oncosphere in water. In anoplocephalids the embryophore is a distinctive pear-shaped body (*pyriform apparatus*), and in taeniids, it consists of a shell

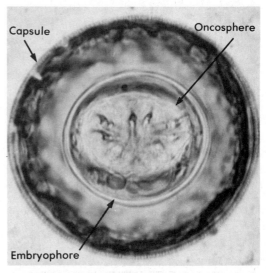

Figure 5–8. Egg of *Hymenolepis diminuta* (Hymenolepidae: Eucestoda) (x900).

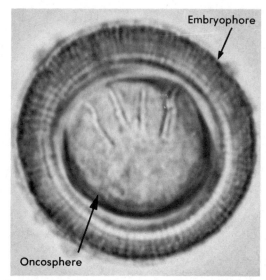

Figure 5–9. Egg of *Hydatigera taeniaeformis* (Taeniidae: Eucestoda) (x2000). The capsule of taeniid eggs is fragile; eggs in fecal smears have usually lost their capsules.

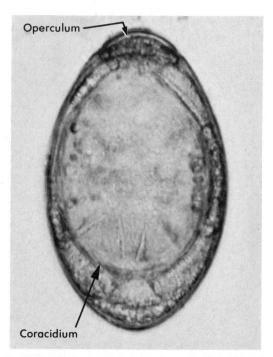

Figure 5–11. Egg of *Spirometra mansonoides* (Diphyllobothriidae: Cotyloda) (x1300). The capsule of diphyllobothriid eggs is operculate; this one contains a fully developed coracidium.

of prismatic blocks. The *capsule* is the outermost covering and is elliptical and operculate in diphyllobothriids, irregularly pyramidal and thick-walled in anoplocephalids, subspherical in hymenolepids, and delicate in taeniids. In fecal preparations, taeniid eggs have usually lost their capsules. The eggs of *Dipylidium* are clustered in packets formed by outpocketings of the uterine wall (see Fig. 12-14).

METACESTODES

Ther term *metacestode* is applied collectively to all cestode stages that parasitize the intermediate host. The oncosphere becomes a

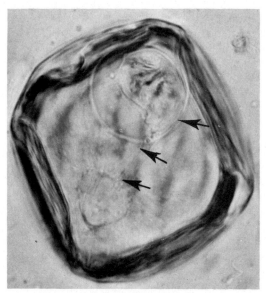

Figure 5–10. Egg of *Moniezia* sp. (Anoplocephalidae: Eucestoda) (x1100). The pear-shaped embryophore (arrows) is typical of anoplocephalid eggs.

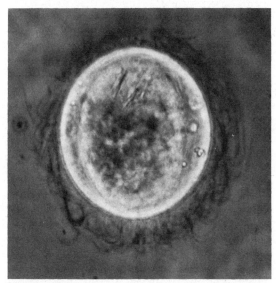

Figure 5–12. Coracidium of *Spirometra mansonoides*, phase contrast electronic flash photomicrograph of the free-swimming organism (x1200); culture provided by Dr. Justus Mueller.

metacestode when it emerges from its embryophore in the lumen and bores into the wall of the intestine. The objective of metacestodal development is to form a scolex and place it where it is likely to be ingested by the proper definitive host. Because this objective has been achieved by adaptation to such diverse hosts as mites and cattle, there is considerably more variety in size and form among the larval cestodes than among the adults. Because it is at this point that uniformity of structure and function gives way to diversity, details of metacestodal development are discussed in connection with the life histories typical of families of cestodes as follows.

FAMILIES OF CESTODES

FAMILY TAENIIDAE

Identification. Adult tapeworms of the genera *Taenia, Multiceps,* and *Hydatigera* measure 10's to 100's of centimeters in length, depending on the species and maturity. The scolex has four suckers and a non-

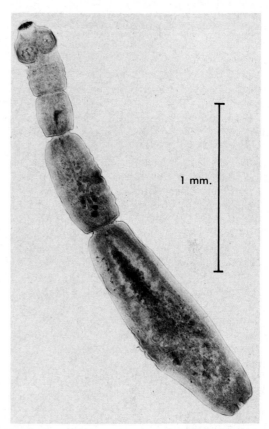

Figure 5–14. *Echinococcus granulosus* (Taeniidae), entire worm (x44).

retractable rostellum armed with two rows of hooks (Fig. 5-13). The segments are more or less rectangular with unilateral genital pores alternating irregularly from one side to the other along the strobila (see Fig. 5-7). The eggs in gravid segments are typical of the family (Fig. 5-9). Differentiation of genera and species is based on number and sizes of rostellar hooks and on morphology of mature segments; this may require the services of an expert (Verster, 1969).

Echinococcus granulosus and *Echinococcus multilocularis* are very small (2 to 8 mm.) and have only four or five segments of which only the terminal segment is gravid (Fig. 5-14). In *E. granulosus,* 45 to 65 testes are generally distributed and the genital pore is located at or posterior to the middle of the segment. In *E. multilocularis,* 17 to 26 testes are found posterior to the genital pore, which is located anterior to the middle of the segment. CAUTION: Human hydatid infection may be acquired by ingesting the eggs of *Echinococcus* spp.; wear gloves and wash carefully.

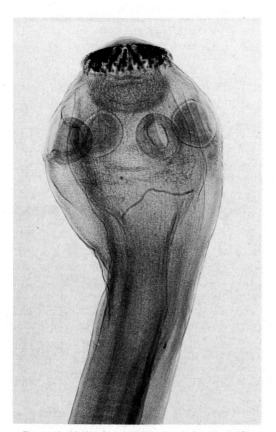

Figure 5–13. Scolex and "neck" of *Taenia* (x40).

Life History. The egg containing the infective taeniid oncosphere is shed in the feces of the carnivorous definitive host. If ingested by a suitable vertebrate intermediate host, usually a species normally taken as prey by the definitive host, the oncosphere hatches, enters the wall of the intestine, and migrates to its organ of predilection, usually the liver and peritoneal membranes or the skeletal and cardiac muscles. Here the oncosphere grows, cavitates, and differentiates into a metacestode that will develop into one or more adult tapeworms when the predator eats its prey. The fully developed metacestode of the family Taeniidae consists of a fluid-filled bladder with one or more scolices and is surrounded by a connective tissue capsule formed by the vertebrate intermediate host. Until the middle of the nineteenth century, the relationship of these bladders to tapeworms was not recognized and they were described and named as distinct species. For example, *Cysticercus cellulosae* was placed in the now defunct phylum Cystica, whereas its parent, *Taenia solium*, was referred to the phylum Vermes. Curiously, this double set of binomial nomenclature is still in use even though the life history of *Cysticercus cellulosae* was elucidated over a century ago. Some corresponding larval and adult names are listed in Table 5-1.

Four basic types of taeniid metacestodes exist: the cysticercus, strobilocercus, coenurus, and hydatid. A *cysticercus* (Fig. 5-15; see

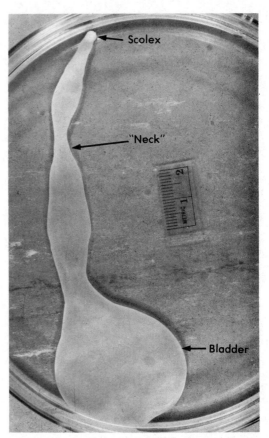

Figure 5–15. Cysticercus of *Taenia hydatigera* (Taeniidae). The bladder of this particular species has an attenuated "neck" region; hence the larval name *Cysticercus tenuicollis.*

Figs. 14-46 and 14-47) consists of a single bladder with one scolex and belongs to the genus *Taenia*. A *strobilocercus* (see Fig. 14-50) is a cysticercus that has already begun to elongate and segment while still in the intermediate host and belongs to the genus *Hydatigera*. A *coenurus* (Fig. 5-16; see Fig. 14-48) consists of a single bladder with many scolices, each with the potential of developing into a mature tapeworm. Coenuri belong to the genus *Multiceps*. Exceptions occur that mar the relationship of metacestode type to genus. For example, although one *Taenia* oncosphere ordinarily develops into only one cysticercus, in some species (e.g., *Taenia crassiceps*) replication by budding leads to the formation of many cysticerci, all contained within a single host cyst (see Fig. 14-49). Such a structure may easily be mistaken for a hydatid cyst by an unwary observer. Many bladders, especially coenuri, branch and ramify extensively, thus giving rise to very complex structures (Fig. 5-17), and teratological malformations, common in taeniid met-

Table 5–1 NAMES OF SOME ADULT AND LARVAL TAENIIDS AND THEIR HOSTS

Adult	Larva
Taenia pisiformis dog	*Cysticercus pisiformis* rabbit
Taenia hydatigera dog	*Cysticercus tenuicollis* sheep, cattle, swine
Taenia krabbei dog, wolf	*Cysticercus tarandi* reindeer
Taenia solium man	*Cysticercus cellulosae* swine, man
Taenia ovis dog	*Cysticercus ovis* sheep
Taeniarhynchus saginatus man	*Cyticercus bovis* cattle
Hydatigera taeniaeformis cat	*Cyticercus fasciolaris* rodents
Multiceps multiceps dog	*Coenurus cerebralis* sheep
Multiceps serialis dog	*Coenurus serialis* rabbit
Echniococcus granulosus dog, wolf	Hydatid cyst sheep, mam others
Echinococcus multilocularis dog, cat, fox	Alveolar hydatid vole, man, others

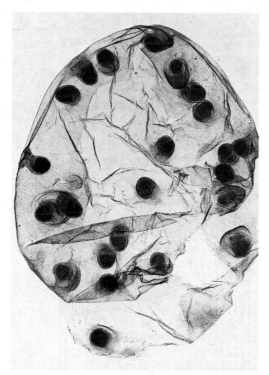

Figure 5–16. A coenurus (x2). Notice the many scolices attached to a rather thin-walled bladder.

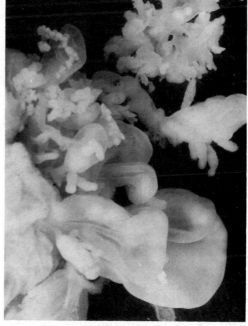

Figure 5–17. A coenurus from the subcutaneous and intermuscular connective tissues of a cottontail rabbit (*Sylvilagus floridanus*) (x2). This bladder displays marked budding and ramification in growth.

acestodes, result in diverse and complex structures that do not conform to any rational classification scheme. Perhaps for these reasons, some very good taxonomists (e.g., Verster,. 1969) lump *Taenia, Multiceps,* and *Hydatigera* together in one rather large genus, *Taenia.* Hydatids belong to the genus *Echinococcus* and are of two kinds, *hydatid cysts* and *alveolar hydatids.*

Hydatid cysts are metacestodes of *Echinococcus granulosus* (Fig. 5-18). Fertile hydatids may grow as large as a man's head. Starting as an oncosphere less than 30 μm in diameter, the metacestode grows very slowly and infrequently exceeds more than a few centimeters in diameter in slaughter animals. The hydatid membrane is surrounded by, but usually not attached to, an inflammatory connective tissue capsule. The space between the host and the parasite generally contains a small volume of clear, colorless or light yellow liquid. Brood capsules, each containing many scolices, develop from the germinal epithelium lining the laminated hydatid membrane (see Fig. 14-51). Some of these rupture, releasing scolices to form a sediment of "hydatid sand" in the hydatid fluid (Fig. 5-19). Endogenous daughter cysts may be found free in the fluid-filled cyst cavity or

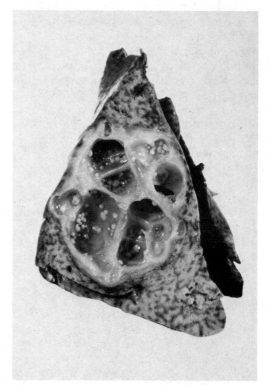

Figure 5–18. A hydatid cyst (*Echinococcus granulosus*) in the liver of a horse (about natural size). This horse displayed no clinical signs of hepatic involvement in spite of the presence of 20 to 30 cysts like the one illustrated.

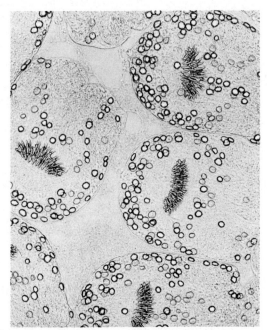

Figure 5–19. "Hydatid sand," i.e., invaginated scolices of *Echinococcus granulosus* found free in the hydatid fluid (x130). This material was recovered from the hydatid cyst of Figure 5–18.

attached to the germinal epithelium. Exogenous daughter cysts are relatively unusual; they may be found in the pericystic space between the hydatid membrane and the host connective tissue capsule. Sterile hydatids lack brood capsules, scolices, and daughter cysts; their identification in cattle and swine is necessarily somewhat presumptive.

Alveolar hydatids are metacestodes of *Echinococcus multilocularis,* a parasite of the dog, fox, and cat (see Figs. 14-45 and 14-52). Alveolar hydatids develop in voles, lemmings, cattle, horses, swine, and man. They are characterized by exogenous budding that does not remain contained within the reactive connective tissue capsule but continuously proliferates and infiltrates surrounding tissue like a malignant neoplasm. Alveolar hydatid infection proves fatal in a few years.

Hydatid Disease

Echinococcus granulosus is a parasite of the dog, wolf, and dingo. Its larva is a hydatid cyst in sheep, swine, cattle, man, moose, caribou, kangaroos, and others. Species vary in their suitability as intermediate hosts; hydatid cysts found in sheep are usually fertile, whereas those in cattle are usually sterile. Subspecies of *E. granulosus* differ in their preferences for intermediate hosts. For ex-

ample, *E. granulosus granulosus* hydatids belong to the subspecies adapted to sheep and man, whereas *E. g. equinus* is the subspecies found in horses, asses, and mules. The hydatid membrane may bud off daughter cysts either internally or externally and the whole structure occupies progressively more space as it grows, but hydatid cysts do not infiltrate, in contrast to alveolar hydatids. Pathogenic effects of hydatid cysts include pressure atrophy of surrounding organs and allergic reactions to hydatid fluid leaks. Rupture of a fertile hydatid cyst may scatter bits of germinative membrane, scolices, and brood capsules throughout the pleural or peritoneal cavity and result in multiple hydatidosis. Pulmonary hydatid cysts may rupture into a bronchus, the contents may be coughed up, and the lesion healed. Hydatid cysts that remain intact eventually die and degenerate, but the course is protracted.

Echinococcus granulosus is endemic in North and South America, England, Africa, the Middle East, Australia, and New Zealand. *Echinococcus multilocularis* is endemic in North Central Europe, Alaska, Canada, and central United States as far south as Illinois and Nebraska (Ballard and Vande Vusse, 1983)

Both *E. granulosus* and *E. multilocularis* tend to establish sylvatic cycles when suitable predator-prey relationships exist in the wildlife population of a region. Thus, *Echinococcus granulosus* cycles are maintained among wild ruminants and wolves in the Canadian North Woods and among wallabies and dingoes in Australia, and natural nidi of *E. multilocularis* are maintained in various rodents and foxes. The sylvatic cycle reaches man through his domesticated animals. Dogs that scavenge the entrails of wild game infected with *Echinococcus* become direct sources of hydatid infection to man and his domestic animals. Contamination of pastures with the feces of infected wild carnivorans also results in hydatid infection of domestic ruminants and swine. The establishment of a pastoral cycle may then result from the feeding of uncooked offal from these domestic animals to dogs and, in the case of *Echinococcus multilocularis,* to cats (Fig. 5-20).

The direct source of human infection is, in most instances, the domestic dog or cat, and scrupulous hygiene is the first line of defense. Periodic anthelmintic medication of dogs or cats, depending on the species of tapeworm involved, carries the threat one step further away. In the case of a well-established sylvatic cycle, this is about as far as it is practicable to go. *Echinococcus* infection

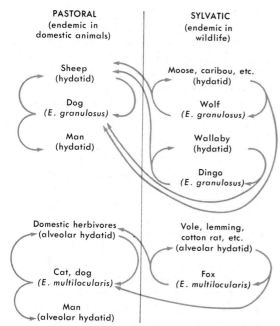

Figure 5–20. Pastoral and sylvatic cycles of *Echinococcus granulosus* and *E. multilocularis*.

may be reduced to insignificant incidence in cases where it is limited to a pastoral cycle and thus exposed to manipulation by man. Destruction of all stray dogs, regimented anthelmintic medication of the rest, and prohibition on the feeding of uncooked offal to dogs and cats are mandatory.

A campaign against hydatid disease has been in effect in Iceland since 1864. At the outset, about one out of six or seven people and virtually all aged slaughter sheep and cattle harbored hydatid cysts, and about one fourth of the dogs were infected with the adult worm. By 1900, the human infection rate had fallen dramatically and has now almost reached the point of extinction. The campaign, devised by Dr. Harald Krabbe of the Royal Veterinary and Agricultural University of Copenhagen, consisted of alerting the public to the need to observe strict hygiene in dealing with dogs, destroying all cysts and infected offal, and mandatory anthelmintic medication of all dogs (Palsson, 1976). Thus, salutary results in *Echinococcus* control can be achieved in a century or so, provided there is no sylvatic cycle to complicate the issue. In Australia, for example, a sylvatic cycle involving kangaroos and *Canis dingo* would have to be considered in any eradication attempt. "Obviously the denial of sheep offal to domestic dogs will not eliminate infection if dogs have access to macropods in dingo infested areas" (Herd

and Coman, 1975). In the United States, *E. granulosus* appears to be most prevalent in sheep-raising areas of Utah (Loveless *et al.*, 1978), and California. In California, the spread of echinococcosis appears to be related to a quaint transhumant form of husbandry in which bands of sheep migrate from place to place under the control of contract Basque shepherds from Spain and France. These shepherds, for the most part, are ignorant of the epidemiology of hydatid disease and feed their dogs mostly on dead sheep (Araujo *et al.*, 1975). Cysticercosis and coenurosis are discussed in Chapter 8.

The metacestodes of all of the following eucestode families are *cysticercoids* of one kind or another; the Mesocestidae have an additional metacestode called a *tetrathyridium*. A cysticercoid may be thought of as a cysticercus that is small enough to fit into the body of an arthropod; it is small and solid rather than cavitated, but has an inverted scolex.

FAMILY ANOPLOCEPHALIDAE

Identification. *Moniezia* spp. have unarmed scolices with four large suckers and very wide segments with bilateral genitalia; they are found in the small intestine of cattle, sheep, and goats. Interproglottidal glands at the posterior margin of each segment extend the full width of *M. expansa* but occupy only the midzone of the *M. benedeni* segment (Fig. 5-21).

Thysanosoma actinoides and *Wyominia tetoni* are found in the bile ducts and small intestine of mountain sheep and goats. *T. actinoides* has wide segments with bilateral genitalia and a *fringe* of outgrowths at the posterior border of each segment. *Wyominia tetoni* resembles *T. actinoides* but segments are not fringed.

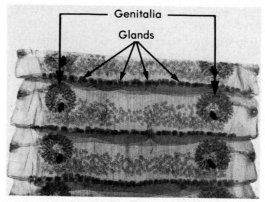

Figure 5–21. Mature segments of *Moniezia expansa* (Anoplocephalidae) (x5).

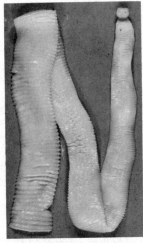
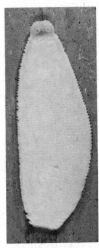

Anoplocephala magna   A. perfoliata

Figure 5–22. *Anoplocephala magna* (3/8 natural size) and *A. perfoliata* (3/4 natural size).

Thysaniezia, Stilesia, and *Avitellina* are exotic anoplocephalids of ruminants.

Anoplocephala magna (Fig. 5-22) and *Paranoplocephala mammilana* (Fig. 5-1) are relatively harmless parasites of the small intestine of horses. *Anoplocephala perfoliata* (Figs. 5-4 and 5-22) is found mainly in the cecum but tends also to cluster in the ileum near the ileocecal valve, where it is associated with ulceration and reactive inflammation of the ileal wall.

Life History. Free-living oribatid mites serve as hosts for cysticercoids of the family Anoplocephalidae, which includes all of the adult tapeworms of horses, cattle, sheep, and goats. The definitive host inadvertently ingests the infected mites while grazing.

FAMILY DIPYLIDIIDAE

Identification. *Dipylidium caninum, Diplopylidium,* and *Joyeuxiella.* The scolex has four suckers and a retractable rostellum armed with several circles of thornlike hooks (Fig. 5-2). Segments are shaped like cucumber seeds and have bilateral genital pores (see Fig. 12-12). The genital apertures of *Dipylidium caninum* lie slightly behind (i.e., away from the scolex) the middle of the segment and each egg capsule may contain from 5 to 30 eggs (see Fig. 12-14). The genital apertures of the Middle Eastern, African, and Australasian parasites *Diplopylidium* and *Joyeuxiella* lie before (i.e., toward the scolex) the middle of the segment and each capsule contains a single egg.

Life History. Cysticercoids of *Dipylidium*

caninum develop in fleas (*Ctenocephalides* spp.) and biting lice (*Trichodectes canis*), and the dog acquires this tapeworm while nipping its insects. Children may also become infected in this way. Cysticercoids of *Diplopylidium* and *Joyeuxiella* develop in coprophagous beetles; reptiles and small mammals serve as second intermediate hosts.

FAMILY HYMENOLEPIDAE

The family Hymenolepidae contains many species that occur in birds and two mammalian parasites. *Hymenolepis diminuta* adults are found in the small intestine of rodents, dogs, and man; the metacestode is a cysticercoid in fleas, flour beetles, fleas, and other insects (Fig. 5-23). *Hymenolepis nana* is also a parasite of rodents and man and its metacestode is a cysticercoid in fleas and flour beetles or in the intestinal mucosa of its definitive host. *Hymenolepis nana* is able to complete its life history within the intestinal tract of a mouse or a man. Some of the eggs hatch within the intestine and burrow into the mucous membrane to form cysticercoids that later re-enter the lumen to complete their development as mature tapeworms. The rest of the eggs pass out with the feces to await ingestion by flour beetles or fleas, in which the cysticercoids develop. Thus, the life history of *H. diminuta* requires fleas, flour beetles, or other insects as intermediate hosts, whereas that of *H. nana* does not. Because the eggs discharged in feces are infective to man, *H. nana* infection in laboratory rodent stocks constitutes something of a health hazard to personnel. Be-

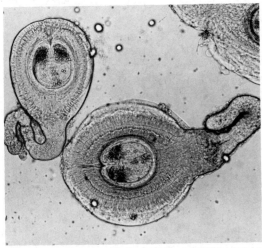

Figure 5–23. Cysticercoids of *Hymenolepis diminuta* (x90).

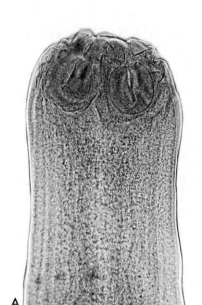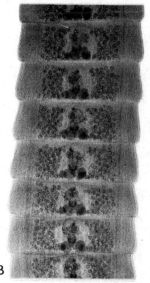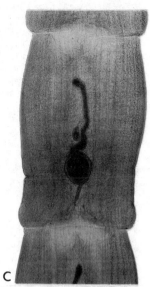

Figure 5–24. *Mesocestoides* sp. A. Scolex (x108). B. Mature segments (x16). C. Gravid segments (x16).

cause *H. diminuta* infection requires ingestion of an infected insect, human infection with this tapeworm is less probable but nevertheless occurs. Hymenolepids have three testes and a single ovary; *H. nana* has a single circle of hooks on its scolex, whereas *H. diminuta* has no hooks.

FAMILY MESOCESTIDAE

Identification. The scolex of *Mesocestoides* has four suckers but no hooks; mature segments have a mediodorsal genital pore and eggs accumulate in a special, thick-walled parauterine organ as the segments mature (Fig. 5-24). Gravid segments detach from the strobila and carry their relatively small burden of oncospheres to the outside world.

Life History. The complete life history of *Mesocestoides* has yet to be worked out. The metacestode infective for the definitive host is called a *tetrathyridium,* and is found in the peritoneal cavity of mammals and reptiles and in the lungs of birds. A "cysticercoidlike" larval stage is hypothesized to precede the tetrathyridium, possibly developing from the oncosphere in a coprophilic insect.

FAMILY DIPHYLLOBOTHRIIDAE

Identification. The scolex of *Diphyllobothrium latum* and *Spirometra mansonoides* has two slitlike grooves (Fig. 5-5). Mature segments are broader than long (Figs. 5-6 and 5-25). The uterus consists of a spiral tube with four to eight loops on each side and opens to the

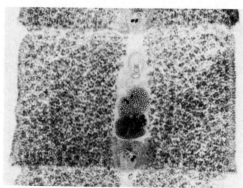

Figure 5–25. Mature segment of *Diphyllobothrium latum* (x60).

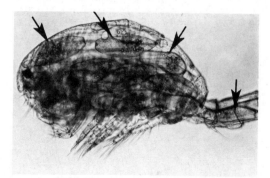

Figure 5–26. Copepod (*Cyclops vernalis*) with body cavity filled with procercoids of *Spirometra mansonoides;* electronic flash photomicrograph of living organisms (x70).

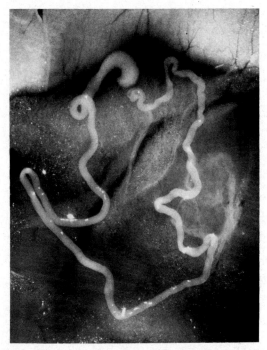

Figure 5–27. *Spirometra mansonoides* plerocercoid larva in the subcutaneous tissues of a white mouse. Photograph by Dr. Robert Smith (about twice natural size); culture provided by Dr. Justus Mueller.

outside through a midventral uterine pore behind the genital pore. The reproductive organs are concentrated at the centers of the segments (Fig. 5-25). Operculated eggs (see Fig. 12-15) are discharged through the uterine pore.

Life History. Whereas eucestode metacestodal development involves only one intermediate host, diphyllobothriids require at least two, of which the first is a crustacean and the second is usually also aquatic or at least amphibious. The coracidium (oncosphere with ciliated embryophore), when in-gested by copepods of the genera *Cyclops* and *Diaptomus,* develops into a solid wormlike *procercoid* within the body cavity of these crustaceans (Fig. 5-26). When the infected copepod is ingested by a fish, the procercoid enters its musculature and develops into a *plerocercoid* (Fig. 5-27). A most remarkable feature of diphyllobothriid life histories is the ability of this plerocercoid to parasitize a series of predatory paratenic hosts until one is found that is suitable for development into the adult stage. Thus, when a pike eats an infected minnow, the plerocercoids merely invade the muscles of the pike, but when a man, a dog, or a cat eats the pike, the plerocercoid matures into an adult tapeworm.

REFERENCES

Araujo, F. P., Schwabe, C. W., Sawyer, J. C., and Davis, W. G. (1975): Hydatid disease transmission in California; a study of the Basque connection. Am. J. Epidemiology, *102,* 291-302.

Ballard, N. B., and Vande Vusse, F. J. (1983): *Echinococcus multilocularis* in Illinois and Nebraska. J. Parasitol., *69,* 790-791.

Herd, R. P., and Coman, B. J. (1975): Transmission of *Echinococcus granulosus granulosus* from kangaroos to domestic dogs. Australian Vet. J., *51,* 591.

Loveless, R. M., Anderson, F. L., Ramsay, M. J., and Hedelius, R. K. (1978): *Echinococcus granulosus* in dogs and sheep in central Utah, 1971-1976. Am. J. Vet. Res., *39,* 499-502.

Palsson, P. A. (1976): Echinococcosis and its elimination in Iceland. Hist. Med. Vet. *1,* 4-10.

Verster, A. (1969): A taxonomic revision of the genus *Taenia* Linnaeus, 1758. Onderstepoort J. Vet. Res., *36,* 3-58.

Wardle, R. A., and McLeod, J. A. (1952): The Zoology of Tapeworms. Minneapolis, University of Minnesota Press.

Wardle, R. A., McLeod, J. A., and Radinovsky, S. (1974): Advances in the Zoology of Tapeworms. Minneapolis, University of Minnesota Press.

6

NEMATODES

MORPHOLOGY

Body form is remarkably constant among nematodes, a fact that may simplify the anatomy lesson but somewhat aggravates the difficulties of identification and taxonomic classification. It is helpful in understanding nematode anatomy and physiology to appreciate the significance of their unique high turgor pressure method of maintaining sufficient corporeal rigidity to permit rapid locomotion by sinusoidal undulation. Crofton (1966) brilliantly expounded these relationships in his book *Nematodes,* and the following represents a summary of his exposition.

Nematodes have a relatively large body cavity (*pseudocoelom*) containing fluid under pressure that varies up to one-half atmosphere above that of the surrounding medium. The body cuticle contains inelastic fibers so arranged that an increase in internal pressure causes an increase in length but minimal change in diameter. This *anisometric* cuticle and high internal pressure thus maintain a relatively constant body diameter. Nematodes do not have a circular muscle layer; all of the somatic musculature is oriented longitudinally and divided into dorsal and ventral fields by lateral expansions of the hypodermis, the *lateral chords.* A muscle cell of either field is connected by a cytoplasmic process to its respective (dorsal or ventral) median nerve. Thus, dorsal and ventral flexion of the body are made possible by independent contraction of the corresponding muscle field, and longitudinal waves of contraction result in the sinusoidal pattern that is characteristic of nematode locomotion.

The high internal pressure also exerts its influence on the structure and organization of the internal organs. In order to fill the lumen of the intestine with food, some sort of pump is essential to overcome the tendency of the pseudocoelomic fluid pressure to collapse it, and most nematodes have a well-developed muscular esophagus for this purpose. Defecation, on the other hand, is accomplished by the contraction of a *dilator ani* muscle (there is no sphincter) that opens the end of the digestive tube and allows it to empty.

The basic *excretory system* consists of paired unicellular glands with a common midventral excretory pore in the neck region and ducts that, in some forms, run nearly the full length of the body in the substance of the lateral chords.

Male nematodes are smaller than the females of their species. Their caudal ends may terminate in a cuticular expansion supported by muscular rays. This so-called *copulatory bursa* reaches its highest development among the strongylids and is used to grasp the female (Fig. 6-1). The *copulatory spicules,* used to dilate the vulva of the female, are cuticular structures that develop by sclerotization of folds of the dorsal wall of the cloaca. Spicules are often paired, but some species have only one (e.g., *Trichuris*) or none (e.g., *Aspiculuris*); they vary greatly in size and shape among species and are often used as diag-

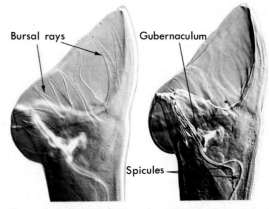

Figure 6–1. Surficial (left) and sagittal (right) aspects of the copulatory bursa of *Cyathostomum labiatum,* a typical member of the order Strongylida (x64).

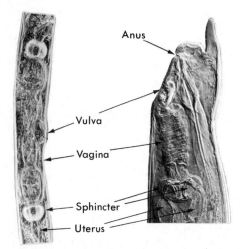

Figure 6-2. Ovijectors of a representative of the superfamily Trichostrongyloidea (left) and of the superfamily Strongyloidea (right) (x64).

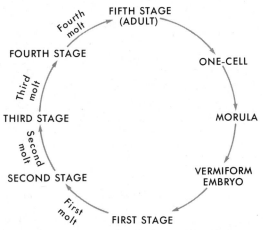

Figure 6–3. Stages and transitions in the ontogenetic development of a nematode.

nostic characters. In many species, accessory sclerotizations of the cloacal wall serve as guides for the spicules; a spicule guide in the dorsal wall is called a *gubernaculum,* and one located in the ventral wall is called a *telamon.* The primary male reproductive organs consist of a single convoluted tube with regions structurally and functionally differentiated as *testis, seminal vesicle,* and *vas deferens.* The terminal portion of the vas deferens with its strong muscular coat is called the *ejaculatory duct;* this empties into the *cloaca.*

The female reproductive system is also tubular and usually has two branches (i.e., *didelphic*) but may be *monodelphic* or even *multidelphic.* Regions structurally and functionally differentiated as *ovary, oviduct, uterus,* and *vagina* communicate through the *vulva* with the exterior. The vulva is ventral in position and may be located near the oral end (*opisthodelphic*), caudal end (*prodelphic*), or close to the middle of the body (*amphidelphic*); the location and special anatomical features of the vulva are useful in identification (Fig. 6-2). In female strongylids, a muscular ovijector regulates the discharge of eggs from the uterus. The eggs contained in the terminal portion of the uterus are valuable aids in identifying nematodes. See Chapter 12 for illustrations of nematode eggs.

LIFE HISTORIES

All rational control efforts are based upon an understanding of the life history and behavior of both host and parasite. A general outline of the ontogenetic development of a nematode is portrayed in Figure 6-3. What

appears to be a rich and confusing diversity of life histories among various orders of nematodes can all be related and rationalized according to this basic pattern. Embryonic development is, of course, a continuous process with change accompanying every cell division. The stages "one-cell," "morula," and "vermiform embryo" are arbitrarily chosen from this continuum because they are stages of egg development most frequently encountered in diagnostic procedures. The difference between a vermiform embryo and a first stage larva is that the former contains only cell clusters as organ primordia, whereas the latter displays clearly recogniz-

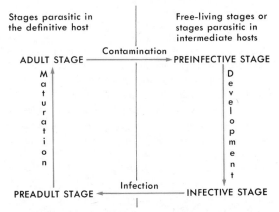

Figure 6–4. A generalization of nematode life histories emphasizing the stages and transitions of greatest importance to diagnosis, treatment, and control. As employed here, the term PREADULT STAGE refers to all stages of parasitic larval development from entry of the parasite into the host to the attainment of sexual maturity. *Maturation* represents the length of time required for this transition. Similarly, PREINFECTIVE STAGE represents all developmental stages leading up to the infective stage and *Development* represents the time required for that transition.

able organs such as esophagus, intestine, and excretory glands. A microfilaria is an example of a vermiform embryo; it develops into a larva only after it has been ingested by a mosquito. Each stage is separated from the next by a molt marked by metamorphosis of the larva and *ecdysis* or casting off the cuticle of the preceding stage.

The nematode life history can also be generalized from the standpoint of the important events related to diagnosis. treatment, and control. Figure 6-4 represents these events as four stages (ADULT, PREINFECTIVE, INFECTIVE, PREADULT) separated by four transitions (*Contamination, Development, Infection, Maturation*). In mastering the details of any particular nematode life history, the process of integrating these two schemes is a profitable intellectual exercise.

CLASS SECERNENTEA (PHASMIDIA)

Order Rhabditida

The order Rhabditida is a very large group of small nematodes with *rhabditoid* or *rhabditiform* esophagus consisting of *corpus, isthmus,* and *bulb* (Fig. 6-5). Many species are free-living or are parasites of lower vertebrate or invertebrate animals. Only three genera of the order Rhabditida, *Rhabditis* (syn., *Pelodera*), *Micronema,* and *Strongyloides,* parasitize domestic animals.

Rhabditis (*Pelodera*)

Rhabditis (*Pelodera*) *strongyloides* is a free-living inhabitant of decaying organic matter but occasionally produces a pruritic, hyperemic dermatitis of cattle, swine, dogs, and rodents that have been exposed to an excess of the nematode's normal habitat. Damp straw bedding has been repeatedly incriminated in canine dermatitis caused by this parasite. Diagnosis is based on finding nematode larvae with a rhabditiform esophagus in skin scrapings (Fig. 6-6); sometimes adults are also present. If *R. strongyloides* larvae are placed on nutrient agar, they will develop into adults in a day or so; these adults are 1 to 2 mm. long and will promptly fill the Petri dish with their offspring.

Micronema

Micronema deletrix has been identified in a nasal tumor, maxillary granulomas, brain, and kidney of horses and in the brain of a

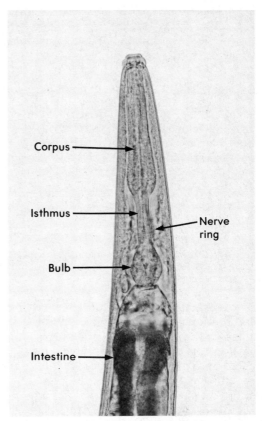

Figure 6–5. Anterior end of a *Strongyloides papillosus* free-living adult with a typical rhabditiform esophagus (x430).

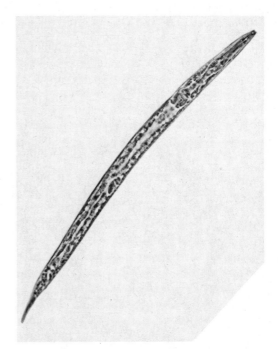

Figure 6–6. *Rhabditis strongyloides* rhabditiform larva from a nutrient agar culture. The culture was grown from scrapings of an acute erythematous dermatitis affecting a dog (x250).

child. Infection of the brain with *M. deletrix* was found in a Quarter Horse mare with clinical signs resembling those of viral encephalitis (Jordan *et al.*, 1975).

Strongyloides

Strongyloides is a very aberrant genus in terms of morphology and life history. Be careful not to confuse the genus name *Strongyloides* with the species name of *Rhabditis* *strongyloides* or with the superfamily name Strongyloidea. Also be warned that the adjective "strongyloid," as used by many authors, is more likely to refer to properties of members of the superfamily Strongyloidea than to those of the genus *Strongyloides*. The ubiquitous prefix derives from the Greek word *strongylos*, meaning round, compact (Webster's, 1976), and apparently has great appeal to taxonomists of every stripe. "Strongyl-" has not been restricted to the christen-

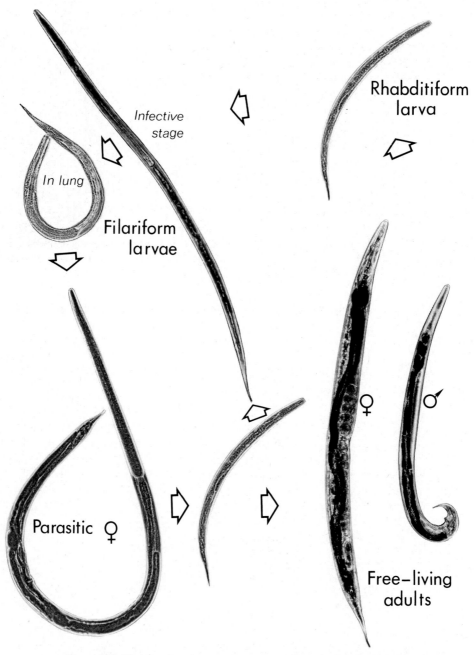

Figure 6–7. Life stages of *Strongyloides stercoralis.* Not to same scale.

ing of worms but has been applied to such diverse animals as sponges (*Strongylophora*), bugs (*Strongylodemas*), and fish (*Strongyliscus*), among upwards of eighty others.

Life History. Many parasites have free-living stages in their life histories, but *Strongyloides* is unique among parasites of domestic animals in having alternate free-living and parasitic *generations*. Parasitic males do not exist, and parasitic females contain no male gonads. The filariform parasitic female produces eggs by mitotic parthenogenesis, and the larvae that hatch from these eggs are termed *homogonic* rhabditiform larvae to distinguish them from the *heterogonic* offspring of the free-living, sexual generation. Homogonic rhabditiform larvae in the external environment may develop through two molts into infective filariform larvae or through four molts into free-living males and females. If the filariform larva enters a suitable host, usually by penetrating its skin, development proceeds through third and fourth molts to the filariform parasitic female. Thus, there are five stages separated by four molts in both parasitic and free-living generations. The free-living rhabditiform males and females mate to produce heterogonic rhabditiform larvae that, with minor exceptions, develop only into infective filariform larvae (Basir, 1950; Triantophyllou and Moncol, 1977). The life history of *Strongyloides* is portrayed in Figure 6-7.

Identification. The tiny parasitic female lies deep in the mucosal crypts of the alimentary tract, particularly the small intestine. *The esophagus is nearly cylindrical and at least one-fourth as long as the body* (Fig. 6-8). Other small nematodes in this location include members of the superfamily Trichostrongyloidea, which have a very much shorter esophagus, and *Trichinella* and *Capillaria*, both of which have a *stichosome esophgagus* (see Trichuroidea and Figures 6-61 and 6-62). The egg, rhabditiform larva, and infective filariform larva are the stages most important in diagnostic procedures. The free-living adults (Figs. 6-5 and 6-7) frequently develop in cultures of feces from *Strongyloides*-infected animals.

Prominent species of *Strongyloides* parasitizing domestic animals and man include *S. stercoralis* of man, dog, and cat; *S. papillosus* of ruminants; *S. ransomi* of swine; *S. westeri* of horses; *S. fuelleborni* of African and Asian primates and of man; *S. cebus* of American primates; and *S. ratti* and *S. venezuelensis* of rats. Thus, all species of domestic animals have a species of *Strongyloides*, as do many

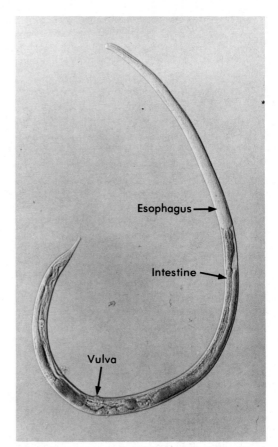

Figure 6–8. *Strongyloides stercoralis* parasitic female (x95).

species of wild mammals and birds (Little, 1966).

Importance. *Strongyloides* infections are moderate and asymptomatic in most individuals of all domestic species and when disease does occur, it is usually confined to massively challenged neonates and nurslings. *Strongyloides papillosus*, for example, although almost universally prevalent in ruminants, rarely causes detectable illness even though the newborn calves, lambs, and kids acquire infective larvae at a tender age in their dam's milk. Transmammary infection also occurs with *S. ransomi* of swine and *S. westeri* of horses. Piglets heavily infected with *S. ransomi* suffer debilitating dysentery, rapid emaciation, anemia, and stunting, starting only a few days after birth (Moncol and Batte, 1966). In like manner, foals begin to shed *S. westeri* eggs about two weeks after birth and may have diarrhea at this time (Enigk *et al.*, 1974; Lyons *et al.*, 1969).

Strongyloides stercoralis infection in dogs may be asymptomatic, or it may cause any grade of clinical illness. Serious cases exhibit signs of bronchopneumonia and severe watery or mucous diarrhea that may easily be confused with the generalized viral diseases of puppyhood. In massive invasions, the lungs of young pups may be sprinkled with petechial and ecchymotic hemorrhages caused by migrating larvae breaking out of the alveolar capillaries. The prepatent period is about one week. The epidemiological role of the dog in human *S. stercoralis* infection has actually been documented by only one report of natural transmission from dog to man (Georgi and Sprinkle, 1974) but the potential hazard to human health should always be taken into account in dealing with infected dogs.

Strongyloides stercoralis infection in man is unique in its chronicity. Once contracted, this infection may persist for decades or for life, now as a slumbering asymptomatic and non-patent infection, again as a bout of abdominal pain with diarrhea or of intensely pruritic "creeping eruption," and sometimes as a catastrophic terminal illness precipitated by massive infection. In at least some cases of human *S. stercoralis* infection, development to the infective filariform larval stage occurs within the patient's digestive tract. These infective larvae may reinvade the host by penetrating either the wall of the bowel (internal autoinfection) or the perianal skin (external autoinfection). Autoinfection accounts for the extreme chronicity of strongyloidiasis in man and, in part, for the explosive development of massive disseminated infection (hyperinfection) that may overwhelm pa-

tients suffering from depressed cell-mediated immunity. Hyperinfection with *S. stercoralis* has caused the deaths of many persons suffering immune deficiency diseases or undergoing immunosuppressive therapy (Dwork *et al.*, 1975). For further details, see Georgi, 1982.

Order Strongylida

Morphology. The *stoma* presents important diagnostic characters that are the same for both male and female and are usually sufficient for generic identification. Strongyloids have well-developed buccal capsules that are, in many cases, armed with teeth (Fig. 6-9). Ancylostomatoids also have well-developed buccal capsules but these are permanently flexed dorsally and armed on their ventral (leading) edge with formidable pointed *teeth* or rounded *cutting plates* (Fig. 6-10). In the Trichostrongyloidea, the buccal capsule is usually reduced in size but may be equipped with a tooth or lancet in bloodsucking species (Fig. 6-11). In the typical metastrongyloid, the buccal capsule is absent.

Male nematodes of the order Strongylida have a caudal copulatory bursa that consists of dorsal, lateral, and ventral expansions of the body cuticle (*lobes*) supported by muscular processes called *rays* (Fig. 6-12). The dorsal lobe contains one ray that is usually median in position and variously branched. The lateral lobes each contain an *externodorsal ray* adjacent to the dorsal lobe and three rays arising in a group, the posterolateral, the

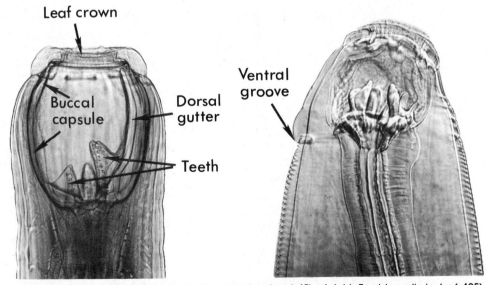

Figure 6–9. Family Strongylidae. At left, *Strongylus equinus* (x45); at right, *Ternidens diminutus* (x125).

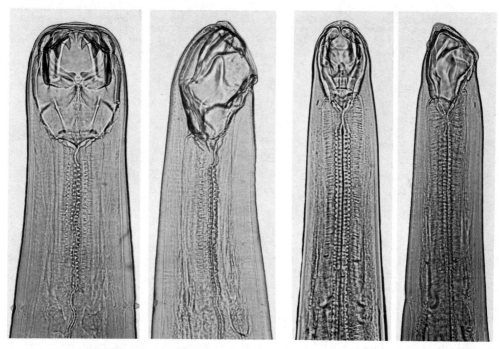

Ancylostoma caninum   *Uncinaria stenocephala*

Figure 6–10. Dorsoventral and lateral aspects of the buccal and esophageal regions of *Ancylostoma caninum* (x100) and *Uncinaria stenocephala* (x160).

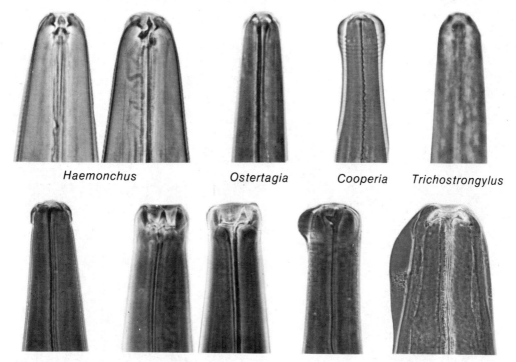

Haemonchus   *Ostertagia*   *Cooperia*   *Trichostrongylus*

Hyostrongylus   *Amidostomum*   *Nematodirus*   *Dictyocaulus*

Figure 6–11. Stomas of eight genera of the superfamily Trichostrongyloidea (from J. H. Whitlock, 1960). *Amidostomum* is a parasite of geese and ducks but not of mammals; its large, toothed buccal capsule is not typical of trichostrongyloids.

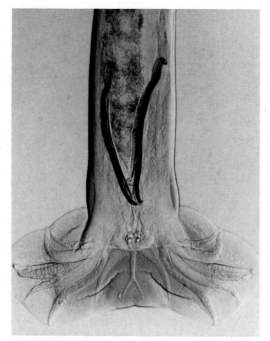

Figure 6-12. Bursa and spicules of *Ostertagia* (x150).

mediolateral, and the anterolateral, respectively. The ventral lobes each contain two rays. The disposition and configuration of these rays are used in classification and identification of strongylids. In typical members of the superfamilies Strongyloidea and Ancylostomatoidea, the dorsal and lateral lobes are about equally developed (Fig. 6-1); in Trichostrongyloidea, the lateral lobes predominate (Fig. 6-12); and in Metastrongyloidea, the bursa tends to be reduced (see Figs. 6-30 and 6-32). In some metastrongyloids (e.g., *Filaroides*), the bursa is completely absent (Fig. 6-31).

The *spicules* of males of the superfamilies Strongyloidea and Ancylostomatoidea tend to be long, thin, and flexible (Figs. 6-1 and 6-13), whereas those of the Trichostrongyloidea are usually short and frequently twisted (Figs. 6-12, 6-13, 6-15, 6-16, and 6-18). However, the spicules of *Nematodirus* (Fig. 6-13) and *Mecistocirrus* (Fig. 6-14), both trichostrongyloids, are long and thin and thus resemble strongyloid spicules. In the Metastrongyloidea, spicules vary so widely in size and shape that generalization is unprofitable.

The strongylid uterus has two horns and is equipped with a well-developed muscular *ovijector* (Fig. 6-2). In typical trichostrongyloids and ancylostomatoids, the vulva is located near the middle of the body and the two horns of the uterus extend in opposite directions (amphidelphic). In strongyloids and metastrongyloids, the vulva is typically

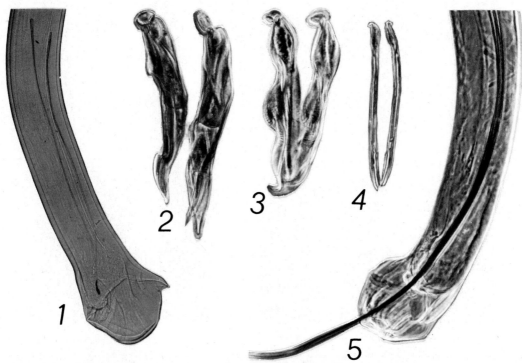

Figure 6-13. Spicules of Ancylostomatoidea: *1 Ancylostoma tubaeform* and Trichostrongyloidea, *2 Trichostrongylus*, *3 Cooperia*, *4 Ostertagia*, *5 Nematodirus* (2 to 5 from J. H. Whitlock, 1960).

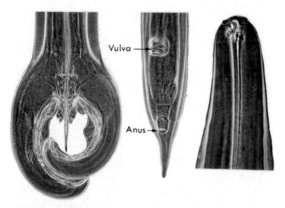

Figure 6–14. *Mecistocirrus* (from J. H. Whitlock, 1960).

located close to the anus and both horns of the uterus extend anteriorly (prodelphic).

Life History. The life histories of superfamilies Strongyloidea, Trichstrongyloidea, and Ancylostomatoidea are typically direct, with free-living microbivorous first and second larval stages and infective third larval stage. Females of all three superfamilies lay typical "strongyle eggs" (see Figs. 12-23 and 12-34), i.e., eggs with smooth-surfaced, ellipsoidal shell containing an embryo in the morula stage of development. The morula develops into a first stage larva that hatches from the egg within a day or two. After feeding, this larva undergoes its first molt to become a second stage larva. Both first and second stage larvae remain in the feces, where they feed on bacteria. In the second molt, the cuticle of the second stage is temporarily retained as a protective "sheath" about the infective third stage larva and will not be shed until this larva enters a suitable host. In about one week, these "sheathed" third stage larvae begin to migrate out of the fecal mass and into the water film covering the surrounding soil particles and vegetation. Infection occurs when these "sheathed larvae" are ingested by grazing animals. Variations on this basic life history pattern are discussed below in connection with the several genera.

Various representatives of the superfamily Metastrongyloidea lay eggs in all stages of development from a single cell (e.g., *Aelurostrongylus*) to an egg containing a first stage larva (e.g., *Filaroides*). However, sufficient development occurs within the host so that the form found in the feces is either a first stage larva or an egg containing a first stage larva. Metastrongyloids typically require a molluscan or annelid intermediate host for development from the first stage to the infective third stage, and infection of the definitive

host occurs through ingestion of snails, slugs, or earthworms containing infective third stage larvae. *Filaroides osleri* and *F. hirthi*, both of which are directly infective to the dog in the first larval stage, form important exceptions to this rule.

Superfamily Trichostrongyloidea

Trichostrongyloid nematodes are especially common and pathogenic in grazing ruminants, but swine, horses, cats, and birds also host important species. The abomasum and small intestine are the usual locations in ruminants, but one aberrant species, *Dictyocaulus*, reaches maturity in the air passages. It is sufficient, for practical purposes of effective treatment and control, to identify trichostrongyloids at the generic level of the older classification schemes (e.g., Yorke and Maplestone, 1926).

Trichostrongylus

Identification. Very small, threadlike worms less than 7 mm. long, without cephalic inflations and virtually without buccal capsule; spicules short, twisted and usually pointed (Figs. 6-11 and 6-15). *Trichostrongylus axei* parasitizes the

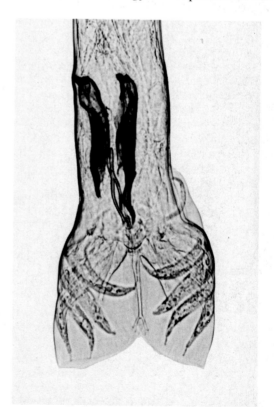

Figure 6–15. Bursa and spicules of *Trichostrongylus* (x375).

simple stomach or abomasum of a wide range of hosts including ruminants, horses, and leporids; other species are parasites of the small intestine of ruminants and display a higher order of host specificity. Even heavy infections with *Trichostrongylus* will be overlooked on necropsy examination unless care is taken to carefully examine washings or scrapings of the stomach and the first 6 meters of the small intestine, preferably with a hand lens or stereoscopic microscope. *Trichostrongylus* is most likely to be confused with *Strongyloides* or with the smaller species of *Cooperia*.

Importance. *Trichostrongylus* infections are often asymptomatic, but when present in large numbers (i.e., over 10,000), these parasites are capable of producing protracted and debilitating watery diarrhea, especially in stressed or malnourished sheep, cattle, and goats. At first, the feces remain semisolid but soon become watery and dark green in color ("black scours"), staining the fleece of the hind quarters. Some of the feces accumulate in pea- to egg-sized masses ("dags") that dangle from the fleece and grow by accretion as fluid feces continue to pour over and dry on them. The resulting foul condition tends to attract blowflies like *Lucilia cuprina* and result in myiasis. Egg counts rarely exceed 5000 eggs per gram because *Trichostrongylus* is a very small worm that lays few eggs and because the feces are greatly diluted with water. Necropsy examination reveals a wasted carcass without obvious lesions even in the affected small intestine and the parasites themselves are easy to overlook. Protracted diarrhea is sufficient to account for the weakness and emaciation typically observed in trichostrongylosis, but it is important to remember that less than massive burdens of *Trichostronglyus* do not usually cause serious illness in well-nourished, unstressed ruminants. Therefore, it may be important to consider the quality of the environment and animal husbandry in identifying the ultimate causes of particular outbreaks.

Ostertagia

Identification. Usually less than 14 mm. long and brownish in color, Ostertagia *has a short, broad buccal cavity (Fig. 6-11) and short, two- or three-pronged spicules* (Figs. 6-12 and 6-16). Ostertagia spp. *are found in the abomasum of ruminants.* Ostertagia *displays remarkable resistance to cadaverous putrefaction and*

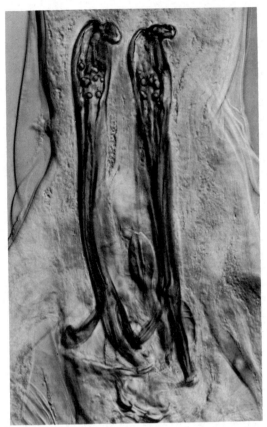

Figure 6–16. Spicules of *Ostertagia ostertagi* (x450).

may be found still alive in a "ripe post" after *Haemonchus* has quite disintegrated. The tip of the tail of the mature female *Ostertagia* is usually annulated (Fig. 6-17) and the eggs in the amphidelphic ovijector are typical strongyle eggs. One species, *O. (Marshallagia) marshalli*, produces huge eggs that might be confused with those of *Nematodirus* (see Fig. 12-23).

Life History. "Type I" or "summer" ostertagiosis usually occurs in pastured young cattle, the worms maturing without first passing through a developmental arrest ("latent phase"). "Type II" or "winter" ostertagiosis typically occurs in late winter when larvae that have remained in arrested development since fall once again become metabolically active and proceed to develop into adults. Such behavior is part and parcel of the normal mechanism employed by *Ostertagia* and many other trichostrongyloids for overwintering but, when mistimed or overdone to such an extent as to overome the compensatory mechanisms of the host, leads to winter ostertagiosis.

Importance. *Ostertagia ostertagi* causes chronic abomasitis in young cattle, a disease

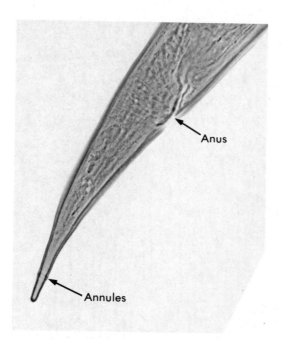

Figure 6–17. Tail of female *Ostertagia* (x425).

marked by profuse, watery diarrhea, anemia, and hypoproteinemia manifested clinically as submaxillary edema. The animal is typically hidebound and emaciated. The appetite remains intact, which seems paradoxical in view of the advanced pathological changes taking place in the abomasum. The hydrogen ion concentration of the gastric juice approaches neutrality. Necropsy examination reveals a wasted carcass with depletion of fat depots typical of extreme malnutrition. The rumen, reticulum, and omasum may be full of good feed but the alimentary tract from the cardia onwards is virtually empty owing to malfunction of the abomasum; the animal has starved to death in the midst of plenty. The "Morocco leather" appearance of the abomasal mucosa is pathognomonic; the whole mucosa is studded with grayish white, pinhead- to pea-sized nodules with a worm protruding from a small opening at the summit of each. *Ostertagia* spp. of sheep and goats may also cause serious endemic disease is certain localities.

Haemonchus

Identification. Up to 30 mm. in length, these parasites of the abomasum of ruminants have a buccal cavity armed with a lancet (see Fig. 6-11). The male has an asymmetrical dorsal ray in its bursa (Fig. 6-18) and short, wedge-shaped spicules. The white, egg-filled uterus of the female spirals around blood-filled gut, giving rise to the so-called "barber pole effect." The vulva is located about a quarter body length from the tail and may or may not be guarded by variously shaped cuticular inflations ("vulvar flaps"); the prevalence of various vulvar flap configurations varies among species and subspecies of *Haemonchus* (Fig. 6-19).

Importance. At peak infection, naturally acquired populations of *Haemonchus contortus* may remove one fifth of the circulating erythrocyte volume per day from lambs and may average one tenth of the circulating erythrocyte volume per day over the course of nonfatal infections lasting two months. These are round figures drawn from observations of a flock of 100 to 175 lambs with erythrocyte loss estimated by the whole-body radioiron retention technique (Georgi, 1964; Georgi and Whitlock, 1965). The pathogenic effects of *H. contortus* result from the inability of the host to compensate for blood loss. If the amount of loss is small and restitution by the host complete, no measurable illness results. "It is doubtful, indeed, whether in such circumstances (i.e., satisfactory nutrition) infection with up to 500 worms has any effect on growth or wool production" (Clunies Ross and Gordon, 1936). However, if the rate of blood loss exceeds the host's hematopoietic capacity, either because the challenge is overwhelming or because the response is handicapped by poor nutrition, defective pheno-

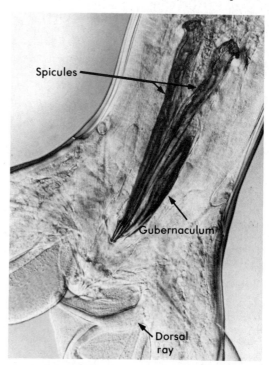

Figure 6–18. Spicules of *Haemonchus* (x140).

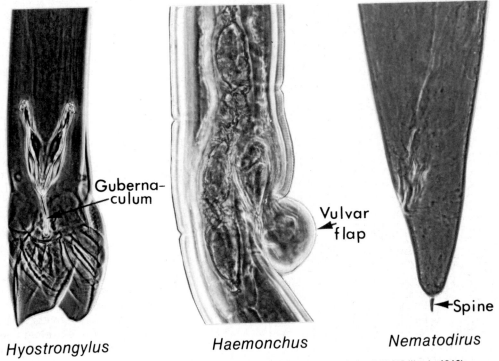

Figure 6–19. Three genera of the superfamily Trichostrongyloidea (from J. H. Whitlock, 1960).

type, or stress, a progressive anemia leads rapidly to death. The cardinal sign of haemonchosis is pallor of the skin and mucous membranes; a hematocrit reading of less than 15 per cent is always accompanied by extreme weakness and shortness of breath and warrants a grave prognosis. Loss of plasma protein results in anasarca frequently manifested externally as submaxillary edema ("bottle jaw"). The appetite typically remains good and, in acute outbreaks, affected animals may not have lost appreciable weight; feces are well formed, diarrhea occurring only in infections complicated by the presence of *Trichostrongylus, Cooperia,* and the like. Lambs are most often the most seriously affected members of a flock but older sheep under stress may also suffer fatal anemia. Individual older ewes may succumb, in late spring, to overwhelming challenge imposed by hordes of larvae simultaneously emerging from developmental arrest. High egg counts, 10,000 eggs per gram or higher, are typical of haemonchosis.

Mecistocirrus

Identification. Like *Haemonchus,* except that the vulva is close to the anus and the spicules are long and thin (see Fig. 6-14), *Mecistocirrus is a parasite of the abomasum of ruminants and the stomach of pigs in Central America, India, and the Far East.*

Cooperia

Identification. Parasites of the small intestine of ruminants, species of Cooperia are less than 9 mm. long, the cuticle of the stomal region is transversely striated and slightly inflated, the buccal cavity is very small, the spicules are short and blunted at their tips, and the dorsal ray of the bursa is lyre-shaped (see Figs. 6-11 and 6-13; Figs. 6-20 and 6-21). Cooperia is most likely to be confused with *Trichostrongylus* or *Strongyloides* because of similarity in size and location in the host.

Importance. The relationship of *Cooperia* spp. to disease production is similar to that presented for *Trichostrongylus* above.

Nematodirus

Identification. Species of *Nematodirus* vary considerably in size; the largest grows to a length of 25 mm. *The cuticle of the stomal region is transversely striated and may be inflated, the stoma is armed with a dorsal, triangular tooth (Fig. 6-11), the neck is usually coiled, the spicules are long and thin (Fig. 6-13), the uterus contains*

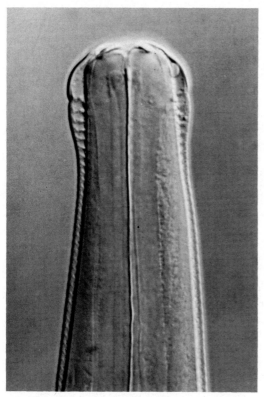

Figure 6–20. Stomal end of *Cooperia* (x690).

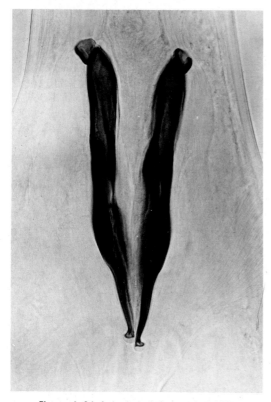

Figure 6–21. Spicules of *Cooperia* (x380).

very large eggs (Fig. 12-23), and the female has a spine at the tip of her tail (Fig. 6-19).

Life History. The life history and epidemiology of *N. battus* are distinctly different from most other trichostrongyloids. The infective larva develops within the egg, and these cold-resistant eggs instead of carrier infections perpetuate the infection from one grazing season to the next. In fact, the eggs must first be subjected to freezing before the larvae will hatch, thus limiting *N. battus* to one generation per year and tending to generate a single wave of infection in late spring. As a result, the severity of infection is directly proportional to the previous year's pasture contamination, and timing of the outbreak is dependent on weather favorable for mass hatching of eggs.

Importance. Although *Nematodirus* spp. infections are usually not associated with clinical disease, *N. battus* causes a specific strongylosis that is characterized by very restricted seasonal incidence and by extremely severe and debilitating diarrhea. Most of the lamb flock display a sudden loss of thrift quickly followed by profuse diarrhea. Deaths begin from two days to two weeks after onset of clinical signs and continue for several weeks, after which survivors gradually recover; mortality may reach 20 per cent in particularly severe outbreaks. Egg counts average 600 and rarely exceed 3000 eggs per gram of feces. Necropsy reveals a dehydrated carcass, enlarged, pale, edematous mesenteric lymph glands, and mild, catarrhal enteritis but very little else in the way of lesions; a count of 10,000 *N. battus* worms is considered significant (Thomas and Stevens, 1956).

Hyostrongylus

Identification. A parasite of the stomach of swine, *H. rubidus* is less than 9 mm. long and has a small, annular buccal collar, short spicules with two points, and a long narrow gubernaculum (Figs. 6-11 and 6-19).

Ollulanus

Identification. *A parasite of the stomach of the pig and cat, O. tricuspis is minute (less than 1 mm. long); the anterior end is rolled up, the vulva is near the anus, the female tail terminates in three or more sharp points, and the spicules are short, equal, and bifurcated.*

Life History. *Ollulanus tricuspis* is viviparous and the larvae develop to maturity in the stomach; a rare example of a nematode capable of completing its life history within a single host. Ingestion of vomitus from an infected host is the most likely means of transmission of *O. tricuspis*.

Dictyocaulus

Identification. Up to 80 mm. long, white adult Dictyocaulus worms are found in the respiratory passages of ruminants and horses. The buccal cavity is small, the bursa somewhat reduced, the spicules short and granular in appearance, the vulva is near the middle of the body, and the eggs contain a first stage larva when laid (see Fig. 6-11; Fig. 6-22).

Life History. Adult *Dictyocaulus* live in the lumen of the bronchial tree, where they cause chronic bronchitis and localized occlusion of the bronchial tree with atelectasis. *Dictyocaulus viviparus* is the only nematode that reaches maturity in the lungs of cattle. The freshly laid egg contains a vermiform embryo that usually hatches before being eliminated in the feces. The free-living stages probably derive their energy from stored food materials instead of from ingested bacteria because they are able to develop to the doubly ensheathed infective stage in aerated clean water, and because the characteristic "food granules" in the intestinal cells of the first stage larva become less conspicuous and finally disappear as development proceeds. Development to the infective stage requires about five days under optimum conditions. When ingested, the infective larvae migrate by way of the mesenteric lymph nodes and thoracic duct and arrive in the lungs about five days later (Jarrett *et al.*, 1957). Egg laying starts about four weeks after infection.

Importance. As a group, the lungworms are well adapted parasites and, in reasonable numbers, impose only a mild burden on their hosts. Light infections with *D. viviparus* are borne without obvious physiological embarrassment; calves cough occasionally and may breathe slightly faster than normal. Heavier infections lead to partial or complete obstruction of the air passages and clinical disease develops in proportion to the degree of obstruction. A progressive increase in respiration rate starts at about the fifth day after ingestion of several thousand infective larvae and the animal coughs occasionally. During the third week, respirations become forced and reach a rate of 100 per minute. Auscultation reveals harsh bronchial sounds and occasional crepitation. *Until the fourth week, no larvae are shed in the feces, and the diagnosis rests entirely on the history and clinical signs.* During the fourth week, first stage larvae appear in the feces and the severity of the clinical signs reaches a maximum. The respiratory rate exceeds 100 per minute, coughing is frequent, crepitation and harsh bronchial sounds can be heard, and air hunger becomes acute; the calves don't feed because they can't spare the time needed for breathing! Clinical improvement can be noted in survivors after the fifth week.

Dictyocaulus filaria has a life history similar to that of *D. viviparus* (Daubney, 1920). However, unless unusually large infections are acquired, the clinical signs are usually mild. Most cases of severe clinical illness associated with *D. filaria* are complicated by the presence of less obvious but more pathogenic parasites in the alimentary tract.

Dictyocaulus arnfieldi is a relatively well-adapted parasite of donkeys (*Equus asinus*) but tends to be quite pathogenic in horses. Where this parasite is endemic, it is hazardous to pasture horses and donkeys together.

SUPERFAMILY STRONGYLOIDEA

Morphology. Strongyloids tend to be larger and stouter-bodied than trichostrongyloids, and most of them have a large buccal cavity

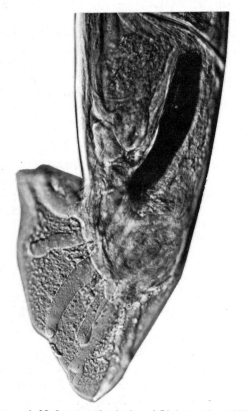

Figure 6–22. Bursa and spicules of *Dictyocaulus* (x168).

surrounded by a sclerotized wall (buccal capsule) that is usually rigid but may be jointed or thin and flexible. The stomal structures of strongyloids are sufficiently distinct to permit identification of species with occasional reference to other characters. Greater dependence must be placed on these other characters when it is impossible to examine both dorsal and lateral aspects of the stoma, as is the case with permanently mounted specimens.

The buccal cavity of strongyloids is large and directed anteriorly (see Fig. 6-9). The stomal opening is surrounded by a row or two of what appear to be leaves or palings of a stockade, depending on the imagination of the observer; these are called *leaf crowns* and much is made of them in the taxonomy of strongyloids. The duct of the dorsal esophageal gland is carried to the rim of the buccal capsule in a sclerotized ridge (*dorsal gutter*) on the inner wall of the buccal capsule. Teeth, when present, lie at the base of the buccal cavity, where they lacerate the plug of mucous membrane that is drawn into the buccal cavity by the sucking action of the muscular esophagus. The copulatory bursa is well developed, the spicules long and thin (see Fig. 6-1). The vulva is close to the anus and the uterus prodelphic in most strongyloids (see Fig. 6-2).

Life History. Strongyloid life histories are typical of the order but significant variations occur in certain groups. For example, *Syngamus*, the "gapeworm" of domestic and wild birds, and *Stephanurus*, the "kidney worm" of swine, use earthworms as paratenic hosts.

FAMILY STRONGYLIDAE

Subfamily Strongylinae

Identification. Members of the subfamily Strongylinae, often referred to as "large strongyles," are chiefly parasites of the large intestine of equines (*Strongylus*, *Triodontophorus*, *Oesophogodontus*, and *Craterostomum*) and elephants (*Decrusia*, *Equinurbia*, and *Choniangium*). Identification of genera and species of strongylin parasites of horses is a matter of comparing the microscopic appearance of the stomal region of specimens with Figures 13-7 and 13-10. There are two leaf crowns but, because the elements of each are similar in size and number, the two crowns appear as one.

Importance. *Strongylus vulgaris*, *S. edentatus*, and *S. equinus* are among the most destructive parasites of the horse. All three are

bloodsuckers as adult worms in the cecum and colon but, even more important, their larvae undergo migrations that inflict even greater damage, especially in foals and yearlings. *Triodontophorus* spp. appear, by the ferocious teeth at the base of their buccal cavities (see Fig. 13-7), to be bloodsucking parasites. Clusters of *T. tenuicollis* worms cause localized ulceration of the colonic mucous membrane. The biology and control of equine strongyles is discussed in Chapter 9.

Subfamily Cyathostominae

Identification. These "small strongyles" are parasites of the large intestine of horses, elephants, pigs, and marsupials, and there is a multitude of them. About 40 species of cyathostomes parasitize the cecum and colon of horses and it is commonplace to find as many as 15 or 20 of these species infecting an individual host at the same time. Cyathostomins have somewhat smaller buccal cavities than strongylins; all have distinct inner and outer leaf crowns the elements of which differ in size and number. In some species, the inner leaf crown elements are inconspicuous and can be seen only in well cleared specimens (e.g., *Cylicolcyclus nassatus*, Fig. 13-12). Identification of species of equine cyathostomes can be accomplished by comparing dorsal and lateral aspects of the buccal regions of fresh or cleared, fixed specimens with Figures 13-8 to 13-18, which include all of the more common species.

Importance. From 75 to 100 per cent of the eggs passed in the feces of naturally infected horses are produced by the small strongyles because these greatly outnumber the large strongyles both in numbers of species and in numbers of individuals. Cyathostomin larvae do not migrate beyond the mucous membrane of the colon and so their pathogenic effects are considerably less dramatic than those inflicted by the larvae of *Strongylus* spp. Heavy infections may be responsible for cases of severe and persistent diarrhea, however. Massive invasions of the bright red fourth stage larvae of *Cylicocyclus insigne* riddling the mucosa of the large intestine are particularly impressive in this regard. Mirck (1977) described verminous enteritis in young horses and ponies in which large numbers of fourth and early fifth stage cyathostomins are discharged in the feces. This form of *cyathostominosis* occurs in the Netherlands from November to May, is characterized by watery diarrhea associated with severe in-

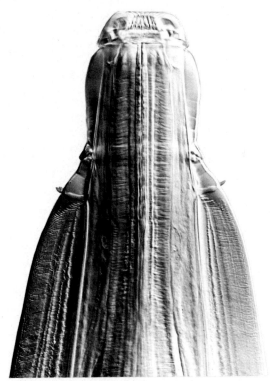

Figure 6–23. *Oesophagostomum columbianum*, dorso-ventral view of buccal and anterior esophageal regions (x168).

flammation of the mucous membrane of the cecum and colon, and often terminates fatally. Most of the worms are immature, and egg counts are therefore misleadingly low. Anthelmintic therapy has no influence on the course of the disease or on the number of worms being passed in the feces. Apparently, the larvae encysted in the mucosa are unaffected by currently available anthelmintic medication. There are many more larvae than can be accommodated as adult parasites and, as they mature, many are swept out with the manure.

Subfamily Oesophagostominae

Identification. There is a transverse fold of cuticle ("ventral groove," see Fig. 6-9) on the ventral side of the body just posterior to the buccal cavity. The buccal cavity varies in size from small (e.g., *Oesophagostomum columbianum*, Fig. 6-23) to very large (e.g., *Chabertia ovina*, Fig. 6-24). Oesophagostomins are parasites of the large intestines of ruminants (*Oesophagostomum columbianum*, *Oe. venulosum*, *Oe. radiatum*, and *Chabertia ovina*), swine (*Oe. dentatum*, *Oe. pudendotectus*), and primates (*Conoweberia* spp. and *Ternidens deminutus*).

Importance. Oesophagostomins are called "nodular worms" because their parasitic larvae tend to become encapsulated by a somewhat excessive reactive inflammation on the part of the previously sensitized host. Acute inflammation may lead to clinical disease characterized by fetid diarrhea, which may be fatal. The nodules later caseate and calcify and severe involvement may interfere mechanically with normal intestinal motility. Clinical signs in ruminants and swine are usually associated with these reactions to the larval stages in the wall of the bowel and not to adult worms in the lumen. Therefore, clinical disease is likely to be associated with nonpatent infection and diagnosis must depend on correct interpretation of clinical signs or postmortem findings. The feces are watery, dark, and very fetid; weakness is marked and emaciation rapid. Necropsy examination conducted during an outbreak of nodular worm disease reveals an inflamed intestine studded with active nodules filled with creamy pus, each containing a living larva (Fig. 6-25). Caseated and calcified nodules should not be held accountable for current acute parasitic enteritis but may occasionally cause intussusception or other mechanical abnormality.

Conoweberia apiostomum, C. stephanostomum, and *Ternidens deminutus* are pathogenic, especially in recently captured primates suffering the unaccustomed stresses of confinement and transportation. Acute and chronic disease syndromes caused by *Oe. stephanostomum* occurred in gorillas from the thirteenth to fortieth days after capture (Rousselot and Pellissier, 1952). The chronic syndrome consisted or intermittent diarrhea,

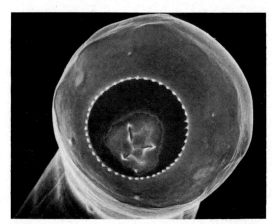

Figure 6–24. *Chabertia ovina*, head-on. The oral end of the esophagus with its triradiate lumen is visible at the base of the buccal cavity (S.E.M. x100).

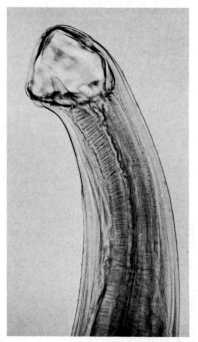

Figure 6–26. *Bunostomum* sp. (x100).

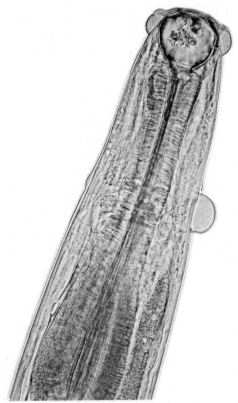

Figure 6–25. *Oesophagostomum radiatum* fourth stage larva from a nodule in the intestinal wall of a calf (x250). *Oesophagostomum* spp. fourth stage larvae are unusual in having relatively larger buccal cavities than the adult stage.

paleness of the mucous membranes, and the presence of eggs in the feces. In the acute form, the gorilla refuses to eat or nibbles a little and suffers some diarrhea but very soon passes only small quantities of glairy mucus streaked with blood, much like that observed in acute amebic dysentery of man. The gorilla remains either lying down or sitting with both hands on its head in an attitude of human desperation.

Superfamily Ancylostomatoidea

FAMILY ANCYLOSTOMATIDAE

Identification. Adult hookworms are bloodsucking parasites of the small intestine. All have a large buccal cavity that is directed obliquely dorsally; the anterior end of the worm is thus "hooked." The ventral margin of the stoma is guarded by pointed "teeth" in the subfamily Ancylostominae and by smoothly rounded "plates" in the subfamily Bunostominae (see Fig. 6-10). Within the subfamily Ancylostominae, *Ancylostoma ca-*

ninum and *A. tubaeforme*, parasites of dogs and cats, respectively, have three such teeth on either side of the midline; *A. duodenale* of man has two, and *A. braziliense* of dogs and cats has one. Genera in the subfamily Bunostominae include *Bunostomum* in ruminants, *Necator* and *Globocephalus* in primates and swine, *Uncinaria* and *Arthrocephalus* in carnivorans, *Bathmostomum* in elephants, and *Grammocephalus* in elephants and rhinoceroses (see Fig. 6-10; Figs. 6-26 and 6-27).

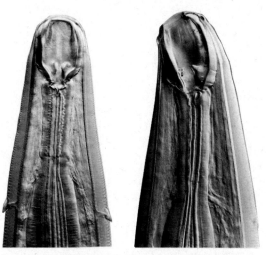

Figure 6–27. *Globocephalus urosubulatus,* a hookworm of swine; dorsal (left) and lateral (right) aspects (x100). Specimen provided by Dr. E. I. Braide.

Life History. Infection occurs either by ingestion of or skin penetration by infective larvae, which then undergo more or less extensive migrations through the tissues of the host before developing into adult hookworms in the small intestine. The details of these migrations are of great importance in effective medication and control and are presented in connection with epidemiology and control of *Ancylostoma caninum* in Chapter 7.

Hookworm Disease

The principal importance of hookworms attaches to their ability to cause anemia, especially in man and dog. Hookworm disease varies in severity from asymptomatic infection to rapidly fatal exsanguination, depending on the magnitude of the challenge and the resistance of the host.

Magnitude of challenge is determined by the virulence and number of hookworms. Virulence depends on the species of hookworm involved. *Ancylostoma caninum* is much more pathogenic for dogs than *A. braziliense* or *Uncinaria stenocephala* because it sucks much more blood. The number of hookworms infecting a particular host depends very heavily on the degree of exposure to infective larvae. Exposure, in turn, depends on the extent to which infected hosts have contaminated the environment by shedding eggs in their feces, and on the suitability of the substrate (gravel and sand are ideal), temperature, and moisture for development and survival of infective larvae.

Host resistance is resolvable into two abilities: (1) The ability to limit the number of hookworms maturing in the small intestine is influenced by age, premunition, and acquired immunity. As dogs grow older, they become more resistant to hookworms whether or not they experience infection. Immunity acquired from previous infection confers increased resistance, but this is difficult to disentangle from the influences of advancing age and from the marked inhibition of further infection exerted by a residual population of hookworms (premunition). (2) The ability to compensate for blood loss caused by hookworms is influenced by the hematopoietic capacity and state of nutrition of the individual, and by the presence or absence of other stresses.

Because hookworm infection is common and the females are prodigious egg layers, populations of infective larvae are likely to bloom whenever the weather becomes favorable for their development and survival. Therefore, most frank hookworm disease cases occur during the late spring, summer, and early autumn in temperate climates, particularly when mild weather is accompanied by adequate rainfall. The infective challenge may become overwhelming in carelessly managed kennels and pet shops where feces are allowed to accumulate long enough to allow infective larvae to develop. Unpaved runs are particularly favorable for the perpetuation of the parasite because the feces mixes with the soil. This not only makes sanitation difficult but provides more favorable cultural conditions, especially when the soil is light, open-textured, and well drained.

The following clinical forms of canine hookworm disease may be distinguished:

Peracute ancylostomosis results from the passage of infective larvae from dam to nursing pups in the milk. Transmammary infection of very young pups with as few as 50 to 100 adult *A. caninum* may prove fatal. Typically, the pups appear healthy and sleek the first week, then sicken and deteriorate rapidly the second week. The visible mucosae are very pale, and the soft to liquid feces are very dark in color because the blood shed by the hookworms in the small intestine has been partially digested on the way out. The worms do not lay eggs until the sixteenth day of infection, so diagnosis must rest on the clinical signs of disease. Prognosis is guarded to poor with or without treatment.

Acute ancylostomosis results from sudden exposure of susceptible older pups to large numbers of infective larvae; even mature dogs may be overwhelmed if exposure is sufficiently great. Usually, many eggs will be found in the feces of affected animals but clinical signs may precede the appearance of eggs by about four days in particularly heavy infections.

Chronic (compensated) ancylostomiasis is usually asymptomatic and diagnosis rests on the presence of hookworm eggs in the feces and measurable reductions in erythrocyte count, blood hemoglobin, or packed cell volume. Occasionally, however, incomplete adjustment between parasite and host produces a state of chronic ill health.

Secondary (decompensated) ancylostomosis usually involves older dogs with more ailing them than just hookworms. The cardinal sign is again profound anemia, usually in a malnourished or even emaciated animal. The hookworms may indeed kill the dog, but it is important in this case to recognize that they play a secondary role. An accurate diagnosis, for example, of "malnutrition with secondary ancylostomosis" logically leads to effective therapy.

Cutaneous Larva Migrans

"Creeping eruption" (human cutaneous larva migrans) is a linear, tortuous, erythematous, and intensely pruritic eruption of the human skin usually caused by migration of a nematode larva (Kirby-Smith et al., 1926). *Ancylostoma braziliense* larvae are most frequently involved in the typical, protracted cases, especially in the coastal regions of the southeastern United States (White and Dove, 1926). Accidental sporadic, or experimental cases involving *A. caninum, Uncinaria stenocephala, Bunostomum phlebotomum, Strongyloides stercoralis,* and *Gnathostoma* spp. have also been reported, and the larvae of those species that normally mature in man (*A. duodenale, A. ceylonicum,* and *Necator americanus*) produce a transient but otherwise typical creeping eruption in previously sensitized individuals (Beaver, 1956). It should also be noted that larvae of *Gasterophilus* and *Hypoderma* also migrate in human skin (James, 1947), producing a clinical condition quite properly termed cutaneous larva migrans.

Probably no nematode larva capable of penetrating the skin is above suspicion in individual cases, but the epidemiological importance of any particular species depends on many influences beyond its intrinsic capabilities. For example, the etiological prominence of *A. braziliense* may have much to do with the defecation behavior of dogs and cats, as may be surmised from the following description of circumstances surrounding infection, lesions and symptoms by Kirby-Smith and colleagues (1926):

At least 50 per cent of the cases of creeping eruption seen by the senior author are believed to have originated at the beach, the probable origin being traced to the soft damp sand in front of the beach buildings at points slightly above the high water mark. Such patients reported with lesions varying in numbers. They were not the most extensively infected ones. Persons with hundreds of lesions definitely attributed the origin of their infection to contact with damp sand when they were wet with perspiration while working: repairing an automobile, doing brick work, or making plumbing connectons underneath houses, etc.

The most recent visible lesion is a very narrow erythematous formation along the course traveled by the worm. Soon a slightly raised line representing the location of the burrow can be palpated. This line becomes visibly elevated, more or less continuous and vesicular. Sometimes bullae are formed. The surface of the lesion dries, resulting in a thin crust, When the parasite travels it moves from a fraction of an inch to several inches a day, advancing, as a rule, more rapidly at night.

To some patients the itching sensation resulting from infection is almost intolerable, while others endure it with less suffering. The severity of the lesions, too, is more pronounced in some than in others.

The severity and persistence of the lesions are at least partly related to hypersensitivity resulting from previous exposure. The lungs may be invaded, but intestinal infection with mature worms ensues only in cases involving those species that are normal parasites of man.

FAMILY STEPHANURIDAE

Identification. Stephanurus dentatus is a stout (up to 2 by 40 mm.) parasite of the hepatic, renal, and perirenal tissues, axial musculature, and spinal canal of swine and sometimes of cattle. The buccal cavity is cup-shaped and directed straight forward with 6 to 10 triangular teeth at its base; the gut is convoluted, the spicules equal and short, and the bursa reduced (Fig. 6-28). Earthworms serve as intermediate hosts. For further details, see Chapter 10.

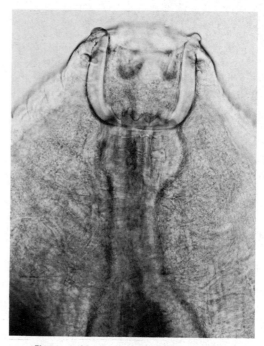

Figure 6–28. *Stephanurus dentatus* (x108).

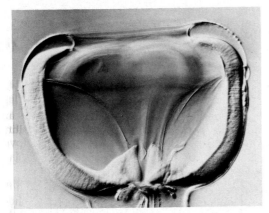

Figure 6–29. *Cyathostoma* (family Syngamidae) buccal capsule (x110).

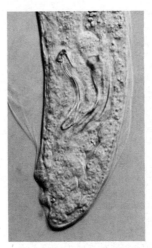

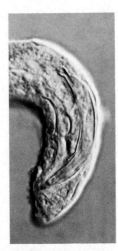

Figure 6–31. *Filaroides hirthi* (left) and *F. milksi* right); caudal ends of male worms (x1050). The spicules of *F. hirthi* are shorter, are broader in relation to their length, and have broader knobs for the attachment of the retractor muscles than the spicules of *F. milksi*.

FAMILY SYNGAMIDAE

Identification. The family Syngamidae includes the genera *Syngamus*, *Mammomonogamus*, and *Cyathostoma* (not *Cyathostomum*), all parasites of the upper respiratory tract. All three have large buccal capsules (Fig. 6-29), and males and females of *Syngamus* and *Mammomonogamus* are fused permanently *in copula*. Earthworms serve as intermediate hosts.

Superfamily Metastrongyloidea

Metastrongyloids are parasites of the respiratory, vascular, and nervous systems of mammals. Most species whose life histories have been investigated require a snail or slug intermediate host, but *Metastrongylus* spp. develop to the infective stage in earthworms, and *Filaroides osleri* and *F. hirthi* infect their definitive hosts directly. The copulatory

bursa is of the basic strongylid pattern but has suffered varying degrees of reduction in the evolution of different families. For example, the bursa is best developed in the family Metastrongylidae (Fig. 6-30) but reduced to mere papillae in the Family Filaroididae (Fig. 6-31). The vulva is close to the anus except in the family Crenosomatidae, in which it is located in the midregion of the body. The diversity of structure and biology displayed by members of the superfamily Metastrongyloidea makes further generalization precarious; it seems doubtful that this superfamily is monophyletic.

FAMILY METASTRONGYLIDAE

The family Metastrongylidae contains only one genus, *Metastrongylus*, all species of which are large white parasites of the bronchi and bronchioles of swine.

Identification. The mouth is flanked by a pair of trilobed lips, the spicules are long and thin, the bursa is well developed, and the vulva is near the anus (Fig. 6-30). When passed in the feces of infected swine, the egg contains a larva (see Fig. 12-34).

Life History. Oviparous females lay eggs containing first stage larvae. These do not hatch or develop into infective larvae unless they are ingested by an earthworm. *Metastrongylus* spp. are of only modest pathological and economic importance. It was once supposed that they acted as vectors of swine influenza virus, but substantial proof for this idea is lacking (Wallace, 1977).

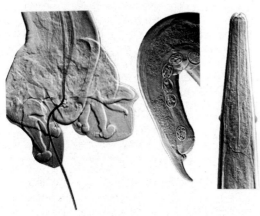

Figure 6–30. *Metastrongylus apri* (x168).

FAMILY PROTOSTRONGYLIDAE

Identification. *Protostrongylids have a well-developed bursa, spicule and spicule guide; the vulva is near the anus* (Figs. 6-32 and 6-33).

Life History. The *oviparous protostrongylid* females deposit *unsegmented* eggs in the surrounding lung, vascular, or neural tissues. These eggs develop into first stage larvae before they appear in the feces (see Fig. 12-26). If these first stage larvae are ingested by any of a wide range of snails and slugs, they develop in these intermediate hosts into doubly ensheathed third stage infective larvae. The protostrongylids considered here are all parasites of sheep and goats.

Protostrongylus

Protostrongylus rufescens lives in the smaller bronchioles where they may cause localized lesions. Males of this brownish-red species can be distinguished from *Dictyocaulus filaria* by their longer, comblike spicules (Fig. 6-32). The female *Protostrongylus* is prodelphic, whereas the female *Dictyocaulus* is amphidelphic.

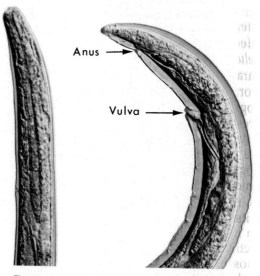

Figure 6–33. *Muellerius capillaris* female (x425).

Muellerius

Muellerius capillaris (Fig. 6-33) is a tiny species so deeply embedded in lung tissue or reactive nodules that specimens are extremely difficult to dissect out intact. Antemortem diagnosis is less difficult because the active first stage larvae are easily separated from the host's feces by the Baermann technique and are not difficult to distinguish from those of *Protostrongylus* and *Dictyocaulus* (see Fig. 12-26). Unfortunately, however, the larvae of *Muellerius* cannot be reliably distinguished from those of *Parelaphostrongylus* (see below). *Muellerius* is nonpathogenic at the levels of infection usually encountered in nature and agriculture.

Parelaphostrongylus

Parelaphostrongylus tenuis is normally a parasite of the meninges of the white-tailed deer, *Odocoileus virginianus*, in which species it rarely if ever causes disease. In abnormal hosts such as sheep, goats, moose, caribou, reindeer, wapiti, and mule deer, however, *P. tenuis* tends to invade the nervous tissue proper, causing serious or fatal neurological disease (Mayhew *et al.*, 1976).

METASTRONGYLOID PARASITES OF CARNIVORANS

The wild carnivorans of North America host a rich and diverse array of metastrongyloid nematodes, some of which may be communicated to domesticated dogs and cats

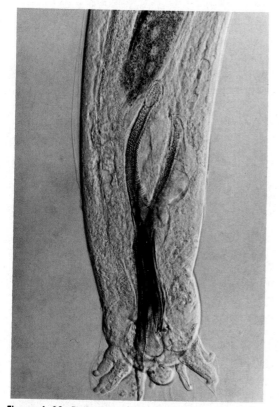

Figure 6–32. *Protostrongylus rufescens,* bursa and spicules of male (x168).

from time to time. Of these, a few have become well established as endemic parasites of the dog and cat. Most metastrongyloid nematodes require a molluscan or annelid intermediate host for development of the infective third stage larvae. This is true of *Aelurostrongylus abstrusus*, a rather common parasite of rural cats, and of the fox lungworm *Crenosoma vulpis*, which also infects dogs occasionally. *Filaroides osleri* and *F. hirthi* present two important exceptions to this rule; larvated eggs in the uteri of these parasites are infective when fed experimentally to dogs. Thus, *F. osleri* and *F. hirthi* are nearly unique among parasites of domestic animals in not requiring a period of development outside the definitive host or in the body of an intermediate host before reaching the infective stage. *Ollulanus tricuspis*, a rare trichostrongylid parasite of cats and pigs, and *Probstmayria vivipara*, the lesser equine pinworm, are the only other nematode parasites of domestic animals that have this capability.

FAMILY CRENOSOMATIDAE

Identification. Crenosomatids have well-developed bursae with a large dorsal ray, the uterus is amphidelphic with a prominent ovijectoral sphincter, and the cuticle is thrown into crenated folds, especially anteriorly (Fig. 6-34). *Crenosoma vulpis* is less than 16 mm. long and is found in the bronchi and bronchioles of foxes (*Vulpes fulva*), wolves (*Canis lupus*), raccoons (*Procyon lotor*), and dogs. *Troglostrongylus* spp. are parasites of Felidae.

Life History. The *ovoviviparous* females deposit first stage larvae or thin-shelled eggs containing first stage larvae. These ascend the trachea and descend the alimentary tract to exit in the host's feces and develop into infective third stage larvae in snails and slugs. The definitive host becomes infected by ingesting infected molluscs; the prepatent period is 19 days (Wetzel, 1940).

FAMILY ANGIOSTRONGYLIDAE

The angiostrongylid bursa may be somewhat reduced but the rays conform to the typical strongylid pattern and are well defined; the vulva is near the anus and the uterus is prodelphic. Aelurostrongylus abstrusus is a parasite of the lung parenchyma of cats, *Gurltia paralysans* is a parasite of the leptomeningeal veins of South American cats, and *Angiostrongylus* spp. are parasites of the lungs and blood vessels of canids and rodents.

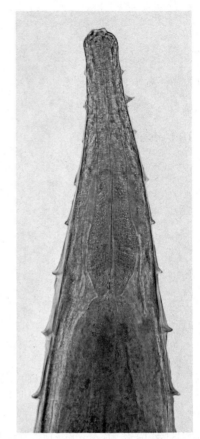

Figure 6–34. *Crenosoma* sp. from the lung of a bear (x250).

Aelurostrongylus abstrusus

Life History. The *oviparous* female of *Aelurostrongylus abstrusus* deposits unsegmented eggs in "nests" in the lung parenchyma; these appear as small, grayish-white subpleural nodules. In histological sections or squash preparations of such nodules (Fig. 14-70), all degrees of development from one-celled eggs to hatched first stage larvae are in evidence. The first stage larvae are carried up the tracheobronchial tree and swallowed, and appear in the cat's feces (see Fig. 12-20). These larvae are very active and are readily demonstrated by the Baermann technique. Further development occurs only if these first stage larvae enter any of a wide variety of snails and slugs (Hobmaier and Hobmaier, 1935; Blaisdell, 1952). Two molts without cuticle shedding occur in the mollusc's foot tissues so that the infective larvae, which develop in two to five weeks, are enclosed in two sheaths. Cats may be infected experimentally by feeding them snails containing third stage larvae but the natural mode of infection is probably through predation of paratenic hosts that normally eat snails. Mice and possibly birds may serve as paratenic hosts; the third stage larvae merely encyst in their tissues and undergo no further development until they are ingested by a cat. Larvae appear in the cat's feces five to six weeks after infection.

Importance. Many cases of *A. abstrusus* infection are free of clinical signs but coughing and anorexia may be associated with moderate infections. Severe infections are manifested by cough, dyspnea, and polypnea; these may terminate fatally (Blaisdell, 1952).

FAMILY FILAROIDIDAE

Identification. The bursal lobes are reduced to mere papillae, the spicules are short and arcuate; the vulva is preanal, and the uterus is prodelphic; the body cuticle is inflated to form a diaphanous teguminal sheath (Fig. 6-31). Do not confuse the family Filaroididae with the very distantly related superfamily Filarioidea.

Life History. The *ovoviviparous* females deposit delicate, thin-shelled eggs containing first stage larvae that hatch before being voided in the host's feces. Unlike other metastrongyloids, most or all of which require a molluscan or annelid intermediate to develop

into the infective third larval stage, *Filaroides* spp. are directly infective as first stage larva, and development through all five stages is completed in the lung tissue of the dog. Infection is acquired through the ingestion of regurgitated stomach contents, lung tissue, or feces of infected dogs.

Adult *F. osleri* worms occur in nodules in the trachea and bronchi of dogs and certain wild canids such as the Australian dingo (Fig. 6-35). The first clue to the transmission of *F. osleri* was reported by Urquhart and colleagues (1954), who isolated 300 larvae from feces, fed them to a six week old pup, and then sacrificed the pup (prematurely, as will be seen) at 60 days after infection. Although they found only one worm with developing eggs immediately exterior to a tracheal cartilage, they correctly concluded that the life history was direct. Later, John Dorrington, a South African veterinary practitioner, reported success in transmitting *F. osleri* infection to dogs by feeding them first stage larvae obtained from female worms (Dorrington, 1968). Like so many original observations in science, these reports were credited by very few parasitologists, so firm was the belief that all metastrongyloids must develop to the infective stage in an intermediate host. However, the infectivity of first stage *F. osleri* larvae for dogs was eventually confirmed by

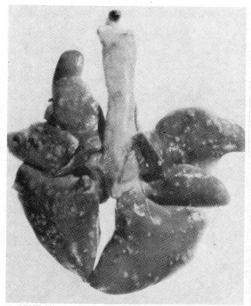
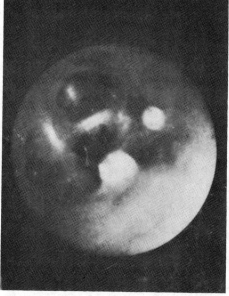

Figure 6–35. Lesions of *Filaroides* spp. At left, the lung of a dog with *Filaroides hirthi* infection. Foci of inflammatory reaction to dead and dying worms are scattered over the lungs. Live *F. hirthi* worms excite little if any tissue reaction and, because they are so very small, are scarcely visible to the unaided eye. At right, early *F. osleri* nodules near the tracheal bifurcation of a dog photographed through a fiberoptic endoscope by Dr. James Zimmer.

other investigators (Dunsmore and Spratt, 1976; Polley and Creighton, 1977) and demonstrated to hold true for *F. hirthi* as well (Georgi, 1976a). It has been postulated that transmission of *F. osleri* occurs directly from parent dingoes to their pups during the period of regurgitative feeding (Dunsmore and Spratt, 1976) and from bitches to their pups by salivary contamination during licking (Dorrington, 1968).

Filaroides hirthi, like *F. osleri*, is infective in the first larval stage and requires no period of development outside the host (Georgi, 1976a). Transmission has been shown to occur among cagemate puppies through the ingestion of first stage larvae in freshly passed feces, and it has been hypothesized that transmission from brood bitches to their litters occurs by the same mechanism after the fourth or fifth week of the nursing period (Georgi *et al.*, 1979a). First stage larvae arrive in the lungs as early as six hours after oral infection, traveling by way of the hepatic portal circulation, the mesenteric lymphatic drainage, or both. Molts occur at one, two, six, and nine days in the lung tissue, and larvae can be demonstrated in the feces by zinc sulfate flotation (S.G. 1.18) at 32 to 35 days after infection (Georgi *et al.*, 1977; Georgi *et al.*, 1979b).

Importance. *Filaroides osleri* infection develops slowly. Nodule formation can be detected with the bronchoscope at about two months and larvae can first be demonstrated in the feces by zinc sulfate flotation (S.G. 1.18) at six to seven months after experimental feeding of larvae (see Fig. 12-8). Milks (1916) summarized the clinical signs manifested by his three cases of *F. osleri* infection as follows:

The only common symptom . . . was the spasmodic attack of a hard, dry cough which could be started by exercise or exposure to cold air. These attacks could not be started by pressure upon the larynx as in most cases of bronchitis. The dogs would cough several times and finally retch after which the attack would usually cease . . . the disease runs a very chronic course and does not materially interfere with the health of the animal until the knots become so numerous as to seriously obstruct the air passages.

Filaroides osleri displays rather low prevalence in spite of its worldwide distribution; it tends to become entrenched in breeding stock and resists all efforts to expel it. The presence of *F. osleri* destroys a kennel's reputation.

Filaroides hirthi is important because the lesions it induces in the lungs of dogs used in toxicological research interfere with the interpretation of experiments (Fig. 6-35; see Figs. 14-71 and 14-72). In 1973, Hirth and Hottendorf described pathological changes in commercially reared beagle dogs that were associated with *F. hirthi*. The presence of these minute lungworms in the alveoli and bronchioles evoked a focal granulomatous reaction and other pulmonary changes, including some that resembled drug-induced and neoplastic lesions. As Hirth as indicated more recently, "It is possible that some reports of toxic and carcinogenic effects of test substances in Beagle dogs may have been based on false interpretation of the lesions caused by this lungworm" (Hirth, 1977). Usually, *F. hirthi* infection is not attended by clinical signs of disease, and antemortem diagnosis is based on demonstrating first stage larvae in the feces (see Fig. 12-8), although very severe infections may be suspected from radiographic changes (Rendano *et al.*, 1979). However, fatal cases of hyperinfection with this parasite have developed in severely stressed and immune deficient animals (Craig *et al.*, 1978; August *et al.*, 1980). Several cases have come to my attention of fatal *F. hirthi* hyperinfection in dogs experimentlly maintained on corticosteroids for long periods. However, because all of these have occurred in commercial pharmaceutical laboratories observing strict proprietary secrecy, the particulars are not available.

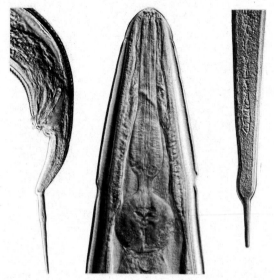

Figure 6–36. *Passalurus ambiguus* tail of male (left), stomal end (center), and tail of female (right) (×168).

Order Oxyurida

Although the order Oxyurida is named for *Oxyuris equi*, the common and unusually large pinworm of the horse, most pinworms are very much smaller than *O. equi*. The oxyurid esophagus has a more or less spherical bulb immediately anterior to its junction with the intestine; this bulb often has a valve in its lumen (Fig. 6-36). One or both sexes have a long, tapering tail and it is for this that they are called pinworms. All oxyurids are highly host-specific parasites of the large intestine.

Enterobius vermicularis

This small (up to 13 mm. long) pinworm of man and great apes still enjoys an extensive distribution among civilized man despite cooking and washing, the nemeses of many of his other parasites (see Fig 13-16). Infection rates vary up to 40 per cent, depending on age and race. White elementary school children display the greatest intensity and prevalence of infection. The gravid *E. vermicularis* female migrates through the anal opening to cement her eggs to the host's perianal skin. The eggs develop to the infective stage within hours and are ready to reinfect the host by contamination of the hands or to infect other individuals by contamination of bedclothing or other fomites, or even by becoming airborne on dust particles. Infection may be suspected in children that suffer from *pruritus ani* and insomnia. Diagnosis is reached by observing the female worm in the act of depositing her eggs on the perianal skin or by demonstrating the eggs. This can be accomplished by momentarily pressing the adhesive side of a piece of cellophane tape against the anus and then sticking the tape to a slide to prepare it for microscopic examination. The important practical point for veterinarians is that *Enterobius vermicularis* is a parasite of man and apes (apes have other species of *Enterobius* as well), but never of dogs or cats. Occasionally, a physician prescribes euthanasia of the family pet to help control pinworms. The finest tact is required in dealing with such a situation.

Oxyuris equi

Severe infection with third and fourth stage *Oxyuris equi* (Fig. 6-37) may produce significant inflammation of the cecal and colonic mucosa manifested by vague signs of abdominal discomfort. However, the most

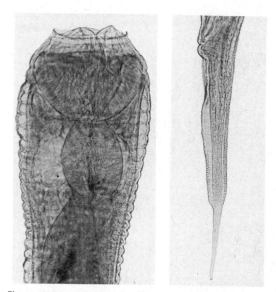

Figure 6–37. *Oxyuris equi* fourth stage larva. At left, the anterior end shows the temporary buccal capsule-like modification of the esophageal corpus that permits attachment to the mucous membrane and at right, the tail (x168).

common affliction perpetrated by *O. equi* on the horse is *pruritus ani* caused by the adhesive egg masses deposited on the perianal skin by the female worm. In its efforts to relieve the itching, the horse will persistently rub its tail against posts, mangers, and the like until the tail head becomes disheveled, bare of hair, or even scarified.

Adult *O. equi* (Fig. 6-38) are found princi-

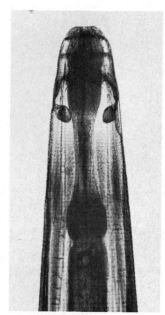

Figure 6–38. *Oxyuris equi* anterior end showing the esophageal bulb (x25).

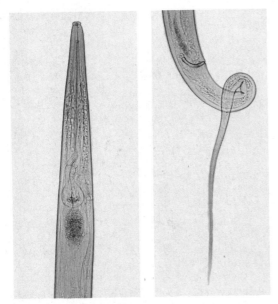

Figure 6-39. *Probstmayria vivipara* adult male anterior end (left) and tail (right) (x108).

containing 8,000 to 60,000 eggs. The eggs develop to the infective stage in four or five days, during which the cementing fluid dries, cracks, and detaches from the skin in flakes. These flakes, which contain large numbers of infective eggs, adhere to mangers, water buckets, walls, and the like, thus contaminating the environment of the stable.

Probstmayria vivipara

This tiny (less than 3 mm. long) pinworm gives birth to infective larvae and is therefore capable of completing its life history within the confines of its host's large intestine (Fig. 6-39).

Skrjabinema

Skrjabinema ovis and *S. caprae*, harmless parasites of sheep and goats, respectively, are 8 to 10 mm. long. The genus name is pronounced ''Skreeyabinema.''

pally in the small colon, although occasional specimens may be found in the large colon. Instead of simply discharging her eggs in the fecal stream, the gravid female *O. equi* migrates down the colon and rectum and out through the anus to cement her eggs in masses to the skin of the anus and its immediate surroundings. These egg masses consist of a tenacious yellowish-gray fluid

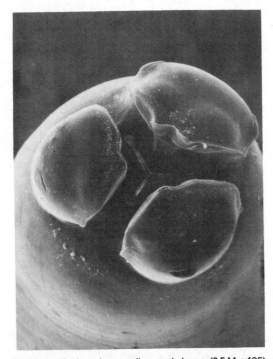

Figure 6-40. *Ascaris suum* lips and stoma (S.E.M. x125).

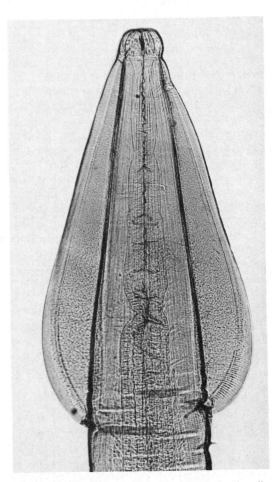

Figure 6-41. *Toxocara cati* stomal end showing the broad cervical alae (x40).

Order Ascaridida

MORPHOLOGY

Ascarids are among the largest and most familiar of nematode parasites infecting domestic animals. The mouth is surrounded by three fleshy lips, one dorsal and two subventral (Fig. 6-40), and the tail of the male is usually curved ventrally. Some genera have lateral cervical alae that make the anterior end of the worm somewhat resemble an arrowhead; hence such generic names as *Toxocara* and *Toxascaris* (Fig. 6-41). Fortunately for the purposes of practical identification, adult ascarids are quite host specific. Thus, *Ascaris suum* infects swine, *Parascaris equorum* infects horses, *Toxocara vitulorum* infects cattle, *T. canis* infects dogs, and *T. cati* infects cats. Dogs and cats also share a second ascarid, *Toxascaris leonina*, which must be distinguished from their respective species of *Toxocara* (see page 268).

Ascarid eggs are relatively thick-walled, contain a single cell when passed in the feces, and are usually sufficiently distinctive to permit identification of the species (see Figs. 12-6, 12-20, 12-32, and 12-34).

LIFE HISTORIES OF ASCARIDS

Development to the infective stage differs only in detail for the various ascarid genera. The single cell develops into an infective larva (Fig. 6-42) inside the egg shell within several days or weeks, depending on the species of worm and the ambient tempera-ture. The infective stage has long been believed to be the second larval stage but recent studies indicate that infectivity is not reached until development has proceeded to the third larval stage. Fortunately, the practical consequences of this controversy are far less important than its theoretical ramifications, so I will simply beg the issue and refer to infective eggs as such without specifying the developmental stage of the larva inside. Ascarid eggs are remarkably resistant to chemical and physical insults, especially after they have arrived at the infective stage. *The single most important fact to remember in relationship to the epidemiology of ascariasis is that the eggs remain infective in soil for many years.* Various ascarid genera display remarkable differences in patterns of intrahost development.

Toxascaris

The simplest form of ascarid life history is displayed by *Toxascaris leonina*, a parasite of canids and felids. The egg of *T. leonina* develops rapidly, usually reaching the infective stage in about one week. When the infective egg is ingested by a suitable definitive host, it hatches in the stomach and the larva invades the mucosa of the small intestine, where it develops and molts before returning to the lumen of the intestine to mature. If the egg is ingested by a rodent or other "unsuitable" animal, the larva hatches and invades the wall of the intestine, where it remains for about a week, but then proceeds to other tissues, where it encysts and remains arrested in the infective stage. Cats and dogs can thus acquire *T. leonina* infection by ingesting infective eggs or rodents with infective larvae encysted in their tissues. These relationships are presented diagrammatically in Figure 6-43.

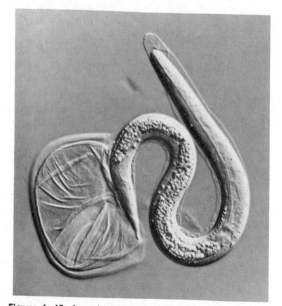

Figure 6–42. *Ascaris suum* mechanically hatched infective larva with retained cuticle of previous stage (x520).

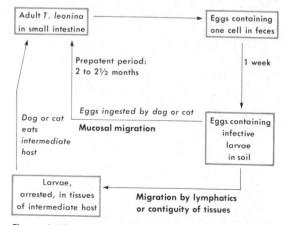

Figure 6–43. Alternative life histories of *Toxascaris leonina*.

Ascaris and Parascaris

Ascaris suum is a ubiquitous and pathogenic parasite of swine. Long considered to be a variety of the morphologically indistinguishable human ascarid *A. lumbricoides*, *A. suum* is considered a distinct species by most contemporary authors. However, *A. lumbricoides* can mature in swine and *A. suum* can mature in man. Although the eggs of both species will hatch and their larvae will migrate extensively in a wide range of hosts, the infective egg in polluted soil or stuck to the mammary skin of the sow is the key element in the epidemiology of *Ascaris* infection. The infective egg hatches in the stomach and small intestine, releasing the larva which enters the wall of the intestine and proceeds to the liver, arriving there in a matter of hours, by way of the portal vein. After tunneling about in the liver for several days, the larva arrives in a pulmonary capillary by way of the caudal vena cava, heart, and pulmonary artery. At this point, the larva either may remain in the circulation to be carried to the somatic tissues or may lodge temporarily in the pulmonary capillary and then break out into an alveolus. In the case of *A. suum*, the latter course appears to be much more probable because the larva will typically proceed up the bronchial tree and trachea to the pharynx, there to be swallowed, and will arrive once again in the small intestine, where it will mature. The pathogenetic consequences of this larval itinerary are considered in Chapter 10.

Parascaris equorum, the very large ascarid parasite of the horse, resembles *Ascaris suum* both epidemiologically and with respect to the route adopted by its larvae in migrating through the tissues. The durable infective egg is the key element in epidemiology of *P. equorum* infection. These eggs accumulate as an ever-increasing reservoir of infection in polluted soils and they stick by their sticky shell coats to the teats and udder of the brood mare and wait there for the foal to be born. *Parascaris equorum* is considered at greater length in Chapter 9.

Toxocara

Toxocara canis. The adolescent wanderings of nematode larvae are influenced not only by their intrinsic capabilities for penetrating tissues and responding to various chemical and physical stimuli but also by the suitability of the host invaded. If a *Toxocara canis* egg hatches in a dog's stomach, the larva invades the bowel wall and arrives in a pulmonary capillary by the same route outlined above for *Ascaris suum*. Unlike *A. suum*, however, the *T. canis* larva is considerably more prone to remain in the circulation than to break into the alveolus, especially if its host is a mature dog. If the larva fails to enter the alveolus, it will be returned to the heart by the pulmonary veins and carried away by the systemic circulation, perhaps to lodge in a kidney or some other somatic tissue where it will encyst as an arrested infective larva. The direction taken at the alveolus is crucial in determining whether the larva will undergo a *tracheal migration* and develop to sexual maturity or a *somatic migration* to remain arrested as an infective larva in that particular dog. The probability of tracheal migration is high in a newborn puppy but by the time the pup is one or two months old, the probability that a newly hatched *T. canis* larva will develop into an adult ascarid *in that particular pup* has fallen to a very low level and remains so indefinitely. During the same period of the pup's life, the probability of somatic migration progressively increases and arrested infective larvae accumulate in the tissues.

Somatic migration also accounts for the accumulation of arrested infective *T. canis* larvae in the tissues of a wide range of other paratenic intermediate hosts, including rodents, sheep, pig, monkey, man, and earthworm. If a mouse with arrested infective larvae in its tissues is eaten by a dog, somatic migration is not observed and, in some instances at least, development proceeds to maturity in the alimentary tract (Sprent, 1958); the mouse has not only saved the larvae but apparently changed them too. Migration and encystment in paratenic hosts and exploitation of the prey-predator relationship is an epidemiological norm for carnivoran ascarids in general. *Toxocara cati* and *Toxascaris leonina* can both be transmitted in this manner, as can ascarid parasites of certain wild carnivorans such as *Baylisascaris procyonis* of the raccoon *Procyon lotor*. *Baylisascaris* larvae grow larger as they migrate and tend to invade the central nervous system of intermediate hosts. These properties render them very pathogenic to woodchucks, rabbits, ground squirrels, chickens, partridges, pigeons, and man (Roth *et al.*, 1982; Kazacos, 1983).

As important as infected intermediate hosts may be to the epidemiology of carnivoran ascarids, the most important arrested *T. canis* larvae are those to be found in the

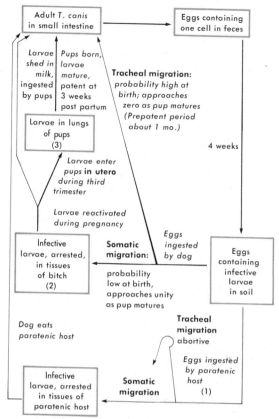

Figure 6–44. Alternative life histories of *Toxocara canis.*
(1) A *paratenic host* is any in which a larval parasite may survive and remain infective for its definitive host without undergoing development. Any of a wide range of animal species including rodents, sheep, pig, monkey, man, earthworm, and adult dog may serve as paratenic host for *T. canis* larvae. (2) Arrested infective larvae are also found in the tissues of male dogs but these are supposed to be of little if any epidemiological importance. (3) The larvae that have entered the pups through the placenta molt once in the fetuses but defer further development until after birth (Sprent, 1958).

tissues of the female of the definitive host species itself. Transmission of infection from bitch to pups occurs by way of both placenta and mammary gland. During the last trimester of pregnancy, arrested larvae are reactivated and migrate from the tissues of the bitch to the pups in utero (Fülleborn, 1921). After parturition, reactivated larvae are also shed in the milk. The alternative life histories of *T. canis* are summarized in Figure 6-44.

Toxocara cati. The migration patterns of *T. cati* differ qualitatively from those of *T. canis* in that (1) prenatal infection via the placenta does not occur and (2) the probability of tracheal migration in egg infections remains high throughout the cat's life. Neonatal infection via the mammary glands is an important route of infection in kittens (Swerczek *et al.*, 1971), and infected paratenic hosts

unquestionably represent an important reservoir of infection for adult cats, at least those with well-developed predatory habits. In both of these latter cases, the infective larvae adopt a much more conservative migration pattern than when they first hatched. Migration and arrested development in the paratenic host appear in some way to satisfy the larval wanderlust and, although a small proportion of the larvae may wander as before, the majority develop to maturity after a sojourn in the wall of the stomach (i.e., a *mucosal migration;* Sprent, 1956).

It follows from these considerations that somatic migration with accumulation of arrested larvae of *T. cati* in the tissues of cats must occur only, or at least principally, in egg infections. Because cats ordinarily display little tendency to ingest feces or soil, many authors have discounted the significance of egg infections in the epidemiology of *T. cati.* However, when one reflects on the perpetual self-grooming that cats indulge in, it is plain enough how infective *T. cati* eggs might be conveyed to their stomachs from time to time. The alternative life histories of *T. cati* are summarized diagrammatically in Figure 6-45.

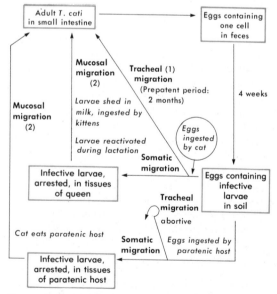

Figure 6–45. Alternative life histories of *Toxocara cati.*
(1) The probability that ingestion of infective eggs will lead to patent infection remains substantial throughout the life of the cat. (2) Larvae that have already undergone somatic migration in a paratenic host, including the queen, satisfy their histotrophic requirements with a mucosal migration (Sprent, 1956; Swerczek *et al.*, 1971). The relative epidemiological importance of these alternatives will depend on the kind of environment, the abundance of suitable paratenic hosts, and the sex and habits of the cats.

IMPORTANCE

Adult Ascarids

Heavy infection with adult ascarids causes moderate enteritis and subnormal growth through interference with digestion and absorption of nutrients. Ascaridosis produces a malnourished, undersized, sickly individual with little stamina and reduced resistance to disease; its haircoat is dull, its skin dry and leathery, and its abdomen too large for its frame. It is not unusual to find a half pailful of *P. equorum* in the small intestine of a foal, a sufficient mass of parasites to actually compete with the host for nutrients. Occasionally, adult *P. equorum* perforate the bowel wall and cause fatal peritonitis.

Heavy prenatal *Toxocara canis* infections cause severe abdominal discomfort in nursling pups. The pups whimper and shriek almost continuously and adopt a peculiar straddle-legged posture of the hind limbs when standing or walking. Alarming numbers of immature and adult worms may appear in the feces or vomitus. Death may result from rupture or obstruction of the intestine as the ascarids, reacting to some irritant, thrash about and become tangled into knots. Obstruction of the bile or pancreatic duct occasionally provides prize exhibits for pathology museums.

Larval Ascarids

In their migrations through various tissues, ascarid larvae at first inflict only mechanical damage, but hypersensitivity rapidly develops and allergic inflammation with eosinophilic inflammation characterizes the host reaction to subsequent invasions. In pig livers, the inflammation heals by fibrosis, giving rise to the so-called *milk spot* lesions that cause the organ to be condemned by meat inspectors as unfit for human consumption. Contrary to the teachings of histologists who argue that because the interlobular septa appear formidable under the microscope, pig liver must necessarily be tough, pig liver is in fact very tender, and the losses caused by *Ascaris suum* larvae must be measured in gastronomic as well as economic terms.

The lesions of early migrations in the lungs are likewise mechanical in nature and, once again, the initial focal hemorrhages are followed by hyperemia, edema, and eosinophilic infiltration as hypersensitivity develops. In young pigs, extensive lung lesions give rise to severe respiratory embarrassment. Breathing is rapid, shallow, and marked by audible expiratory efforts ("thumps") and coughing; pigs may die.

Human Toxocarosis (Visceral Larva Migrans). The widespread distribution of dog feces and the prevalence of *T. canis* eggs therein led Fülleborn (1921) to wonder about the pathological significance in man of nodules containing larvae of this parasite. These nodules occurred principally in the liver, lungs, kidneys, and brain. Beaver and colleagues (1952) recognized the etiological role of *T. canis* larvae in cases of sustained eosinophilia (above 50 per cent), pneumonitis, and hepatomegaly in children under three years of age and dubbed the conditon "visceral larva migrans." As a horrible sequela occurring at 3 to 13 years, the larvae may produce granulomatous retinitis. Misdiagnosis of *T. canis*-induced granulomatous retinitis as retinoblastoma has prompted the unnecessary enucleation of children's eyes in at least 36 reported cases.

The typical epidemiological situation involves a toddler eating soil that is heavily contaminated with infective *T. canis* eggs. Such soil is likely to be found wherever dogs habitually defecate and, in particularly high concentration, in the nests of maternal bitches and their litters. The soil of public parks in cities tends to be heavily contaminated with infective *T. canis* egs (Woodruff and Burg, 1973; Dubin *et al.*, 1975). Dirt eating is often considered to be a manifestation of depraved appetite (i.e., pica) resulting from dietary deficiency or emotional insecurity, but reliance should not be placed on even well-nourished, well-adjusted babies forgoing whatever delicacies may be at hand. Children must not be allowed to play where dogs habitually defecate and dog feces must never be used to fertilize vegetable gardens. Because ascarid eggs remain infective in soils for years, *T. canis* contamination and the hazard of visceral larva migrans tends to be cumulative. *Toxocara cati* is only somewhat less important than *T. canis* as a cause of human visceral larva migrans, and cases have been reported of infection of children with adult *T. cati* (Wiseman and Lovel, 1969; Van Reyn *et al.*, 1978). The veterinary profession has a clear responsibility to identify and eliminate *T. canis* and *T. cati* infection at every opportunity, and to provide the public with objective scientific information regarding the epidemiology and prevention of human toxocarosis. Pet raccoons and their ascarids have recently been shown to cause a particularly serious form of human visceral larva migrans (Kazacos, 1983).

Order Spirurida

The order Spirurida contains two suborders: Camallanina and Spirurina. Members of both suborders require either an insect or a crustacean intermediate host for development to the infective stage. The definitive host acquires spirurid infection by ingesting infected arthropods or paratenic hosts that have fed on such arthropods.

SUBORDER CAMALLANINA

Dracunculus

The suborder Camallanina contains only one genus of veterinary significance, *Drancululus*, a parasite of the subcutaneous tissues of carnivorans and man (Fig. 6-46). The female *Dracunculus* is very large (up to 120 cm.) and the male is smaller (up to 40 mm.). When a female has been fertilized, the anus and vulva atrophy and a shallow ulcer forms in the host's skin at the location of the anterior end of the worm. When water wets this ulcer, the female projects her body and prolapses a length of uterus, which then bursts to discharge a horde of larvae (Fig. 6-47). Then she retires to await the next wetting. A primitive technique for extracting *Dracunculus* consists of wetting the ulcer to lure the worm out far enough to grasp it and then winding it up on a stick a little at a time. The winding takes days because if the worm is broken in the process, a severe reaction may develop. Surgical excision is the modern treatment of choice. If they are ingested by a copepod of the genus *Cyclops*, the larvae that are discharged into the water develop to the infective third larval stage in about three weeks. The definitive host becomes infected by ingesting these *Cyclops* in the drinking water. Two species of *Dracunculus* are *D. medinensis*, a parasite of man in the Middle East and India, and *D. insignis*, a parasite of

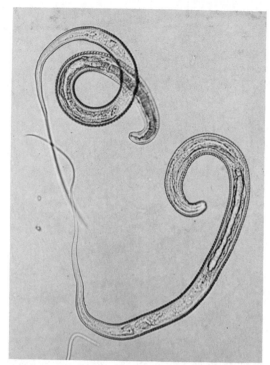

Figure 6–47. *Dracunculus insignis* first stage larvae (x250).

the raccoons and other carnivorans, including the dog and cat, in North America.

SUBORDER SPIRURINA

The suborder Spirurina contains ten superfamilies, of which six are of interest as parasites of domestic animals. The stoma and surrounding structures of spirurins are distinctive; comparison of specimens with the illustrations of this section should suffice for generic identification.

SUPERFAMILY GNATHOSTOMATOIDEA

Gnathostoma has a doughnut-shaped collar of spines surrounding its oral opening (Fig. 6-48). Adult specimens are found in cystic nodules in the stomach walls of wild and domestic carnivorans. Eggs are passed in the one- to two-cell stage and develop to the second larval stage in water. These larvae hatch and develop to the infective third stage only if ingested by copepods (*Cyclops*). A variety of amphibians, snakes, and fishes may serve as paratenic hosts and convey the gnathostome from the copepod to the definitive host. The migrations of gnathostome larvae in the liver and other organs of the definitive host are destructive. The cystic

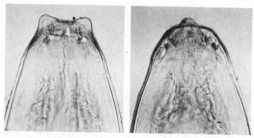

Figure 6–46. *Dracunculus insignis* from the axillary connective tissue of a dog. At left is the lateral aspect of the stomal end and at right the dorsoventral aspect (x150).

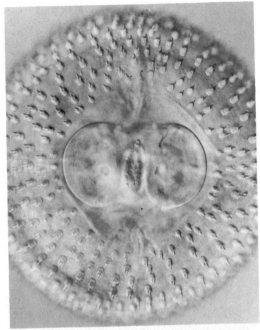

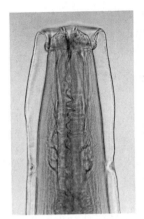
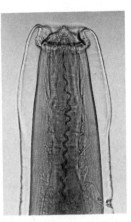

Figure 6–49. *Physaloptera* sp. At left the dorsoventral and at right the lateral aspects of the anterior extremity (x100).

tive stage in various coprophagous beetles. The mouth is flanked by *pseudolabia* and surrounded by a cuticular collar (Figs. 6-49 and 6-50).

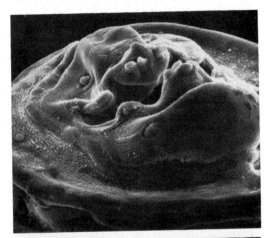

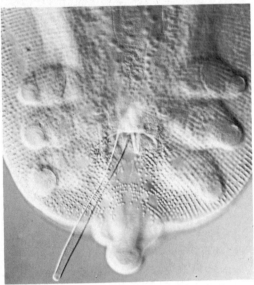

Figure 6–48. *Gnathostoma* stomal end (upper) and caudal extremity of male (lower) (x140).

nodules housing adult *G. spinigerum* may break open into the peritoneal cavity with fatal outcome. Larvae of *G. spinigerum* ingested by human beings tend to wander aimlessly without maturing.

SUPERFAMILY PHYSALOPTEROIDEA

Physaloptera spp. are parasites of the stomach of carnivorans. The female worm lays thick-walled eggs that develop to the infec-

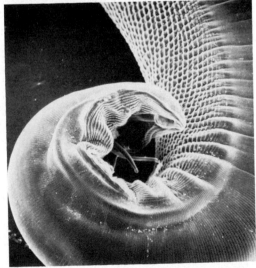

Figure 6–50. *Physaloptera* sp. stoma (upper, x400) and caudal extremity of male (lower, x80).

SUPERFAMILY THELAZIOIDEA

Family Pneumospiruridae

Pneumospirurids are parasites of the lungs of wild carnivorans and appear occasionally in domestic dogs and cats. *Pneumospirura* and *Metathelazia* are representative genera.

Family Thelaziidae

Thelazia spp. (see Fig. 6-51) are parasites of the conjunctival sacs of domestic animals. The female worm deposits thin-shelled eggs containing larvae that develop to the infective stage in the face fly *Musca autumnalis*. *Thelazia* spp. apparently do little harm to cattle and horses in North America.

SUPERFAMILY SPIRUROIDEA

Gongylonema (see Fig. 13-26) is covered with wartlike cuticular bosses, especially near the anterior end. *Gongylonema* is usually found woven into a remarkably regular sinusoidal tract in the mucous membrane of the host's esophagus (*G. pulchrum*) or rumen (*G. verrucosum*). Eggs containing first stage larvae are passed on the host's feces and, if ingested by a dung beetle or a cockroach,

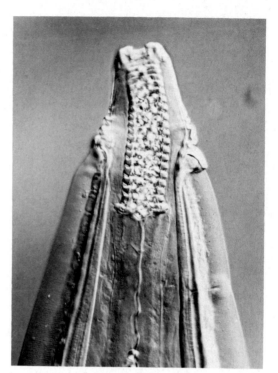

Figure 6–52. *Physocephalus sexalatus* (×168).

develop to the infective stage in about a month. The definitive host becomes infected by ingesting the infected insect. *Gongylonema* spp. are harmless.

Spirocerca lupi is found in fibrous nodules in the wall of the esophagus or stomach (see Figs. 14-80, 14-81 and 14-82). The very small (12 by 30 μm) egg contains a vermiform embryo when shed in the feces (see Figs. 12-6 and 14-83). If ingested by a coprophagous beetle, this vermiform embryo develops into a larva capable of infecting dogs and a broad range of paratenic hosts, including lizards, chickens, and mice. When infective larvae are ingested by a dog, they migrate in the adventitia of the visceral arteries and aorta to the walls of the esophagus and stomach. Some go astray and encyst in ectopic locations, but reproductive adults are normally found in cystic nodules that communicate with the lumen of the esophagus or stomach through fistulas. Dysphagia and vomiting, esophageal neoplasia, aortic aneurysm or rupture, and secondary pulmonary osteoarthropathy may be associated with chronic *S. lupi* infection.

Other examples of spiruroids are *Ascarops* and *Physocephalus* (Fig. 6-52), parasites of swine, and *Streptopharagus* (see Fig. 13-16), a parasite of primates.

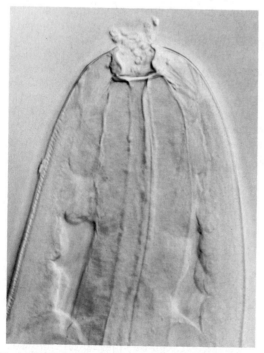

Figure 6–51. *Thelazia* sp. from the conjunctival sac of a horse (×365).

SUPERFAMILY HABRONEMATOIDEA

Draschia megastoma, Habronema muscae, and *H. microstoma* are parasites of the equine stomach, where the adult worms stay remarkably close to the *margo plicatus. Draschia megastoma* is about 13 mm. long and has a funnel shaped buccal cavity, whereas *Habronema* spp. are larger (22 to 25 mm.) and have cylindrical buccal cavities (Fig. 6-53). The left spicule of *H. muscae* is five times as long as the right one, whereas only a twofold disparity exists between the spicules of *H. microstoma. Draschia megastoma* excites the formation by the host of fibrous nodules riddled with intercommunicating galleries filled with a creamy puslike material in which the worms live. *Habronema* spp. are not associated with nodules. Larvae hatch from the tiny eggs (see Fig. 12-32) soon after they are laid. If ingested by maggots (*Musca domestica* for *D. megastoma* and *H. muscae; Stomoxys calcitrans* for *H. microstoma*), these develop to the infective third stage larvae in a little more than a week. The infective larvae migrate to the head of the fly and collect in the labium. When a fly alights on a warm, wet surface such as the muzzle, ocular conjunctiva, or cutaneous wounds of a horse, the larvae change hosts. Those larvae that are swallowed presumably complete their life histories, whereas those that enter wounds have probably reached an impasse. However, from a veterinary standpoint, these aberrant larvae are extremely important because of the granulomas they induce.

Although *Draschia* and *Habronema* are unimportant as stomach parasites, their larvae are responsible for persistent cutaneous granulomas called cutaneous habronemiasis and a variety of colloquial names ("swamp cancer," "bursatti," "summer sores," "esponja"). These granulomas develop in minor wounds and in areas of skin subjected to more or less continuous wetting. In pastured horses, the skin adjacent to the medial canthus of the eye may be drenched in tears stimulated by the presence of flies and also very attractive to them. Typical cutaneous habronemiasis lesions are characterized by an initial rapid production of granulation tissue that steadfastly refuses to resolve during fly season, by the subsequent appearance of caseocalcareous nodules in this granulation tissue, and by the presence of *Draschia* or *Habronema* larvae. Pruritus is intense and secondary injury may result from the horse's efforts to find relief. Habronemic conjunctivitis usually assumes the form of an ulcerated nodule containing caseocalcareous foci and situated near the medial canthus. Such nodules tend to abrade the cornea and must be removed surgically to prevent or alleviate keratitis (Underwood, 1936).

SUPERFAMILY FILARIOIDEA

Filarioids include some of the most important nematode parasites of man in tropical climates. *Wuchereria bancrofti* and *Brugia malayi* cause the acute lymphangitis and chronic elephantiasis of bancroftian filariasis and *Onchocerca volvulus* causes the ophthalmitis of "river blindness." All filarioids are transmitted by blood-sucking insects in which vermiform embryos called *microfilariae* develop into infective third stage larvae. The microfilariae either circulate in the blood of the definitive host (e.g., *Wuchereria, Brugia, Dirofilaria, Dipetalonema, Setaria*) or accumulate in the dermal connective tissues (e.g., *Onchocerca, Elaeophora*). In either case, the microfilariae are ingested and the infective larvae deposited when the insect feeds on the definitive host.

Dirofilaria

Dirofilaria immitis, the canine heartworm, is by far the most important filarioid parasite of domestic animals in North America. Adults are normally found in the caval veins and right heart. When defunct, they are carried to the lungs, where they occlude the pulmonary arterial branches and produce infarcts. The stoma of these large (up to 30 cm. long), white worms is very plain (Fig. 6-54).

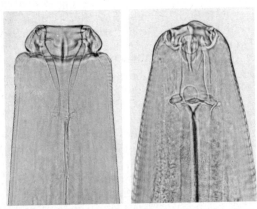

Figure 6–53. *Draschia megastoma* (left, x150) and *Habronema muscae* (right, x250).

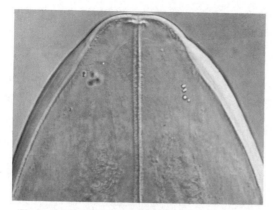

Figure 6–54. *Dirofilaria immitis*, stomal end (x150).

Endemic areas exist in all parts of the United States (Rothstein, 1963). Heartworm infection is particularly common along the Atlantic and Gulf Coasts where salt marsh mosquitoes are prevalent, and in some localities, half the dogs examined will be found to be infected. A lower prevalence is encountered in the Midwest and North Central States. Even Minnesota contains endemic areas.

The life history, as outlined in Figure 6–55, may involve many species of mosquitoes as intermediate hosts. Today, mosquito-borne diseases such as malaria and filarial infections are popularly viewed as tropical diseases but,

not too long ago, malaria came with every summer in the United States. Malaria disappeared when the population density of suitable mosquitoes fell below the level necessary for transmission of the malarial plasmodia. Reduction in mosquitoes came with the drainage of swamps for agricultural purposes, with the construction of roads, and to some extent, with intentional efforts at mosquito abatement. Heartworm manages to remain endemic and even spread in regions where malaria has disappeared, possibly because this parasite is less discriminating in its choice of mosquito hosts. In any case, only when mosquito populations are sufficiently reduced will heartworm disappear.

The six to seven month prepatent period is free of any evidence of infection; the developing and migration worms cause no disturbance. The patent period, when microfilariae (see Fig. 12-40) may be detected in the circulating blood, is the time of clinical illness. In the conventional view, the physiological burden imposed on the host is attributed in part to the physical obstruction of vessels, heart chambers, and valves by the adult worms and in part to the development of a progressive pulmonary endarteritis and obstructive fibrosis leading to pulmonary hypertension and right heart failure (Adcock, 1961). Repeated embolisms of the finer arterial branches by defunct adults with infarction and inflammatory response eventually lead to permanent damage of the vascular bed. However, obstruction of capillaries by microfilariae may also play a part in the pathogenesis of heartworm disease. Jackson and colleagues (1966) found that dogs with no signs of disease harbored an average of 25 worms and that about 50 worms were associated with moderate to severe heartworm disease. In dogs with signs of acute hepatic failure, about 100 worms were concentrated in the venae cavae and right atrium. Dogs with typical heartworm disease fatigue easily, cough, and appear unthrifty. Decompensation of the right heart leads to chronic venous congestion with hepatic cirrhosis and ascites. Pulmonary embolism precipitates acute episodes of respiratory distress during which blood and worms from ruptured vessels may be coughed up. Postcaval occlusion causes sudden collapse followed by death within a few days from acute hepatic insufficiency. A surgical procedure has been devised for relieving the caval occlusion by way of a jugular vein (Jackson *et al.*, 1962, 1977).

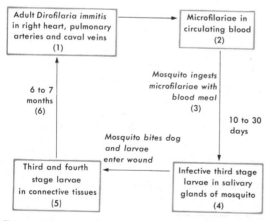

Figure 6–55. Life history of *Dirofilaria immitis*, the canine heartworm. (1) Adult heartworms may survive as long as five years. (2) Microfilariae survive up to two years. (3) About half of the species of North American mosquitoes are possible intermediate hosts but significant vector roles have been demonstrated for only a few. (4) Larval development occurs in the Malpighian tubules, after which infective larvae migrate to the salivary glands of the mosquito. (5) Third and fourth stage larvae remain in the connective tissues for about four months. After the final molt, the immature adults (fifth stage) migrate to the right heart, apparently by way of the venous circulation. (6) After reaching the right heart, the fifth stages mature and start producing microfilariae in two or three months.

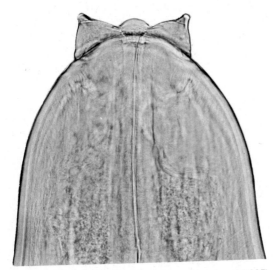

Figure 6–56. *Setaria labiatopapillosa,* stomal end (x225).

Setaria

Setaria labiatopapillosa (Fig. 6-56) and *S. equina* (Fig. 6-57) are large white parasites of the serous membranes of cattle and horses, respectively. Microfilariae of *Setaria* spp. show up on blood smears, and the adult parasites are likely to be encountered during abdominal surgery or on the killing floor or necropsy table. Migrating *Setaria* larvae occasionally invade the central nervous system and cause serious neurological disease, especially when they find themselves in other than their normal host species.

Onchocerca

Onchocerca adults, although large, are likely to escape notice because they are intricately

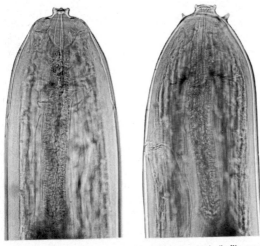

Figure 6–57. *Setaria equina,* dorsoventral (left) and lateral (right) aspects of the stomal end (x50).

woven into connective tissues (e.g., nuchal ligament) and virtually impossible to extricate intact. The microfilariae frequently appear in skin biopsy material (see Fig. 12-41). In a random survey of pastured horses in Tompkins County, New York, eight of 12 horses yielded from one to 3000 *O. cervicalis* microfilariae per biopsy specimen, a piece of skin weighing on the order of 15 mg (Georgi, 1976b). Microfilarial pityriasis, summer mange, equine dhobie itch, and plica polonica are colloquial names for an intensely pruritic dermatitis conventionally ascribed to microfilariae of *Onchocerca cervicalis,* but see "Queensland itch," page 9.

Parafilaria

"Summer Bleeding." "Summer bleeding" is caused by *Parafilaria multipapillosa* in horses and *P. bovicola* in cattle. These parasites live in the subcutaneous and intermuscular connective tissues and, when sexually mature, produce crops of pea sized nodules that bleed through a tiny pore. The blood escapes in fine drops, runs off in streaks along the hairs, and dries in brown crusts. Eggs and microfilariae of *Parafilaria* may be demonstrated in this material but never in samples from the circulation. Active bleeding occurs only during daylight hours and especially when horses are exposed to direct sunshine. Baumann (1946) reported that affected horses would, as a rule, immediately stop bleeding when brought into the stable, only to start again when led back out into the sunshine. He rarely observed bleeding during cool weather. The activity of the lesions observed by Baumann suggests an adaptation on the part of *Parafilaria* to the habits of flies that feed on blood, are active in warm weather, and avoid shade. It has been shown that *P. multipapillosa* develops in the fat body of *Haematobia atripalpis* (Gnedina and Osipov, 1960).

Dipetalonema

Adult specimens of *Dipetalonema* are most likely to be encountered as parasites of the peritoneal cavity of monkeys, in which they are very common (Fig. 6-58). The canine parasite *D. reconditum* has, as its species name suggests, been viewed by few human beings. This is because it is small, usually few in number, and lies inconspicuously in the connective tissues. The microfilariae of *D. reconditum,* on the other hand, are rather commonly seen (see Fig. 12-40). *Dipetalonema*

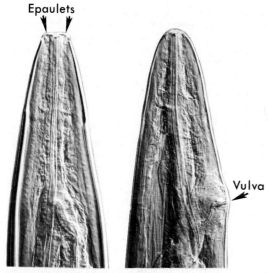

Figure 6–58. *Dipetalonema* sp. from the peritoneal cavity of a monkey. At left the dorsoventral and at right the lateral aspects of the stomal end (x110).

reconditum develops from microfilaria to infective third stage larva in the flea *Ctenocephalides.*

Elaeophora

Microfilariae of *Elaeophora schneideri,* the arterial worm of deer, elk, and domestic sheep, produce patches of moist, exudative dermatitis with crust formation on the polls and faces of sheep sent to summer range above 6000 ft. (1828 meters) in New Mexico, Arizona, and Colorado. Adults, up to 120 mm. long, are found in the carotid, iliac, and mesenteric arteries. Tabanids are cyclodevelopmental hosts.

Stephanofilaria

Adults and microfilariae of *Stephanofilaria stilesi,* a very small (less than 6 mm. long) filariid, are found in dermatitic lesions on the ventral abdomen of cattle. The infective larvae of *S. stilesi* develop in the horn fly *Haematobia irritans.*

CLASS ADENOPHOREA (APHASMIDIA)

Order Enoplida

SUPERFAMILY DIOCTOPHYMATOIDEA

Dioctophyme

Dioctophyme renale, the ''giant kidney worm'' of carnivorans, swine, and sometimes man, is one of the largest species of nematodes. Mink are the principal definitive hosts. The female *D. renale,* which may reach one meter in length and one centimeter in diameter, produces brownish, thick-shelled eggs (68 by 44 μm) with bipolar plugs. Males are somewhat smaller (less than 400 mm.) and have a terminal bell-shaped copulatory bursa and one spicule. The eggs are passed in the urine in the one-cell stage. If ingested by a branchiobdellid oligochaete annelid worm (*Cambaricola*), itself an external parasite or commensal of crayfish (*Cambarus*), *D. renale* larvae develop and pass through three molts. The definitive host is infected by swallowing either the infected annelid or a catfish serving as paratenic host. In the dog, *D. renale* may be found in the pelvis of the right kidney or free in the abdominal cavity; the latter type of infection is nonpatent.

SUPERFAMILY TRICHUROIDEA

The superfamily Trichuroidea contains some very common parasites of domestic animals. Members of this superfamily are distinguished by their *stichosome esophagus,* which consists of a capillary tube surrounded by the bodies of a single file column of gland cells called *stichocytes* (Figs. 6-59 and 6-60). There are five genera of interest: *Trichinella,*

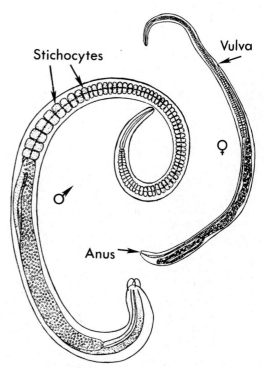

Figure 6–59. *Trichinella spiralis,* not to scale (redrawn from Yorke and Maplestone, 1926).

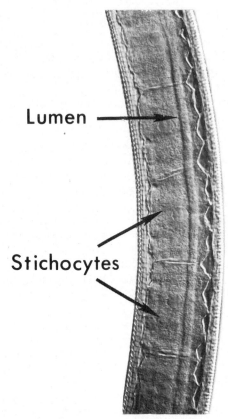

Figure 6–60. A portion of the stichosome esophagus of *Trichuris giraffae* (x168).

Trichuris, Capillaria, Trichosomoides, and *Anatrichosoma.*

Trichinella

Identification. The tiny adults of *Trichinella spiralis* are found embedded in the mucosa of the small intestine of swine, carnivorans, and man. *The male is 1.4 to 1.6 mm. long, lacks spicule or spicular sheath, and presents two small knobs over the cloaca. The female is 3 to 4 mm. long with anus terminal and vulva in midesophageal region; she deposits prelarvae directly into the host's intestinal mucosa* (Fig. 6-59). Males of other trichuroid genera have a single spicule or at least a spicular sheath, which is often spinate (Fig. 6-61), and the females lay eggs with bipolar plugs (see Figs. 12-6, 12-20, and 12-23).

Life History. Predation has provided an efficient channel for the evolutionary development of many parasites. In most instances, the larval parasite lies encysted in the tissues of the prey, and the reproductive adults inhabit the alimentary tract of the predator. The predator becomes infected by eating the prey, and the prey becomes infected by ingesting eggs passed in the feces of the predator. In the unique life history of *Trichinella spiralis,* both adult and larval stages occur in sequence in the same host, the tiny adults lying among the villi of the small intestine, and the larvae curled up in cysts in the striated muscle.

First stage larvae of *T. spiralis,* liberated from their cysts by the digestive enzymes of the host, invade the intestinal mucosa. Both sexes reach maturity about two days after the infected meat is eaten. The male dies after copulation. At five days postinfection, the viviparous females are giving birth to prelarvae (Fig. 6-62), which enter the lymphatics and later the bloodstream to be transported to the muscles (Ali Kahn, 1966). After these prelarvae invade striated muscle cells, they at first lie parallel to the long axes of the fibers and are quite easily overlooked. After two or three weeks they have developed into first stage larvae and roll up in spirals or like pretzels, become enveloped in cysts, and are then infective (see Figs. 12-42 and 14-87). Old cysts containing defunct larvae calcify.

The intestinal (adult) phase of *T. spiralis* infection varies in duration from a little over a week in a dog to three or four months in man. Immunosuppressant therapy, often instituted to ameliorate the tissue reaction to invading larvae, may prolong the lives of the adult female worms. Fortunately, these are accessible to anthelmintic attack. Almost all mammals can be experimentally infected with *T. spiralis,* but only carnivores and om-

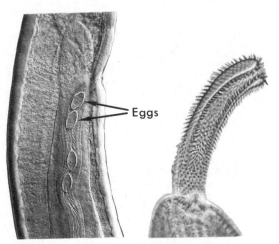

Figure 6–61. *Trichuris discolor* (x84). At left, four eggs are seen in the vagina of a female and at right, the spinate spicular sheath of the male is protruded.

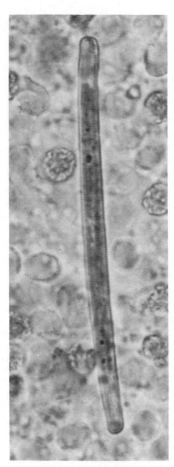

Figure 6–62. *Trichinella spiralis* prelarva demonstrated in the blood of a cat by the Knott technique (x1000).

nivores are likely to become naturally infected. Infection occurs through predation, cannibalism, and carrion feeding; the larvae encysted in muscles are exceptionally resistant to external conditions, including extreme putrefaction. Madsen (1976) considers that *T. spiralis* larvae in the decomposing carcass represent a free-living stage in a special biotope whose function is analogous to that of the species-dispersing, free-living eggs and larvae of other nematodes. Madsen attaches paramount importance to the rotting carcass of carnivores in the epidemiology of *T. spiralis*.

Importance. Human trichinosis usually results from eating raw or undercooked pork, bear, or seal. Properly cooked trichinae are quite harmless, but a sojourn in the oven does not guarantee that the parasites in the center of a large roast will be made more than uncomfortable unless raised to a uniform internal temperature of 77°C. The cut surface of cooked fresh pork should be "white"; any trace of pink demands its return

to the oven or frying pan. Some methods of rapid cooking in microwave ovens do not kill all of the encysted *T. spiralis* at 77°C or even at 82°C, apparently because the meat does not heat uniformly (Kotula *et al.*, 1983). Even roasts that appear to be well-done may contain live larvae when prepared in a microwave oven (Zimmermann, 1983).

Freezing of pork products for several weeks (e.g., at −15°C for 20 days) has long been considered adequate to kill *T. spiralis*. However, this cannot safely be applied to bear strains of the organism, which can withstand storage at −20°C for six months (Worley *et al.*, 1976). In certain countries (e.g., Germany) where the public demands uncooked pork products, meat inspection includes microscopic examination for trichinae in diaphragm muscle squash preparations of every carcass. In the United States, the traditional policy has been instead to persuade the public to cook fresh pork thoroughly and to require manufacturers of "ready-to-eat" products to cook or freeze them according to specifications that assure the destruction of trichinae. The German system works much better; the prevalence of human *T. spiralis* infection in the United States is the highest in the world. This has declined in recent decades, however, possibly owing to an increase in the practice of cooking garbage to be fed to swine, a measure adopted to control vesicular exanthema.

Outbeaks of human clinical trichinosis most often involve small groups of people that have shared uncooked sausage or an undercooked roast from a locally slaughtered pig. However, in one Illinois outbreak, in which 23 of 50 members of an extended Dutch-German family became ill, the source of the *T. spiralis* larvae in the homemade sausage was USDA-inspected pork (Potter *et al.*, 1976). Occasionally, individuals perversely eat completely raw ground meat, a habit more prevalent among beef lovers ("cannibal sandwich") than pork lovers. Neither is safe, however; hamburger often contains a considerable amount of ground pork whether it is supposed to or not. It has been estimated that for man, ingestion of 5 trichina larvae per gram of body weight is fatal, for hogs 10, and for rats 30 (Chandler and Read, 1961). Human trichinosis sufferers may display periorbital edema, myalgia, fever, gastroenteritis, conjunctivitis, pruritus, and skin eruption; eosinophilia usually exceeds 20 per cent.

Clinical trichinosis in domestic animals

may result both from insult inflicted on the intestinal mucosa by the adult worms and from the host's reaction to invasion of skeletal muscles by the larvae. A case of trichinosis in a rural Massachusetts cat caused transient hemorrhagic enteritis, during which adult *Trichinella spiralis* worms were found in the feces and prelarvae were identified in the blood (Fig. 6-62). The phase of muscle invasion was without clinical signs, but eosinophilia persisted for three months (Holzworth and Georgi, 1974). A second case in a three month old kitten is typical of the phase of muscle invasion: the kitten was lying helplessly on its side with limbs extended, showed pain on handling, salivated, breathed superficially, and cried constantly (Hemmert-Halswick and Bugge, 1934). Case reports of trichinosis in dogs and cats are few; one wonders how often it may be overlooked or misdiagnosed.

Trichuris

Identification. The adult body is whip-shaped, the anterior end fine, hairlike, and embedded in the wall of the large intestine; the posterior end stout and lying free in the lumen (Fig. 6-63). The egg is lemon-shaped with a distinct plug at each pole, and contains a single cell when passed in the feces (Fig. 6-61; see Figs. 12-6, 12-20, and 12-23).

Life History. An infective first stage larva develops inside the egg in about one month but does not hatch unless the egg is swallowed by a dog. The infective egg is very resistant, so that dogs in contaminated environments tend to become reinfected after treatment. The prepatent period is two and one-half to three months.

Importance. Most canine whipworm infections are symptomless, but heavy infections cause bouts of diarrhea alternating with periods during which normal stools are passed. The diarrheal feces often contain much mucus and may be flecked with blood. *Trichuris* infection is rare and unimportant in North American cats but interesting for its novelty (Fig. 6-63; see Fig. 12-20). Ruminants and swine are frequently infected but only occasionally made ill by their respective species of *Trichuris*. Individual young cattle with extraordinarily heavy *Trichuris discolor* infections may suffer massive, sometimes fatal hemorrhages into the lumen of the cecum. These cases are rare and other members of the herd are not clinically affected, at least not with *T. discolor*. Perhaps the affected individuals practice peculiar habits that favor ingestion of soil containing *Trichuris* eggs or perhaps they are afflicted with a hemorrhagic diathesis that magnifies the cost of the minor trauma inflicted on the cecal wall by the parasite.

Capillaria

Identification. The adult body is small and although not whip-shaped otherwise somewhat resembles Trichuris and lies partially embedded in mucous membranes (e.g., bronchial, alimentary, vesical) or buried in tissue (e.g., liver) (see Fig. 14-89). The eggs differ from those of *Trichuris* only in detail.

Bronchial Capillariasis. The life history of *Capillaria (Eucoleus) aerophila* may be direct or involve earthworms as facultative intermediate hosts. Infection of dogs and cats is rarely responsible for more than a slight cough, but foxes on fur farms may harbor pathogenic burdens. Hanson (1933) described the disease in foxes as insidious and chronic, characterized by a rattling and wheezy respiration with spells of coughing and weakness, and by poor growth, unthrifty fur, failure to shed properly, and death due to bronchopneumonia in heavy infections. Low grade *C. aerophila* infection is common in cats and dogs; diagnosis is based on identifying the rather plump, often asymmetrical, bipolar eggs in the feces or tracheal mucus (see Fig. 12-20). However, cats and dogs infrequently develop the severe degree of

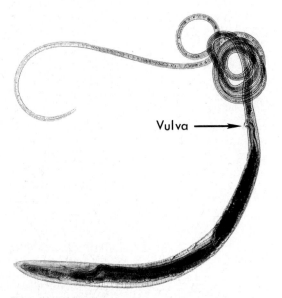

Vulva ⟶

Figure 6–63. *Trichuris* sp. from a cat from Puerto Rico (x11).

infection observed in captive foxes confined to earthen runs.

Urinary Capillariasis. *Capillaria plica* adults weave the anterior portions of their bodies into the mucous membrane of the urinary bladder and other -parts of the urinary tract of dogs, cats, foxes, and wolves. The eggs contain one cell when passed in the urine (see Fig. 12-20). The first stage larva develops in a little over a month but does not hatch unless ingested by an earthworm, which serves as paratenic host. The definitive host becomes infected by eating earthworms that have first stage larvae in their tissues, and eggs first appear in the urine about two months later. Enigk (1950) claimed that *C. plica* infection caused growth impairment in young foxes, but dogs and cats appear to bear their usually modest worm burdens without inconvenience. *Capillaria feliscati* is a parasite of the urinary bladder of the cat and resembles *C. plica* in its biological properties.

Trichosomoides

Trichosomoides crassicauda is a parasite of the urinary bladder of rats. The tiny male *T. crassicauda* lives inside the uterus of its mate (Fig. 6-64). Infection is usually transmitted from mother rats to their offspring prior to weaning.

Anatrichosoma

Anatrichosoma spp. are 25 X 0.2 mm. trichuroids that burrow in the stratified squamous epithelium of the nasal passages of African monkeys. The female worms deposit 76 X 58 μm, bipolar eggs in these burrows. The fully embryonated eggs reach the surface in the normal course of epithelial regeneration and desquamation. Antemortem diagnosis is based on demonstrating the eggs on nasal swabs (see Fig. 12-36). *Anatrichosoma cutaneum* gives rise to subcutaneous nodules and edema about the joints of the extremities and serpiginous blisters of the palms and soles of monkeys.

MISCELLANEOUS WORMS

Thorny-headed worms, leeches, and tongueworms are not related to the nematodes, nor are they related to each other. I have lumped them together here for want of a logical and convenient alternative.

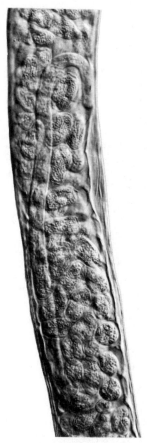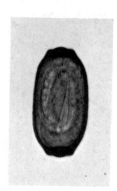

Figure 6–64. *Trichosomoides crassicauda* male in the uterus of a female *T. crassicauda* (left, x168). S. H. Weisbroth, who provided this specimen, has described a Millipore filtration procedure for demonstrating the eggs of *T. crassicauda* (right, x425) in rat urine.

Phylum Acanthocephala

The Acanthocephala, or thorny-headed worms, is a small phylum of highly specialized parasites of the vertebrate digestive tract (Figs. 6-65 and 6-66). The body is normally flattened *in situ* but becomes more or less cylindrical when placed in water, which is the indispensable first step in preparing specimens for identification. The resulting osmotic turgor forces the retractable, spiny attachment organ or *proboscis* out of the body so that the shape and number of spines can be ascertained and the specimen thereby identified (Fig. 6-67). Once the proboscis (and male copulatory bursa) are well protracted, the specimen can be fixed in hot AFA solution (85 parts of 85 per cent ethanol, 10 parts of stock formalin, 5 parts of glacial acetic acid). These technical details are stressed here because, unless specimens are properly

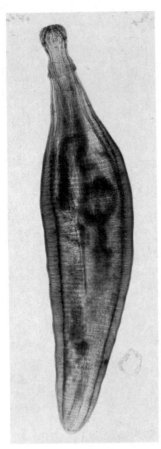

Figure 6–65. *Oncicola* sp. from an Arizona coyote *Canis latrans* (x14). This specimen was provided by Dr. Frances Phillips.

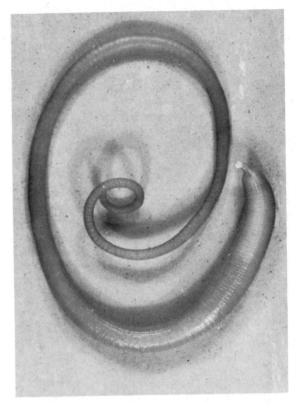

Figure 6–66. *Macracanthorhynchus hirudinaceus* (3/4 natural size).

prepared, even a specialist may not be able to identify them.

Identification. *Acanthocephalans consist of a body and a retractable spiny proboscis by which the parasite attaches itself to the intestinal wall of its host. There is no digestive tract, so that nutrients must be absorbed through the tegument.*

Life History. When the egg is laid, it contains a fully developed larva called an *acanthor* (Fig. 6-68). If the egg is ingested by a suitable arthropod intermediate host, the acanthor develops through an *acanthella* stage (Fig. 6-69) into an encysted infective larva called a *cystacanth* (Fig. 6-70). The cystacanth is capable of re-encysting in a range of vertebrate paratenic hosts should they ingest the infected arthropod. Frequently, the cystacanth even re-encysts in its normal definitive host instead of developing to maturity. For example, *Prosthenorchis elegans* adults may be found in the intestinal lumen of a monkey, and cystacanths of the same parasite may be found encysted in the peritoneal membranes.

Macracanthorhynchus

Macracanthorhynchus hirudinaceus (Fig. 6-66), a large worm by acanthocephalan standards, is a parasite of swine that develops to the acanthor infective stage in May beetles, dung beetles, and water beetles in about three months. Pigs acquire *M. hirudinaceus*

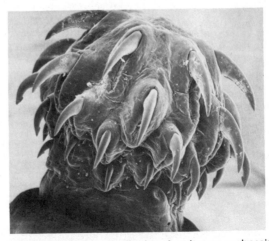

Figure 6–67. *Macracanthorhynchus ingens* proboscis (x125).

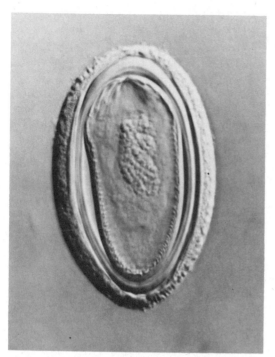

Figure 6–68. *Macracanthorhynchus ingens* egg containing acanthor larva (x660).

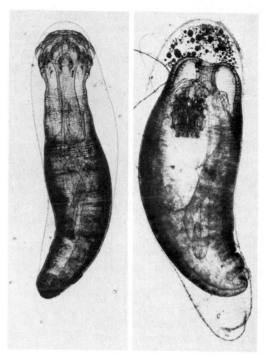

Figure 6–70. *Macracanthorhynchus ingens* cystacanth infective larvae from a *Narceus* millipede (x20).

while rooting for beetle grubs, but the infected adult beetle is also a source of cystacanths. The prepatent period is two to three months. Pigs may display no outward sign of *M. hirudinaceus* infection, or there may be diarrhea and emaciation with evidence of acute abdominal pain, depending on how deeply the proboscis is embedded in the intestinal wall.

Macracanthorhynchus ingens (Fig. 6-67), even larger than *M. hirudinaceus,* is a parasite of the raccoon (*Procyon lotor*) and uses millipedes of the genus *Narceus* as intermediate hosts. These parasites occasionally infect dogs that eat the infected millipedes. To eat a millipede requires extraordinary cunning, frightful taste, great excitement, or utter boredom on the part of the dog because the millipedes give off a potent defensive secretion. The raccoon gets around the secretion problem by rolling the millipede around in the dust before eating it, but few dogs are that clever.

Prosthenorchis

Prosthenorchis spp. are up to 55 mm. long, pink, acanthocephalan parasites of primates. *Prosthenorchis* propagates very successfully in monkey colonies by using cockroaches and certain beetles as intermediate hosts. Monkeys become infected when they eat a cockroach containing the cystacanth larvae of *Prosthenorchis.*

Both chronic and acute disease syndromes have been described for *Prosthenorchis* infection. The chronic course is marked by watery

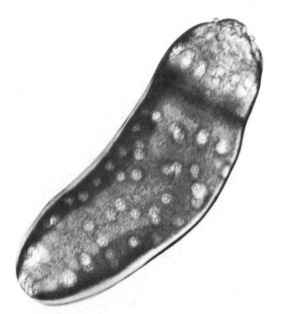

Figure 6–69. *Macracanthorhynchus ingens* acanthella from a *Narceus* millipede (x27).

diarrhea of several months duration with weakness and progressive emaciation. The appetite remains normal until a day or so before death. The acute course is of less than one day's duration and is caused by acute bacterial peritonitis resulting from perforation of the intestinal wall by the proboscis.

Moniliformis

The great length (up to 32 cm.) and pseudosegmentation of the body invite misidentification of this acanthocephalan as a tapeworm. A common parasite of wild rodents, *Moniliformis* uses cockroaches as intermediate hosts.

Oncicola

Oncicola canis (Fig. 6-65), less than 14 mm. long, is a parasite of the dog, coyote, and other canids; it uses the armidillo as paratenic host for cystacanths.

Phylum Annelida
CLASS HIRUDINEA

Leeches are predatory or parasitic worms of the phylum Annelida, which includes the free-living earthworms. Leeches have terminal suckers for locomotion and attachment and move by looping movements like those of an inchworm; they are usually dark or black in color. Bloodsucking species fasten to the skin or oropharyngeal mucous membrane by means of their powerful suckers, pierce the epidermis, and suck blood. A salivary enzyme, hirudin, acts as an anticoagulant and assures a copious flow of blood. In some localities, surface waters abound with bloodsucking leeches that attach to the oropharyngeal or laryngeal mucous membrane when imbibed by the unwary person or animal. Their presence in these locations may cause severe bouts of coughing and choking, during which blood is ejected by the victim. Infection may last several weeks and occasionally causes death. Treatment consists of mechanical removal of the leech.

Phylum Arthropoda

CLASS PENTASTOMIDA

Pentastomids, or "tongueworms," are highly specialized arthropods, as unlikely as

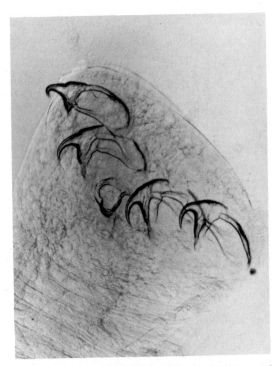

Figure 6–71. Stoma and hooks of a pentastomid nymph from a South American otter (x35).

that may seem. The adult parasites live in the respiratory passages of predacious reptiles, birds, and mammals. Eggs containing four- or six-legged larvae are discharged with the nasal secretions. If ingested by an appropriate intermediate host, usually a member of some species likely to fall prey to the predator in question, these larvae invade the tissues, develop, and encyst in the viscera as nymphs that resemble the adults in all particulars except for mature reproductive organs. The body is annulated and the anterior, subterminal stoma is flanked by two pairs of retractable, hollow fangs or hooks (Fig. 6-71).

Linguatula serrata occurs in the nasal and paranasal sinuses of dogs and cats, where it causes bleeding, catarrhal inflammation, and some impediment to respiration. Cattle, sheep, rabbits, and other animals serve as intermediate hosts; fully developed nymphs, the form infective for carnivorans, are found encysted in the lymph nodes and serous membranes.

REFERENCES

Adcock, J. L. (1961): Pulmonary arterial lesions in canine dirofilariasis. Am. J. Vet. Res., 22 (89), 655-662.

Ali Kahn, Z. (1966): The postembryonic development of *Trichinella spiralis* with special reference to ecdysis. J. Parasitol., 52, 248-259.

August, J. R., Powers, R. D., Bailey, W. S., and Diamond, D. L. (1980): *Filaroides hirthi* in a dog: Fatal hyperinfection suggestive of autoinfection. J. Am. Vet. Med. Assoc., *176*, 331-334.

Basir, M. A. (1950): The morphology and developoment of the sheep nematode, *Strongyloides papillosis* (Wedl, 1856). Can. J. Res. *28*, 173-196.

Baumann, R. (1946): Beobachtungen beim parasitären Sommerbluten der Pferde. Wien. Tierärtzl. Monatschr., *33*, 52-55.

Beaver, P. C., Snyder, C. H., Carreara, G. M., Dent, J. H., and Lafferty, J. W. (1952): Chronic eosinophilia due to visceral larva migrans. Pediatrics, *9*, 7-19.

Blaisdell, K. A. (1952): A study of the cat lungworm, *Aelurostrongylus abstrusus*. Ph.D. thesis, Cornell University.

Chandler, A. C., and Read, C. P. (1961): Introduction to Parasitology, 10th ed. New York, John Wiley and Sons.

Clunies Ross, I. and Gordon, H. McL. (1936): The Internal Parasites and Parasitic Diseases of Sheep. Sydney, Angus and Robertson Ltd.

Craig, T. M., Brown, T. W., Shepstad, D. K., and Williams, G. D. (1978): Fatal *Filaroides hirthi* infection in a dog. J. Am. Vet. Med. Assoc., *172*, 1096-1098.

Crofton, H. D. (1966): Nematodes. London, Hutchinson University Library.

Daubney, R. (1920): The life histories of *Dictyocaulus filaria* (Rud.) and *Dictyocaulus viviparus* (Bloch). J. Comp. Pathol. Therap., *33* (4), 225-226.

Dorrington, J. E. (1968): Studies on *Filaroides osleri* infestation in dogs. Onderstepoort J. Vet. Res., *35* 225-285.

Dubin, S., Segall, S., and Martindale, J. (1975): Contamination of soil in two city parks with canine nematode ova including *Toxocara canis:* A preliminary study. Am. J. Public Health, *65*, 1242-1245.

Dunsmore, J. D., and Spratt, D. M. (1976): The life cycle of *Filaroides osleri* in the dingo. Abstract of paper presented at the meeting of the Australian Society of Parasitology. Melbourne, Australia.

Dwork, K. G., Jaffe, J. R., and Lieberman, H. D. (1975): Strongyloidiasis with massive hyperinfection. N.Y.S. J. Med., *75* (8), 1230-1234.

Enigk, K. (1950): Die Biologie von *Capillaria plica* (Trichuroidea:Nematodes). Zeitschr. für Tropenmed. u. Parasitol., *1* (4), 560-571.

Enigk, K., Dey-Hazra, A., and Batke, J. (1974): Zur Klinischen Bedeutung und Behandlung des galaktogen erworbenen *Strongyloides* -Befalls der Fohlen. Deutsche Tierärztliche Wochenschrift, *81*, 605-607.

Fülleborn, F. (1921): Askarisinfektion durch Verzehren eingekapselter Larven und ubergelungene intrauterine Askarisinfektion. Arch. Schiffs. u. Tropenhyg., *25*, 367-375.

Georgi, J. R. (1964): Estimation of parasitic blood loss by whole-body counting. Am. J. Vet. Res, *25* (104), 246-250.

Georgi, J. R. (1976a): *Filaroides hirthi:* Experimental transmission among Beagle dogs through ingestion of first stage larvae. Science, *194*, 735.

Georgi, J. R. (1976b): Letter to the Editor: Accessions of the Laboratory of Parasitology for 1975. Cornell Vet., *66* (4), 604-615.

Georgi, J. R. (1982): Strongyloidiasis, in Handbook Series in Zoonoses, Section C: Parasitic Zoonoses Vol. II, M. G. Schultz, ed., CRC Press, Florida.

Georgi, J. R., and Sprinkle, C. L. (1974): A case of human strongyloidosis apparently contracted from asymptomatic colony dogs. Am. J. Trop. Hyg., *23* (5), 899-901.

Georgi, J. R., and Whitlock, J. H. (1965): Erythrocyte loss and restitution in ovine haemonchosis; methods and basic mathematical model. Am. J. Vet. Res., *26* (111), 310-314.

Georgi, J. R., Georgi, M. E., Fahnestock, G. R., and Theodorides, V. J. (1979a): Transmission and control of *Filaroides hirthi*, lungworm infection in dogs. Am. J. Vet. Res., *40*, 829-831.

Georgi, J. R., Fahnestock, G. R., Bohm, M. F. K., and Adsit, J. C. (1979b): The migration and development of *Filaroides hirthi* in dogs. Parasitology, *79*, 39-47.

Georgi, J. R., Georgi, M. E., and Cleveland, D. J. (1977): Patency and transmission of *Filaroides hirthi* infection. Parasitology, *75*, 251-257.

Gnedina, M. P., and Osipov, A. N. (1960): The life cycle of *Parafilaria multipapillosa* (Dondamine and Drouilly, 1878) parasitic in the horse. Doklad. Acad. Nauk SSSR, *131*, 1219.

Hanson, K. B. (1933): Test of the efficacy of single treatments with tracheal brushes in the mechanical removal of lungworms from foxes. J. Am. Vet. Med. Assoc., *82* (1), 12-33.

Hirth, R. S. (1977): *Filaroides hirthi* infection in Beagle dogs used for research. Bull. Soc. Pharm. Environ. Path., *5*, 11-17.

Hirth, R. S., and Hottendorf, G. H. (1973): Lesions produced by a new lungworm in Beagle dogs. Vet. Path., *10*, 385-407.

Hemmert-Halswick, A., and Bugge, G. (1934): Trichinen und Trichinose. Ergebn. Allgem. Path. u. Path. Anat., *28*, 313-392.

Hobmaier, A., and Hobmaier, M. (1935): Intermediate hosts of *Aelurostrongylus abstrusus* of the cat. Proc. Soc. Exp. Biol. Med., *32*, 1641-1647.

Holzworth, J., and Georgi, J. R. (1974): Trichinosis in a cat. J. Am. Vet. Med. Assoc., *165* (2), 186-191.

Jackson, R. F., von Lichtenberg, F., and Otto, G. F. (1962): Occurrence of adult heartworms in the venae cavae of dogs. J. Am. Vet. Med. Assoc., *141* (1), 117-121.

Jackson, R. F., Otto, G. F., Bauman, P. M., Peacock, F., Henricks, W. L., and Maltby, J. H. (1966): Distribution of heartworms in the right side of the heart and adjacent vessels of the dog. J. Am. Vet. Med. Assoc., *149* (5), 515-518.

Jackson, R. F., Seymour, W. G., Growney, P. J., and Otto, G. F. (1977): Surgical treatment of the caval syndrome of canine heartworm disease. J. Am. Vet. Med. Assoc., *171* (10), 1065-1069.

James, M. J. (1947): The Flies That Cause Myiasis in Man. U.S.D.A. Misc. Publication 631.

Jarrett, W. F. H., McIntyre, W. I. M., Jennings, F. W., and Mulligan, W. (1957): The natural history of parasitic bronchitis with notes on prophylaxis and treatment. Vet. Rec., *69* (49), part two, 1329.

Jordan, W. H., Gaafar, S. M., and Carlton, W. W. (1975): *Micronema deletrix* in the brain of a horse. Vet. Med./ Sm. An. Clin., 707-709.

Kazacos, K. R. (1983): Racoon Roundworms (*Baylisascaris procyonis*)—A Cause of Animal and Human Disease. Station Bulletin No. 422, Agr. Expt. Sta., Purdue University.

Kirby-Smith, J. L., Dove, W. E., and White, G. F. (1926): Creeping eruption. Arch. Dermatol. Syphilol., *13*, 137-173.

Kotula, A. W., Murrell, K. D., Acosta-Stein, L., Lamb, L., and Douglas, L. (1983): Destruction of *Trichinella spiralis* during cooking. J. Food Sci., *48*, 765-768.

Little, M. D. (1966a): Comparative morphology of six species of *Srongyloides* (Nematoda) and redefinition of the genus. J. Parasitol. *52* (1), 69-84.

Little, M. D. (1966b): Seven new species of *Strongyloides* (Nematoda) from Louisiana. J. Parasitol. *52* (1), 85-97.

Lyons, E. T., Drudge, J. H., and Tolliver, S. (1969):

Parasites from mare's milk. Blood Horse, 95 (2), 2270-2271.

Madsen, H. (1976): The life cycle of Trichinella spiralis (Owen, 1835) Railliet, 1896 (Syns. T. nativa Britov et Boev, 1972, T. nelsoni Britov et Boev, 1972, T. pseudospiralis (Garkavi, 1972), with remarks on epidemiology and a new diagram. Acta Parasitol. Pol., 24 (14), 143-158.

Mayhew, I. G., deLahunta, A., Georgi, J. R., and Aspros, D. G. (1976): Naturally occuring cerebrospinal parelaphostrongylosis. Cornell Vet., 66 (1), 56-72.

Milks, H. J. (1916): A preliminary report on verminous bronchitis in dogs. Cornell Vet., 6 (1), 50-55.

Mirck, M. H. (1977): Cyathostominose: een vorm van ernstige strongylidose. Tijdschr. Diergeneesk., 102 (15), 932-934.

Moncol, D. J., and Batte, E. G. (1966): Transcolostral infection of newborn pigs with Strongyloides ransomi. Vet. Med./SAC, 61, 583-586.

Polley, L., and Creighton, S. R. (1977): Experimental direct transmission of the lungworm, Filaroides osleri in dogs. Vet. Rec., 100, 136-137.

Potter, M. E., Kruse, M. B., Matthews, M. A., Hill, R. O., and Martin, R. J. (1976): A sausage-associated outbreak of trichinosis in Illinois. Am. J. Public Health, 66 (12), 1194-1196.

Rendano, V. T., Georgi, J. R., Fahnestock, G. R., and King, J. M. (1979): Filaroides hirthi lungworm infection in dogs; its radiographic appearance. Vet. Radiol., 20, 2-9.

Roth, L., Georgi, M. E., King, J. M., and Tennant, B. C. (1982): Parasitic encephalitis due to Baylisascaris sp. in wild and captive woodchucks (Marmota monax). Vet. Pathol., 19, 658-662.

Rothstein, N. (1963): Canine microfilariasis in sentry dogs in the United States. J. Parasitol., 49 (5 Sect. 2), 49.

Rousselot, R., and Pellissier, A. (1952): III. Oesophagostomose nodulaire à Oesophagostomum stephanostomum du gorille et du chimpanzé. Soc. Path. Exotique Bull., 45 (4), 568-574.

Sprent, J. F. A. (1956): The life history and development of Toxocara cati (Schrank, 1788) in the domestic cat. Parasitology. 46 (1-2), 54-58.

Sprent, J. F. A. (1958): Observations on the development of Toxocara canis (Werner, 1782) in the dog. Parasitology, 48 (1-2), 184-209.

Swerczek, T. W., Nielsen, S. W., and Helmbolt, C. F. (1971): Transmammary passage of Toxocara cati in the cat. Am. J. Vet. Res., 32, 89-92.

Thomas, R. J., and Stevens, A. J. (1956): Some observations on Nematodirus disease in Northumberland and Durham. Vet. Rec. 68, 471-475.

Triantophyllou, A. C., and Moncol, D. J. (1977): Cytology, reproduction, and sex determination of Strongyloides ransomi and S. papillosus. J. Parasitol. 63 (6), 961-973.

Underwood, J. R. (1936): Habronemiasis. Veterinary Bulletin, 30 (1), 16-28. Washington, D. C., Office of the Surgeon General, U.S. Army.

Urquhart, G. M., Jarrett, W. H. F., and O'Sullivan, J. G. (1954): Canine tracheo-bronchitis due to infection with Filaroides osleri. Vet. Rec., 66 (10), 143-145.

Van Reyn, F. C., Roberts, T. M., Owen, R., and Beaver, P. C. (1978): Infection of an infant with an adult Toxocara cati. J. Pediatrics, 93, 247-249.

Wallace, G. W. (1977): Swine influenza and lungworms; Editorial. J. Inf. Dis. 135 (3), 490-492.

Wetzel, R. (1940): Zur Biologie des Fuchslungenwurmes Crenosoma vulpis. Archiv fur Wissenschaftl. und Praktische Tierheilk., 75 (6), 445-460.

White, G. F., and Dove, W. E. (1926): Dogs and cats concerned in the causation of creeping eruption. Official Record, USDA, V, No.43.

Wiseman, R. A., and Lovel, T. W. (1969): Human infection with adult Toxocara cati. British Med. J., 4, 454-455.

Woodruff, A. W., and Burg, O. A. (1973): Prevalence of infective ova of Toxocara species in public places. British Med. J., 4, 470-472.

Worley, D. E., Fox, J. C., Winters, J. B., Jacobson, R. H., and Greer, K. R. (1976): Helminth and arthropod parasites of grizzly and black bears in Montana and adjacent areas. Proc. Third Int. Conf. on Bears, U.S.A. and U.S.S.R., June 1974.

Yorke, W., and Maplestone, P. A. (1926): Nematode Parasites of Vertebrates. London, J. and A. Churchill. Reprint, New York, Hafner Publishing Co., 1969.

Zimmermann, W. J. (1983): Evaluation of microwave cooking procedures and ovens for devitalizing trichinae in pork roasts. J. Food Sci., 48, 856-860.

TWO

TREATMENT AND CONTROL OF CLINICAL PARASITISMS

by Jay R. Georgi and Vassilios J. Theodorides

Effective treatment and control of parasites depends on detailed knowledge of the epidemiologically important aspects of their life histories, the behavior patterns and conditions of domestication of their hosts, and the selection and correct application of suitable antiparasitic drugs. Chapters 7 through 10 consider the complex interactions that occur between our principal domestic animals and their respective assemblages of parasites and the measures we take to influence the outcome of these interactions. In each chapter, parasite taxa are taken up in approximately the same order as in Part One, for the sake of consistency.

Intelligent antiparasitic therapy requires not only the selection of an appropriate parasiticide and its correct application, but a clear understanding of the limitations and hazards of chemotherapy. Chapter 11 presents detailed, practical information on the indications, contraindications, dosages, and toxicity of most of the anthelmintic, insecticidal, and antiprotozoal drugs currently available to the North American veterinary practitioner. Before adopting any new or unfamiliar insecticidal, antiprotozoal, or anthelmintic drug, please study the profile of that drug presented in Chapter 11. There you will find useful and important information. The label or package insert is the best source of current information and veterinary practitioners are required by law to use the product only as directed therein. If informational discrepancy exists between this text and the label or insert, be guided by the latter.

Dosages are expressed in milligrams of active substance to be administered per kilogram of body weight of the host, usually abbreviated as "mg. per kg." If we say, for example, that a particular drug is to be administered at 50 mg. per kg. twice daily, we mean that the animal should receive, at approximately 12 hour intervals, 50 milligrams of the drug for each kilogram it weighs; we do not mean that the 50 mg. per kg. dose be divided into 25 mg. per kg. doses. Please excuse us if this appears ridiculously obvious, but it is particularly important that no misinterpretations arise with respect to dosages.

PARASITISM OF DOGS AND CATS

7

The particular objectives of antiparasitic medication and other control measures must be carefully considered in order that the course adopted will prove effective but no more laborious or expensive than necessary.

ARTHROPODS

Control of Insects and Acarids

Entomophobia, a "morbid dread of arthropods," is probably the most common human discomfort inspired by fleas, ticks, and other ectoparasites of dogs and cats. Moreover, several dog and cat ectoparasites will attack people, especially those that share their beds with their pets, so a brief review of the problems that may be experienced by the pet owner is included in the following exposition of ectoparasite control.

FLIES

Control of flies in the environment is discussed in the next chapter.

Myiasis. A *Cuterebra* larva is removed by enlarging its breathing hole in the skin sufficiently to allow it to be extracted with forceps, care being taken not to crush the larva in the process. Tranquilization or sedation facilitates restraint but is rarely necessary. The wound heals rather slowly and sometimes suppurates or even sloughs; this may be due to secondary bacterial infection or leakage of *Cuterebra* antigens into the surrounding tissues during extraction.

Calliphorid myiasis usually involves weakened or paralyzed dogs and may progress unnoticed in long-haired unfortunates to an appalling state in which great areas of skin have been completely eaten away. The condition of the patient can be evaluated accurately and effective treatment undertaken only after the hair has been clipped away and all affected areas bathed. Most of the maggots will be removed in the process; any remaining may be routed by judicious local application of an insecticidal solution such as a pyrethroid or an organophosphate. Any really vigorous application of insecticide might easily kill the debilitated and denuded host.

FLEAS

The control of fleas on dogs and cats is a very difficult task requiring steady, earnest, and energetic application of insecticides to the animals and to the premises frequented by them. Products that contain pyrethrins, carbaryl, propoxur, lindane, chlorfenvinphos, dichlorvos, dioxathion, phosmet, tetrachlorvinphos, and cythioate are all very effective and suitable for application to both animals and premises. Flea collars or medallions may offer continuous protection against flea infestations. We have seen many dogs suffering from flea bite dermatitis that had flea collars around their necks, however.

We suggest initial control of fleas on dogs by dipping or bathing the animal with products containing carbamates and prescribe cythioate twice a week throughout the flea season. The premises are sprayed once a week with 0.5 per cent aqeous solution of malathion. In cats we recommend instillation of two drops of cythioate in the ears twice a week, dusting with carbaryl products, and that a propoxur flea collar be worn during the flea season (Horak, 1976; Miller *et al.,* 1977). Chlorinated hydrocarbons are contraindicated for cats.

Ctenocephalides fleas much prefer dogs and

cats but frequently attack people, especially when deprived of their normal hosts. A home vacated by a dog or cat for several weeks is likely to fairly jump with blood-thirsty fleas so that one's ankles may become covered with them·in a few minutes after entering the building. Unfed fleas may survive for several months, so it is usually impracticable to try to starve them out. A combination of housecleaning and insecticidal attack is in order. Efforts may profitably be concentrated on the places where the dog or cat habitually rests and sleeps because here is where eggs are most likely to be deposited and the development of adult fleas to follow. The human flea *Pulex irritans* is rather indiscriminate in its choice of hosts and therefore is unlikely to display the distinct preference for dog and cat that *Ctenocephalides* does. Rodent fleas will also attack people when their hosts have been exterminated by poisoning or disease. *Xenopsylla cheopis*, the vector of *Yersinia pestis*, attacks man more readily than other rodent fleas when deprived of its normal host.

LICE

Lice (Figs. 7–1 andf 7–2) are readily controlled with carbaryl and dioxathion shampoo, spray, or dip. Usually, two treatments are adequate when applied at an interval of 1 week.

Lice are very host-specific, and exchanges of such fauna between man and dog are always temporary. Occasionally, a particularly coarse-haired dog may be found harboring a substantial population of human

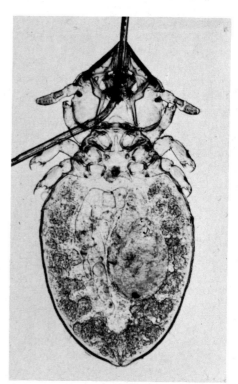

Figure 7–2. *Felicola subrostratus*, the cat louse (x70).

crab lice *Pthirus pubis*, but that comes of sharing a bed with its lousy master; the dog is the victim and not the villain. Crab lice are spread among adult human beings principally through sexual intercourse and, less importantly, through bedding, towels, borrowed clothing, and the like. In young children, crab lice may be found clinging to the eyelashes and eyebrows, these furnishing the nearest approximation to a pubic hair that a child has to offer. Dealing with a family outbreak of crab lice that involves a falsely incriminated dog requires considerable tact.

TICKS

Ticks are controlled by application of such compounds as dichlorvos, lindane, carbaryl, propoxur, chlorfenvinphos, and dioxathion. Dogs in tick-infested areas may need to be sprayed or dipped weekly and wear flea collars containing dichlorvos, carbaryl, or propoxur. Control of *Rhipicephalus sanguineus* in buildings may be achieved by spraying with diazinon.

Rhipicephalus sanguineus ticks infrequently attack man north of Mexico, but because larvae, nymphs, and adults all feed on the dog, enormous populations may build up in homes, kennels, and veterinary hospitals.

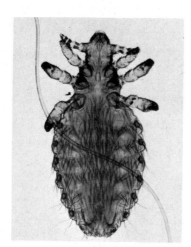

Figure 7–1. *Linognathus setosus*, the sucking lice of dogs (x38).

Originally a tropical species, *R. sanguineus* has taken advantage of central heating to spread into the temperate zones and, unlike *Dermacentor*, does not survive a temperate zone winter outdoors. Dogs in temperate regions therefore usually acquire their *R. sanguineus* ticks in infested premises but infestation may be acquired outdoors in summer. If enduring results are to be achieved, elimination of *R. sanguineus* infestations must include acaricidal treatment both of the dog and of the premises. The latter procedure is a job for a professional exterminator. Ticks are so repulsive to many people that the sight of a platoon of *R. sanguineus* "questing" on a curtain is enough to precipitate an attack of entomophobic shock. It obviously behooves veterinary practitioners to be meticulously careful in preventing and controlling *R. sanguineus* infestations in their hospitals and kennels.

MITES

Sarcoptes. Sarcoptic mange responds readily to 1 per cent lindane dip. The treatment is repeated every week for five or six weeks. The hair should be clipped and all crusty material removed with keratolytic shampoos prior to applying acaricidal compounds. A single application of phosmet is often adequate for the treatment of sarcoptic mange in dogs. A single dermal application of amitraz (0.25 per cent) provided excellent control of both *Demodex* and *Sarcoptes* infestations in dogs (Folz et al., 1978).

Sarcoptes scabiei and other sarcoptiform parasites may temporarily infest people that come into intimate contact with mangy dogs and cats. In this case, acaricidal treatment of the pet is the key to lasting success in curing the people. On the other hand, proper scabies contracted from another human being causes very persistent dermatitis and misery unless effectively treated and, of course, has little or nothing to do with dogs and cats.

Notoedres. *Notoedres cati* infestations are treated with lime sulfur solution. The cat is first bathed and then dipped or washed with a 1:40 solution of lime sulfur in warm water. This treatment is applied weekly for at least six weeks. Malathion dips, 0.5 per cent, are also recommended (Reedy, 1977).

Otodectes. *Otodectes* ear infestations respond to rotenone, methyl phthalate, and thiabendazole (Faulk and Schwirck, 1978). The ear canal should be thoroughly cleaned prior to instillation of the acaricidal solution.

Demodex. *Demodex canis* is susceptible to benzyl benzoate, rotenone, ronnel, and cythioate (Manson et al., 1969). The localized form of demodectic mange may be controlled by applying rotenone ointment or benzyl benzoate lotion. These drugs have very little residual activity and therefore must be applied daily. The treatment of generalized demodectic mange is a challenge and frequently proves to be a frustating experience for the clinician and client alike. A 1 per cent alcoholic solution of rotenone or 1 per cent solution of ronnel (if avalilable) in propylene glycol is applied to one third of the body every day until skin scrapings are negative for *D. canis*. Amitraz (MITABAN) is approved for the control of generalized demodicosis in dogs. Amitraz is applied topically as a 0.25 per cent aqueous suspension at two week intervals for a total of three to six applications. It is recommended that treatment be continued until no viable mites can be found in skin scrapings at two successive treatments. A brood bitch with asymptomatic *D. canis* infection may be bred but a bitch with demodectic mange or a history of demodectic mange should be spayed.

Cheyletiella. *Cheyletiella yasguri* infestations respond to lindane treatments. The dogs are bathed with lindane shampoo weekly for six weeks. *Cheyletiella* is also susceptible to amitraz. The premises should be sprayed with a residual organophosphate insecticide such as diazinon to destroy these rather hardy mites.

Cheyletiella yasguri of dogs and *C. blakei* of cats also attack people, especially those that share their beds with their pets. Curiously, *C. blakei* rarely produces obvious lesions on cats, but the owner may be aware of frequent bites. If *C. blakei* infestation is suspected, one can attempt to collect mites from the fur with a bit of Scotch Tape. However, the diagnosis is more often reached fortuitously when the mites or their eggs are found in a routine fecal flotation. Because cats so religiously groom themselves, a fecal flotation often affords a better sample of what is on the cat's exterior than direct examination does.

PROTOZOANS

AMEBIASIS

Entamoeba histolytica. Very little is known about the treatment of canine amebiasis. In man, metronidazole is the drug of choice in treatment of intestinal and hepatic amebiasis and is therefore a logical choice for treating canine amebiasis. Roberson (1977) suggests oral administration of 50 mg. metronidazole per kg. body weight daily for five days.

GIARDIASIS

Giardia infections in dogs usually respond readily to medication with either metronidazole (50 mg. per kg. orally once a day for five consecutive days) or quinacrine. Quinacrine is administered orally or intramuscularly according to the following schedule: For large breeds, 200 mg. per dog three times on the first day and twice daily during the next six days; for small breeds, 100 mg. per dog twice on the first day and once daily for the next six days; for puppies, 50 mg. per pup twice daily for six days.

Trichomonas infections in puppies may be controlled with metronidazole administered orally at 66 mg. per kg. once daily for five consecutive days (Buckner and Ewing, 1977).

COCCIDIOSIS

Isospora spp. Coccidiosis outbreaks in dogs and cats can be controlled with sulfonamide drugs. Sulfadimethoxine is administered to dogs for the treatment of coccidial enteritis according to the following schedule: 55 mg. per kg. for the first day and 27.5 mg. per kg. for the next four days or until the dog is asymptomatic for at least two days.

Toxoplasma gondii. Dogs and cats clinically ill with toxoplasmosis acquired postnatally may respond to pyrimethamine administered concurrently with standard doses of sulfadiazine or triple sulfonamides. Pyrimethamine is administered orally to human infants at 1 mg. per kg. per day for the first three days and 0.5 mg. per kg. per day thereafter (Jones, 1979). Pyrimethamine causes megaloblastic anemia or leukopenia and therapy should be discontinued if there is no response by 30 days.

A cat shedding oocysts of *Toxoplasma* should be hospitalized to prevent exposure of its owner and treated with sulfadiazine until oocyst shedding ceases. This will happen automatically at the end of 7 to 10 days anyway, so treatment is almost invariably a success. Reinfection, if it occurs, results in a low-grade shedding of short duration, and intercurrent *Isospora* infection may trigger a brief output of *T. gondii* oocysts but, in general, once a cat has passed through a patent *T. gondii* infection, it is a relatively minor source of infection.

Human beings may contract toxoplasmosis either by ingesting sporulated oocysts from the feces of an infected cat or by eating uncooked meat of animals containing *T. gondii* cysts. It is particularly important that pregnant women should be protected from infection because transplacental infection with this parasite can lead to disease and malformation of the developing fetus. "Pregnant women should eat only adequately cooked meat and either leave the cleaning of cat litter pans to someone else or wear disposable gloves" (Frenkel and Dubey, 1972).

BABESIOSIS

Babesia canis infection usually responds to a single intramuscular injection of 3.5 mg. diminazene (BERENIL) per kg., or to subcutaneous injections of 15 mg. phenamidine (GANASEG) per kg. (Roberson 1977; Lewis and Huxsoll, 1977). *Babesia gibsoni* infections are not as readily curable with these drugs as is *B. canis* (Ruff *et al.*, 1973). Unfortunately, these drugs are not available for general use in the United States and, for that reason are not included in Chapter 11. Trypan blue and acridine derivatives (e.g., acriflavin) have also been used in the treatment of babesiosis.

HELMINTHS

Trematodes

SOURCES OF INFECTION

Most trematode parasites of dogs and cats are acquired by eating fish, frogs, or crayfish in or on which the metacercariae of these parasites have encysted (Fig. 7–3). Prevention of infection is equivalent to preventing ingestion of these foods uncooked. Cats become infected with *Platynosomum fastosum* by eating lizards, toads, geckos, and skinks, (Chung *et al.*, 1977; Eckerlin and Leigh, 1962). If the source of infection is not apparent, correct identification of the trematode in question will clarify the situation.

ANTHELMINTIC MEDICATION

Paragonimus kellicotti. Fenbendazole, 50 mg. per kg. for 10 to 14 days, is highly effective against these lung flukes (Dubey *et al.*, 1979). Albendazole, at a dosage rate of

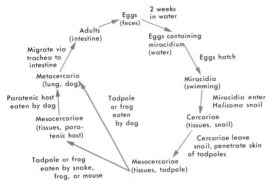

Figure 7–3. Life history of *Alaria canis*. The prepatent period is 35 days. Mesocercariae migrate directly through the diaphragm on their way to the lungs.

25 mg. per kg. twice daily for 14 days is also highly effective. However, neither of these drugs is yet approved by FDA for use in dogs in the United States.

Opisthorchis. Lienert (1962) used hexachlorophene in a single oral dose of 20 mg. per kg. for the treatment of opisthorchiasis in dogs and cats.

Platynosomum. Nitroscanate, 100 mg per kg., and praziquantel, 20 mg per kg., markedly reduced the number of *Platynosomum* eggs passed in the feces of cats (Evans and Green, 1978).

Cestodes

Adult tapeworm infections cause little harm or inconvenience to dogs and cats. It is true that infected dogs frequently sit down and drag their bottoms, but so do uninfected dogs. No doubt a tapeworm segment wandering about the perineum tickles and this phenomenon must certainly be included in the list of etiologies for *pruritus ani*, but distended anal sacs are more frequently to blame. The veterinarian who treats *pruritus ani* by expressing anal sacs will obtain better results than another who prescribes anthelmintics for this condition.

SOURCES OF INFECTION

A tapeworm segment crawling about on their pet's tail or freshly passed feces offends most clients, and the civilized world makes quite a business of poisoning tapeworms. To obtain lasting results, the source of infection must also be dealt with or the segments will reappear and the client may not.

Dipylidium caninum requires only two to three weeks to develop from a cysticercoid

into a segment-shedding tapeworm, so the benefits of anthelmintic therapy are particularly short-lived in its case unless fleas and biting lice are also brought under control.

Taenia, Multiceps, Hydatigera, and *Echinococcus* can only be acquired by a dog or cat eating uncooked meat. The most common sources for dogs are cottontail rabbits (*Taenia pisiformis*) and cattle, sheep, or swine offal (*T. hydatigena*), whereas meadow voles and other rodents (*Hydatigera taeniaeformis*) are the most common source for cats.

Mesocestoides infection results from predation upon snakes, birds, and small mammals. Some clients find it difficult to accept that their civilized pets are using their long, sharp teeth in an atavistic way, especially sportsmen with expensive bird dogs and vegetarians with cats. However, the carnivoran must be denied prey if *Mesocestoides* infection is to be prevented. Most taeniids have about a two month prepatent period but *Mesocestoides* may start discharging segments in little over two weeks after infection, thereby imparting the impression that the anthelmintic has not worked at all. To make matters worse, *M. corti* tapeworms multiply asexually in the intestine of dogs; if this species is not totally eliminated by anthelmintic medication, it will repopulate the intestine even without further exposure (Eckert *et al.,* 1969).

Diphyllobothrium latum and *Spirometra mansonoides* are less obtrusive because these tapeworms do not detach segments but release their eggs more or less continuously through the uterine pores of their mature segments. Therefore, the client is usually unaware of *Diphyllobothrium* and *Spirometra* infection unless a whole tapeworm or a long chain of senile segments is discharged at once. *Diphyllobothrium* infection is acquired by eating uncooked predatory freshwater fish. *Spirometra mansonoides* can be passed experimentally from the copepod through such diverse second intermediate hosts as frogs and mice. In the type locality (Syracuse, N.Y.), *Natrix*, a water snake, is frequently found infected with *S. mansonoides* plerocercoids.

Hymenolepis diminuta occurs rarely in dogs; its large handsome eggs are easily identified (Fig. 12-35).

ANTHELMINTIC MEDICATION

There are many drugs with proven efficacy against the tapeworms affecting dogs and cats. Arecoline salts, dichlorophene, bunamidine, mebendazole, niclosamide, nitroscanate, and praziquantel all show activity against one or more tapeworm genera, but almost all fail against one or another genus.

The preferred cestocidal drug is praziquantel, which, in a single 5 mg. per kg. oral or subcutaneous dose, eliminates 100 per cent of both immature and adult *Taenia hydatigena, T. pisiformis, T. ovis, Hydatigera taeniaeformis, Echinococcus granulosus, E. multilocularis, Mesocestoides corti,* and *Dipylidium caninum* from dogs and cats (Dey-Hazra, 1976; Rommel *et al.,* 1976; Anderson *et al.,* 1978; and Thomas and Gönnert, 1978). Praziquantel at a dosage rate of 7.5 mg. per kg. for two consecutive days eliminated 100 per cent of *Diphyllobothrium erinacei,* and a single dose of 35 mg. per kg. eliminated all *D. latum* from infected cats (Sakamoto, 1977).

Mebendazole, nitroscanate, and bunamidine are active against adult *E. granulosus* but at much higher dosage levels than praziquantel (Gemmell *et al.,* 1975; Boray *et al.,* 1979; Forbes, 1966; Gemmell and Shearer, 1968; Anderson *et al.,* 1975; Trejos *et al.,* 1975). Mebendazole is practically ineffective against *Dipylidium caninum.*

Fenbendazole administered for three days at 50 mg./kg. is effective against *T. pisiformis.*

Bunamidine also displayed a high degree of efficacy against *Mesocestoides corti* (Todd *et al.,* 1978). It is important that any compound employed against *M. corti* possess 100 per cent efficiency because of the ability of this parasite to multiply asexually in the intestine of dogs (Eckert *et al.,* 1969). It is worth noting that manufacturers' dosage recommendations may vary from one country to another. Williams and Keahey (1976) reported sudden death of two German shepherds and an Irish wolfhound that had received 50 mg. per kg. of bunamidine hydrochloride. King (1976) explained that these deaths were due to drug overdosage. In Canada, the regular dosage of bunamidine hydrochloride is 30 mg. per kg. up to a maximum of 600 mg. for dogs weighing over 20 kg.

Nematodes

ASCARIDS

SOURCES OF INFECTION

Soil Pollution. *Toxocara* and *Toxascaris* eggs are very resistant to environmental adversity and remain infective for years, especially in poorly drained clay and silt soils, hence their accumulation in soil and filth and the threat they pose to successful dog rearing progress with time. A reasonable explanation for the heavy ascarid infections so frequently encountered in hound pups might be sought in the common practice of chaining the hounds almost permanently to doghouses, a practice particularly conducive to soil pollution. Because the infective eggs are virtually immune to any reasonable measures taken to destroy them, the most effective measure is to entomb them under a concrete or bituminous asphalt slab. Once the slab is installed, and provided feces are not allowed to accumulate for more than a week at a time, the probability of the confined dog ingesting infective ascarid eggs will become quite small. The next best way of decontaminating polluted soil is to replace the top foot or so with fresh gravel.

Contaminated Kennel Areas. All surfaces must first be made physically clean. High pressure washers like those in "car washes" are very effective, and inexpensive mobile units are quite satisfactory. Wood and wire contruction is difficult to clean properly with any kind of equipment or amount of effort. After surfaces are physically clean, they may be mopped or sprayed with 1 per cent sodium hypochlorite (three cups Clorox per gallon of cool water) to strip off the outer protein coat of the ascarid eggs so they won't stick to surfaces and can be rinsed away. The preliminary cleaning is absolutely essential because any appreciable amount of residual organic matter will neutralize the sodium hypochlorite and render it ineffective in stripping the ascarid eggs. Notice that nothing has been said about killing the ascarid eggs. The above treatment does not kill ascarid eggs, it just knocks them loose.

Arrested Larvae in Tissues of Bitches and Queens. Arrested larvae are immune to anthelmintics because they are metabolically inactive. When reactivated, these larvae become moderately susceptible to a few anthelmintics administered frequently and in high dosage (see *Toxocara canis–Free Dogs,* below) but there is still no easy, inexpensive way to get rid of somatic larval burdens.

Paratenic Hosts. Mice and other small paratenic hosts may play a significant role in the epidemiology of *Toxocara* and *Toxascaris* infection, especially as regards predacious cats. If you dissect the mice, voles, moles, shrews, and snakes that your cat drags in, you will find *Toxocara* larvae encysted in most of them. In a rural setting, there is probably little that can be done about this source of infection except to confine the dogs and cats indoors. Rodents are attracted to the abundance of food in kennels and catteries and are not put off by the presence of their ferocious predators; a mouse is quite willing to risk its life for a kibble. There seems to be little information regarding the importance of rodents in transmitting ascarids and other parasites to dogs and cats confined to buildings and outdoor enclosures, but, considering the facts gathered here, an investment in rodent control could be partly written off against the cost of controlling parasites.

ANTHELMINTIC MEDICATION

Many safe and effective anthelmintic drugs are available to North American veterinarians for the treatment and control of ascarid infections of dogs and cats. Piperazine compounds, dichlorvos, toluene, and *n*-butyl chloride are all suitable for administration to dogs and cats in full therapeutic dosage. Diethylcarbamazine, mebendazole, fenbendazole, and pyrantel pamoate, in therapeutic dosage, have also been cleared for dogs. Daily medication with diethylcarbamazine, alone or in combination with styrylpyridinium to control hookworms, may offer an effective means of controlling ascarid infections in dogs subjected to continuous exposure.

SPECIAL CONTROL PROBLEMS

Toxocara canis

Young pups. Piperazine compounds are practically nontoxic yet highly effective against ascarids in the lumen of the alimentary tract. Therefore they are ideally suited to removing *Toxocara canis* as they arrive and develop in the intestinal lumens of perinatally infected pups. Unless heroic measures have been taken to prevent infection (see *Toxocara canis–Free Dogs*, below), pups may be assumed to be infected. Medication should start routinely as early as the second week of life and be repeated every three weeks until the pup is three months old. The standard therapeutic dose is 110 mg. piperazine base per kg. body weight but substantially lower dosages appear on the labels of many proprietary preparations. The reason for this is not clear. If the ascarids receive too little piperazine, they may recover their motility and their place in the small intestine before peristalsis has had a chance to eliminate them. It is better to give the full dose. Special preparations of dichlorvos are also available for pups, but these are more expensive and therefore might be applied more economically to mixed infections of *Toxocara* and *Ancylostoma.*

In breeding situations, the role of the bitch in the epidemiology of *T. canis* is paramount because she harbors that part of the reservoir of infection not contained in the soil. Clients should be advised that bitches that bestow pathogenic *T. canis* burdens on their litters will likely repeat the performance once or twice again even after the uptake of infective eggs has ceased. They should also be made aware that the environment of a bitch with a litter of nurslings is likely to contain veritable clouds of eggs from three weeks postpartum onward and it is during this period that anthelmintic medication and sanitation can be applied most effectively and efficiently. Rather heavy *patent* infections are regularly observed in nursing bitches for a short period beginning about one month after parturition. This has been explained as follows (Sprent, 1961). Some reactivated larvae fail to establish themselves in the pups' intestines and are passed with their feces. Brood bitches eat their pups' feces to clean the nest and, in so doing, afford these jettisoned larvae a second chance to mature.

Toxocara canis–Free Dogs. By *T. canis*–free, we imply that the dogs are devoid of both adult and larval parasites. However, it is nearly impossible to detect small numbers of *T. canis* arrested larvae in the tissues of even a small pup, so the status "*T. canis*–free" is always to be taken *cum grano salis*. The sort of measures required for producing *Toxocara canis*–free dogs and illustrated by the following examples, are usually beyond the resources (and requirements) of commercial breeders.

Griesemer and Gibson (1963) obtained *T. canis*–free pups from colostrum-deprived bitches that were raised in isolation and given daily therapeutic doses of diethylcarbamazine for many months. In addition, three Beagle bitches that had been maintained on wire through several gestations yielded *T. canis*–free litters without anthelmintic medication. In the latter case, the somatic larval burden apparently was eliminated through the placenta over the course of several pregnancies, whereas in the former, somatic contamination of the bitches was precluded by preventing their access to infective eggs from birth.

Bitches with *T. canis* and *Ancylostoma caninum* infections were medicated daily with fenbendazole from the fortieth day of gestation to the fourteenth day of lactation at a dosage rate of 50 mg. per kg. Their pups were found free of both parasites (Düwel and Strasser, 1978). The timing of medication coincided with the period of reactivation and migration of arrested *T. canis* larvae in these parturient females.

Thiabendazole administered orally at 150 mg. per kg. for 20 to 25 days starting when the pups were five days old, controlled prenatal *T. canis* infections (Congdon and Ames, 1973). Yakstis *et al.* (1968) reported that thiabendazole, mixed with pup ration at a concentration of 250 ppm., prevented the establishment of *T. canis* as well as *Ancylostoma, Trichuris,* and *Strongyloides.*

Toxocara cati. Somatic migration of *T. cati* larvae occurs principally in egg infections. Because cats are such ardent self-groomers, infective eggs adhering to fur gain easy access to their interiors and arrested larvae accumulate in the tissues. When reactivated during lactation, these larvae pass to the nurslings, undergo a mucosal migration, and mature, somatic migration in the queen apparently having satisfied their wanderlust (Sprent, 1956; Swerczek, 1971). Because *T. cati* larvae do not cross the placenta, it is theoretically possible to raise *T. cati*–free kittens for experimentation by removing them from their dam by caesarean section or at natural birth but before they have nursed, and raising them artificially. However, if less than absolute *T. cati*–free status is required, administration of an anthelmintic at intervals of three weeks for the first three or four months of life should suffice. Piperazine compounds, dichlorvos, *n*-butyl chloride, and nitroscanate are the preferred anthelmintics for the control of ascarid infections in cats (nitroscanate is not approved by FDA for use in the United States). The role of paratenic hosts in the epidemiology of *T. cati* infection should always be taken into account in planning control measures.

Toxascaris leonina. The restricted mucosal migration of *T. leonina* in dogs and cats precludes the development of somatic larval burdens and the transmission of infection by way of the placenta and mammary gland. Ingestion of infective eggs and paratenic hosts seems to be the only means by which cats and dogs acquire *T. leonina* infection. *Toxascaris leonina* possesses one advantage, however; its eggs develop to the infective stage in only one week as compared with four weeks for *Toxocara* spp. This rapid development might explain the persistence of *T. leonina* infection in reasonably well-sanitized cage colonies of dogs. But, of course, there's always the possibility that mice or other paratenic hosts are to blame.

Hookworms

SOURCES OF INFECTION

Contaminated Environment. From two to eight days are required for the morula in the hookworm egg to develop into an infective third stage larva. Shirt-sleeve temperatures (23 to 30°C) and a moderately moist, well-aerated medium are optimal. Thus, hookworm larvae develop well on shaded areas of well-drained soils but not on heavy, waterlogged soils or where they are exposed to direct sunlight and desiccation. *Ancylostoma* eggs and larvae are destroyed by freezing, whereas those of *Uncinaria* are very resistant to cold. *Ancylostoma caninum* larvae will not develop to the infective stage at temperatures consistently below 15°C. Above the optimum (30°C) development is very rapid and the infective stage may be reached within 48 hours at 37°C, the highest temperature compatible with development (McCoy, 1930). Thus, compared with *Toxocara* eggs, soil pollution by hookworm infective larvae may be viewed as a temporary problem that a good hard freeze will probably solve. During mild weather, sodium borate, broadcast at the rate of 10 lbs. per 100 sq. ft. (0.5 kg. per sq. m.) and raked in, will destroy hookworm larvae in gravel- or loam-surfaced runs. This treatment destroys vegetation as well as hookworm larvae and is therefore unsuitable for lawns. Resinated dichlorvos was reported to interfere with the development of first and second stage larvae of *Ancylostoma caninum* (Kalkofen, 1971).

Paved surfaces, cages, and the like should first be cleaned thoroughly and then mopped or sprayed with 1 per cent sodium hypochlorite solution (Clorox). This solution kills the larvae or at least induces them to cast off their sheaths, after which they are more susceptible to drying and other unfavorable environmental stresses.

Large commercial dog rearing operations make extensive use of wire-bottomed cages and pens to effect the physical separation of the dogs for the bulk of their feces. Anthelmintic medication may be employed to re-

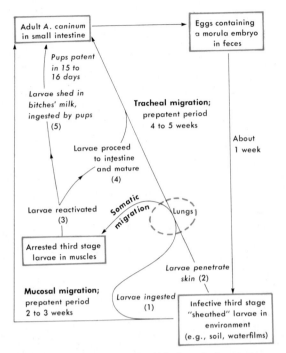

Figure 7–4. Alternative life histories of *Ancylostoma caninum*. (1) Ingested larvae develop principally in the alimentary mucous membrane and start producing eggs in two to three weeks. A portion, however, behave like skin-penetrating larvae. (2) Skin-penetrating larvae are carried by the venous blood flow to the lungs whence they proceed either on a TRACHEAL MIGRATION to maturity in four to five weeks or on a SOMATIC MIGRATION to a state of arrested development in skeletal muscles. Larvae exposed to chilling before infection tend to become arrested in the gut wall (Schad, 1974, 1979, personal communications). (3) Modest numbers of arrested larvae are reactivated more or less continuously and re-embark on their migrations. (4) Larvae reaching the intestine via the lungs mature, provided the intestine is not already occupied by adult *A. caninum*. If adult worms are eliminated by anthelmintic therapy, patent infection will be re-established by reactivated larvae in 23 to 39 days (Little, 1978). (5) Reactivated larvae enter the mammary gland of lactating bitches and are shed in the milk in greatest concentration during the first week of lactation. The prepatent period of transmammary infection in pups is 15 to 16 days.

duce the output of hookworm eggs in the feces and thus limit the degree of contamination of the environment with infective larvae. Therapeutic dosages may be administered periodically or when indicated by positive fecal examinations, or suitable medication may be administered continuously at lower dosage mixed with feed.

Arrested Larvae in Tissues. Currently available anthelmintics, even those administered by parenteral routes, appear to lack significant efficacy against hookworm larvae ar-

rested in the tissues. The arrested larvae of *A. caninum* in the intestinal wall and skeletal muscle tissue of the adult dog population are thus a relatively inaccessible reservoir of infection. This reservoir "leaks" larvae directly or via the lungs to the intestinal lumen of the adult dog, and via the mammary gland to the intestines of the nursling pups (Fig. 7–4).

Little (1978) obtained evidence that larvae are continually migrating from the muscles to the intestine via the lungs. When adult worms were already present in the intestine, few if any of these larvae developed to maturity, but when the adult worms were eliminated by disophenol therapy, these larvae from the muscles were able to mature and start producing eggs in about four weeks. A second course of disophenol then eliminated the new adults and these in turn were replaced by more larvae from the muscles. Why these reactivated larvae from the muscles should require twice as long as newly ingested larvae to mature is unclear. Schad's experiences with arrested *A. caninum* larvae differ somewhat from those of Little. Infective larvae were chilled before being administered orally to dogs. These larvae became arrested in the gut wall instead of the muscle tissue and when reactivated were able to become established in the intestine in the presence of adults (Schad, 1974, 1979, personal communications). Both investigators' findings led to similar practical consequences, however. Practicing veterinarians frequently encounter dogs with hookworm infections that refuse to "clean up" even after repeated wormings with a variety of drugs over the course of many months. This "larva leak" phenomenon provides a plausible explanation for such refractory cases.

Infection of nursling pups occurs via the mammary gland (Kotake, 1929a, 1929b; Stone and Girardeau, 1966, 1968). Formerly, prenatal infection by migration of larvae across the placenta was supposed to account for the occurrence of peracute hookworm disease in two or three week old pups, but meticulous experimentation by Stoye has demonstrated that transplacental infection, if it occurs at all, is overshadowed by transmammary infection, in the case of the hookworm. A bitch exposed to only one substantial oral or percutaneous infection will shed hookworm larvae in her milk for the next three lactations, although the larval output will diminish with each lactation (Stoye, 1973).

ANTHELMINTIC MEDICATION

Thenium closylate and disophenol are specific remedies for canine hookworm infections. Pyrantel pamoate, dichlorvos, mebendazole, fenbendazole, and nitroscanate are effective against hookworms and several other important helminth parasites of the intestinal tract. Two older drugs, n-butyl chloride and toluene, are still available and retain their original efficacy. They should not be set aside completely just because they are old drugs.

Feline hookworm infections may be treated with dichlorvos, disophenol, nitroscanate, n-butyl chloride, and toluene. Particular attention should be paid to ridding young kittens of hookworms.

Primary Ancylostomosis

Treatment is often to little avail in *peracute neonatal ancylostomosis*. Blood transfusion is essential to keep affected pups alive long enough for anthelmintic medication to take effect, and anthelmintic medication must be administered immediately to stop the loss of blood as soon as possible. On no account should anthelmintic therapy be delayed; it is impracticable to attempt replacement of hookworm blood losses by transfusion for any appreciable length of time.

In *acute ancylostomosis* and in *chronic (compensated) ancylostomiasis*, response to simple anthelmintic therapy is usually dramatic, and supportive therapy beyond provision of an adequate diet is unnecessary.

Secondary Ancylostomosis

The efficacy of mebendazole and fenbendazole was dramatically reduced in iron- and protein-deficient rats infected with *Nippostrongylus brasiliensis* (Duncombe *et al.*, 1977a, 1977b). Clinical experience indicates that protein sufficiency is also essential to efficient anthelmintic action against hookworms and other parasites. Cases of *malnutrition with secondary ancylostomosis* and cases that may seem to be adequately nourished but fail to respond to anthelmintic medication should first be given a course of supportive therapy (e.g., high protein diet, ferrous sulfate orally or parenteral iron injections, vitamins, and, if necessary, blood transfusion) and then remedicated with a suitable anthelmintic (e.g., mebendazole, pyrantel pamoate, disophenol).

SPECIFIC CONTROL PROBLEMS

Preventing Peracute Neonatal Ancylostomosis. Routine cage, pen, and run sanitation and periodic anthelmintic medication of all adult dogs are essential to reduce the level of environmental contamination with hookworm larvae. Where neonatal losses have already been experienced, it is essential to examine the visible mucosae of each pup daily from about the seventh day of life until weaning and administer an anthelmintic at the first sign of anemia. Alternatively, antihookworm therapy should begin two weeks after pups are whelped and continue weekly for three months (Kelly, 1977). Bitches that have lost litters may be treated with fenbendazole, 50 mg. per kg. per day from the fortieth day of gestation to the fourteenth day of lactation, to prevent further losses. This treatment attacks the reactivated larvae and is effective but rather expensive.

The Refractory Hookworm Egg-Shedder. In spite of excellent supportive therapy and flawless anthelmintic medication, the "larva leak" phenomenon provides a few highly persistent cases of hookworm infection. Prevention of somatic larval burdens is the key to prevention of such refractory clinical problems because, at present, there seems to be no satisfactory way of handling the dog that persists in shedding hookworm eggs after months of treatment. The intracellular location and metabolic quiescence of arrested *A. caninum* larvae should, it would seem, shelter them from even the most effective anthelmintics. Stoye (1973), however, showed that estrogens stimulate the reactivation of arrested larvae; he induced an outpouring of larvae in the milk of lactating bitches by treatment with estradiol and progesterone. Perhaps a way can be found to combine hormonal and anthelmintic therapy effectively in attacking the somatic burden of *A. caninum* larvae.

Strongyloidiasis

Canine *Strongyloides stercoralis* infection may be asymptomatic or any grade of clinical illness may be associated with it, and it always demands consideration as a possible menace to human health (Georgi and Sprinkle, 1974). Any dog or cat infected with *S. stercoralis* should be isolated from other animals and care should be taken to avoid human infection. Chronic strongyloidiasis tends to be refractory and recurrent; fecal specimens from recognized cases should be examined monthly for *S. stercoralis* larvae for at least six months following apparently successful therapy. In no case should a single negative fecal specimen be accepted as proof of cure, because the numbers of larvae shed in the feces of infected animals may oscillate drastically from day to day (Galliard, 1951a).

No invariable statement of fact can be made regarding the infectivity or virulence of *S. stercoralis*, because geographic strains exist that differ greatly in their infectivity and virulence for different hosts. For example, Galliard (1951b) had no difficulty in producing durable infections in dogs by using 19 strains of *S. stercoralis*, 11 obtained from Europeans infected in different regions of French Indochina (Vietnam) and 8 from natives of Tonkin, but he found dogs quite refractory to strains imported from the West Indies and Africa. Therefore, the actual threat to human health posed by any particular *S. stercoralis*–infected dog is unpredictable and the introduction or emergence of highly virulent strains is always at least a theoretical possibility. Clearly, it is best to play it safe and handle infected dogs with extraordinary caution until it is quite certain that their *S. stercoralis* burdens have been eliminated.

ANTHELMINTIC MEDICATION

Treatment of *S. stercoralis* infection requires patience and a willingness to experiment. Kelly (1977) recommended 100 to 150 mg. thiabendazole per kg. body weight for three days, repeated weekly until larvae disappear from the feces. Continuous feeding of 250 ppm of thiabendazole prevented establishment of *S. stercoralis* in puppies (Yakstis *et al.*, 1968). Dithiazanine iodide is administered for 10 to 12 days at 20 mg. per kg. as an alternative to thiabendazole.

CONTROL MEASURES

The complex life history of *S. stercoralis* is discussed on page 100 and illustrated in Figures 6–7 and 7–5. The epidemiological importance of the heterogonic cycle depends on the degree of contact between the host and the soil, but *S. stercoralis* is able to achieve and maintain high morbidity rates even in colonies that are housed on wire-bottom cages. Homogonic filariform infective larvae can develop from freshly passed rhabditiform larvae within 24 to 36 hours so that cages and pens must be cleaned and sanitized at

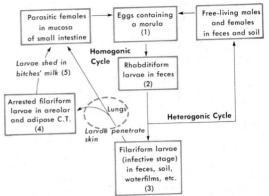

Figure 7–5. Alternative life histories of *Strongyloides stercoralis*. (1) The parasitic female lays eggs in the morula stage of development but the rhabditiform first stage larva hatches within the host and is the form found in fecal specimens. (2) Rhabditiform larvae of the homogonic generation may develop into infective filariform larvae, free-living males, or free-living females. Rhabditiform larvae of the heterogonic generation, on the other hand, develop only into filariform larvae, which, in turn, develop only into parasitic females. (3) Filariform larvae infect the host by penetrating its skin. Ingested filariform larvae, except for those that penetrate the oral and pharyngeal mucosae, are destroyed in the stomach. (4) Larvae reaching the lungs may undergo a tracheal migration and mature in the small intestine or undergo a somatic migration to become arrested larvae in the areolar and adipose connective tissues. (5) Somatic migration and transmammary passage of filariform larvae have been demonstrated experimentally to occur in *S. westeri* in the horse, *S. ransomi* in swine, and *S. papillosus* in sheep, and there is little reason to doubt that *S. stercoralis* behaves in like manner in the dog.

less than 24 hour intervals to break the cycle. Development of somatic arrested larval burdens and transmammary infection of offspring have not been specifically demonstrated to apply to *S. stercoralis* infection in dogs but are well established for several other species of *Strongyloides*. We have observed *S. stercoralis* infection in dam-reared pups but not in their hand-reared littermates, indicating that infection is acquired after birth either from dam's milk, dam's fecal contamination, or both.

The rigor of measures adopted must, as always, be consonant with the objectives of control and the resources of the client. For example, to reliably produce *S. stercoralis*–free experimental pups from infected breeding stock, it is necessary to deliver pups by caesarean section or separate them from their dam immediately at natural birth and rear them artificially on canine milk substitute (e.g., Esbilac). This procedure requires 24 hour attendance and a strong maternal instinct; it can seldom be applied under practical kennel conditions.

Reduction of the level of infection in a breeding colony from the point of sporadic mortalities to the point of asymptomatic, if still prevalent, infection can probably be accomplished by rigorous daily disinfection of cages and pens and monthly or bimonthly administration of a suitable anthelmintic drug. However, *Strongyloides stercoralis* will probably not be driven from the scene either completely or permanently by these measures, thanks to its exceedingly rapid development and the accumulation of arrested larvae in the tissues of bitches. Continued reliance on anthelmintics eventually produces resistant strains. The next step is usually to switch to a different anthelmintic, invariably a more expensive one.

To prevent transmission of *S. stercoralis* from an infected pet to its master requires appropriate anthelmintic medication and monthly Baermann fecal examinations for six months to a year to assure that larval output has been terminated.

WHIPWORMS

Infective *Trichuris vulpis* eggs survive in soil for a long time and dogs kept in contact with contaminated soils tend to become reinfected after treatment. Lasting success in removing these parasites depends on separating the patient from these eggs. However, in emphasizing the need for sanitation, an important possibility may be overlooked. Assuming that the developing parasitic larvae are more resistant to anthelmintic action than the adult worms, it follows that patent infection is almost certain to recur through maturation of immature forms that have survived a dose of anthelmintic. Most canine nematode parasites require only a few weeks to mature, so a second dose of anthelmintic administered two or three weeks after the first theoretically rids the host of the worms that were unaffected by the first treatment. *T. vulpis* differs from the others in requiring about three months to mature, so medication should be routinely repeated three times at monthly intervals to destroy the worms as they mature and prevent them from contaminating the environment.

ANTHELMINTIC MEDICATION

Trichuriasis

In the United States, the preferred drugs for treatment of trichuriasis are mebendazole, fenbendazole, dichlorvos, and glycobiarsol. Overseas, the preferred drug is oxantel, an analogue of pyrantel. Phthalofyne is used in obstinate whipworm infections. Butamisole, an injectable analogue of tetramisole, is also indicated. The rare case of *Trichuris* infection in the cat must be handled on an experimental basis because no drug has been cleared specifically for this purpose; dichlorvos and glycobiarsol are probably suitable.

Capillariasis

Capillariasis, whether bronchial, urinary, or intestinal, is usually asymptomatic but, having identified *Capillaria* eggs in the feces or urine sediment or on a bronchial swab, the modern veterinarian usually feels compelled to medicate. There is no known specific drug for the treatment of *Capillaria* spp. infections. Kelly (1977) suggested levamisole at 2.5 mg. per kg. for five days or a single oral dose of fenbendazole at 50 mg. per kg. as potentially useful drugs for the treatment of these parasitisms in dogs and cats.

Trichinelliasis

Trichinella spiralis infection is infrequently diagnosed in cats and dogs but, because both of these hosts frequently consume uncooked meat in the form of scraps and prey, and the dog displays such a predilection for carrion, it stands to reason that it must in fact be rather common. Treatment of canine and feline trichinosis is experimental; thiabendazole is used in human medicine.

HEARTWORM

ANTHELMINTIC MEDICATION

Different anthelmintics are used to attack three different parasitic stages of *Dirofilaria immitis*, microfilariae in the circulating blood, larvae migrating through the tissues on their way to the heart, and adult worms in the right heart and caval veins. Treatment of a dog with patent heartworm infection consists of first removing the adult parasites with arsenamide and then eliminating the circulating microfilariae with dithiazanine iodide or levamisole later on. Prevention of heartworm infection currently consists of daily administration of diethylcarbamazine to all dogs exposed to the attacks of infected mosquitoes.

Treatment of Heartworm Patients

Adulticide Medication. Arsenamide (thiacetarsamide) is administered intravenously at the rate of 0.1 ml. of 1 per cent buffered solution per pound of body weight (i.e., 2.2

mg. per kg.) twice a day for two days to remove adult heartworms. Some veterinarians believe that the therapeutic efficiency is more consistent if this regimen is extended to three days. The anthelmintic efficiency of arsenamide was observed to vary with the duration of infection. Efficiency was highest at two months, lowest at four months, and thereafter gradually increased (Blair *et al.*, 1982). These observations suggest that, in the case of poor response to arsenamide therapy, it might be wise to wait a few months before trying again.

After arsenamide therapy, heartworms die slowly over a period of days or weeks and are carried by the pulmonary arteries to the lungs, where they lodge and obstruct the circulation temporarily. Eventually, the dead worms are removed by phagocytosis. Probably, if the worms were killed rapidly and simultaneously, treatment would prove more lethal than the heartworms. However, even with the slow kill, the lungs are gravely insulted during the four to six weeks after arsenamide therapy and the dog must not be subjected to stress during this period. An occasional dog will vomit or develop fever and respiratory distress after treatment. If these reactions are more than transitory, arsenamide medication should be discontinued and supportive therapy, administration of steroids, and enforced rest initiated.

Microfilaricide Medication. Microfilaricidal medication should be delayed until at least six weeks after arsenamide therapy. Dithiazanine iodide at 4.4 to 11 mg. per kg. for seven days is recommended for the elimination of circulating microfilariae. Treatment should be initiated at the lower dosage rate and changed to the higher rate only if response is unsatisfactory.

Levamisole is administered orally at 11 mg. per kg. for 6 to 12 days for the elimination of circulating microfilariae. Levamisole is not as yet approved by the FDA for use on dogs.

Ivermectin displays remarkable activity against both microfilariae and migrating larvae but none at all against adult *Dirofilaria immitis* (Blair *et al.*, 1983). Unfortunately, ivermectin is not approved by FDA for use as a microfilaricide in dogs, and field experience is still rather limited at the time of this writing. Please refer to Chapter 11 for a detailed account of ivermectin.

PREVENTION

Prevention of canine heartworm is achieved primarily by daily oral administration of diethylcarbamazine at 6.6 mg. per kg. from the beginning until two months after the end of mosquito activity (Kume *et al.*, 1962a, b, 1964, 1967). In warm climates, where mosquitoes are active the year around, dogs must be dosed daily throughout their lives. Continuous medication is certainly a desperate course of action, but so far there is no practicable alternative. Diethylcarbamazine must not be administered to dogs with microfilaremia because severe or fatal shock-like reactions may ensue (Levine and Diamond, 1967; Kume, 1970). Dogs with patent heartworm infections must therefore undergo the arsenamide-dithiazanine (or levamisole) therapeutic sequence outlined above before being placed on the diethylcarbamazine prophylactic regimen.

METASTRONGYLOID LUNGWORMS

ANTHELMINTIC MEDICATION

Filaroides hirthi. Albendazole administered orally at a dosage rate of 25 mg. per kg. of body weight twice daily for five days killed all but a very small proportion of *F. hirthi* lungworms and sterilized the rest (Georgi *et al.*, 1978). Unfortunately, albendazole still has only limited clearance in the United States at this writing and is not available for general distribution. To date, albendazole medication has been applied only to asymptomatic cases of *F. hirthi* infection and there is no information as to its effect on dogs suffering from hyperinfection with this parasite. In normal dogs with light infections, the killed worms provoke an extensive and persistent tissue reaction which, if multiplied by the enormous numbers involved in hyperinfection, could reasonably be expected to be so severe as to kill the dog. However, hyperinfection apparently results at least in part from depression of cell-mediated immunity, so the reaction to albendazole medication of a dog suffering from *F. hirthi* hyperinfection is unpredictable.

Filaroides osleri. Criteria of successful chemotherapy of *F. osleri* infection include: (1) disappearance of cough and air hunger on exercise, (2) resolution of tracheal and bronchial nodules as demonstrated by bronchoscopy, and (3) cessation of fecal larval output. These criteria have rarely been satisfied and authors disagree as to the efficacy of various treatments. Arsenamide injected intravenously at 2.2 mg. per kg. daily for 21 days has led to resolution of nodules in some but not in all cases (Dietrich, 1962; Dorrington,

1963, 1968). Thiabendazole administered orally at 32 mg. per kg. twice daily for 21 days resulted in resolution of nodules in three dogs but left one of them with a mild cough (Bennett and Beresford-Jones, 1973, Bennett, 1975). Levamisole also showed promise in a clinical trial when administered orally at 7.5 mg. per kg. daily for 10 to 30 days (Darke, 1976). Unfortunately, in none of the above trials were the numbers of animals sufficient nor the opportunities for prolonged observation subsequent to medication adequate to meet the standards of experimental proof. Despite the high anthelmintic efficacy displayed by albendazole against the closely related *F. hirthi,* this drug proved disappointing against *F. osleri* in an experiment described as follows: Three pups received 25 mg. albendazole suspension per kg. body weight orally twice daily for five days 10 to 12 months after artificial infection with *F. osleri.* When necropsied 39 to 66 days later, all were found still infected with reproductively active *F. osleri* worms. Thus, for the present at least, there appears to be no satisfactory anthelmintic medication for *F. osleri* infection.

Aelurostrongylus abstrusus. Levamisole, administered orally to cats at the rate of 8 mg. per kg. three times at two-day intervals, is usually effective in stopping the output of *A. abstrusus* larvae in the feces.

Crenosoma vulpis. Stockdale and Smart (1975) treated *C. vulpis*–infected dogs with a single oral dose of 8 mg. per kg. of levamisole.

CONTROL MEASURES

Filaroides hirthi. The principal objective of *F. hirthi* control is to produce experimental dogs whose lungs are free of worms and tissue reactions to them. Therefore, medication of the prospective experimental animals themselves is contraindicated. Recall that the infective stage of *F. hirthi* is the first stage larva in the freshly passed feces of the infected host and that dogs become infected by eating these feces. One sure way to raise *F. hirthi*–free pups from an infected dam is to remove them by caesarean section and raise them artificially out of contact with all infected dogs, but this is obviously impracticable on a large scale. In order to produce *F. hirthi*–free experimental dogs, two large research Beagle breeding colonies with initial infection rates among marketed dogs of 65 to 100 per cent, cooperated in the following experiment: All stud dogs and all nonpreg-

nant, nonlactating brood bitches were given two courses of albendazole two to four weeks apart, each course consisting of 25 mg. albendazole suspension per kg. body weight orally, twice daily for five days with the objective of eliminating infective first stage larvae from the feces of the bitches. In addition, puppies of treated dams were isolated from puppies of nontreated dams to exclude that source of infection. This program was started in 1978 and has continued to this writing (1983). As of the beginning of 1981, the infection rate among marketed dogs had dropped to 0.2 per cent for one of the colonies, and 24 per cent for the other (Erb and Georgi, 1982).

Filaroides osleri. Infection with this parasite virtually destroys the reputation of a kennel and will continue to do so until an effective anthelmintic or practicable control measures can be devised. As with *F. hirthi,* infection is passed from dog to dog as first stage larvae in fresh feces so that transmission is easy to prevent except in the case of bitches and their litters. Because there is no really effective anthelmintic against *F. osleri,* there is no convenient way of interrupting the flow of infective first stage larvae from feces of the bitch to stomachs of her offspring. The only sure way of raising *F. osleri*–free pups from infected bitches is to remove the pups by caesarean section and raise them artificially and in isolation from all infected dogs. Such expensive and laborious measures might be appropriate in the case of extraordinarily valuable breeding stock but only when the kennel management and staff are people that have great affection for their dogs and exceptional patience and perseverance, because only such people can succeed in raising more than a litter or two "on the bottle."

Aelurostrongylus abstrusus. Infection with this lungworm usually involves individual rural cats that like to hunt. Control consists of preventing the cat's access to infected intermediate hosts. Unfortunately, we cannot specify what these might be, with the exception of a wide range of snails and slugs that few cats would deign to eat anyway. Probably the cats get their *A. abstrusus* infective larvae from paratenic hosts such as mice and voles, but our knowledge of the epidemiology of *A. abstrusus* and other carnivoran metastrongyloids is incomplete.

Crenosoma vulpis. *Crenosoma,* like *Aelurostrongylus,* requires a molluscan intermediate host, and control depends on preventing the dog's access to intermediate hosts.

SPIRUROID NEMATODES

ANTHELMINTIC MEDICATION

Very little is known about the chemotherapy of spiruroid nematodes. Disophenol, 10 mg. per kg., administered twice at an interval of one week was very effective against adult *Spirocerca lupi* (Seneviratna *et al.*, 1966; Chhabra and Singh, 1972). Good therapeutic results were also obtained with diethylcarbamazine, 200 mg. per kg., for 10 or more days (McGaughey, 1950).

REFERENCES

Anderson, F. L., Loveless, R. M., and Jensen, L. A. (1975): Efficacy of bunamidine hydrochloride against immature and mature stages of *Echinococcus granulosus*. Am. J. Vet. Res., *36*, 673-675.

Anderson, F. L., Conder, G. A., and Marsland, W. P. (1978): Efficacy of injectable and tablet formulations of praziquantel against mature *Echinococcus granulosus*. Am. J. Vet. Res., *39*, 1861-1862. Ann., *15*, 256-260.

Bennett, D., and Beresford-Jones, W. P. (1973): Treatment of *Filaroides osleri* infestation in a 16-month old male Yorkshire Terrier with thiabendazole. Vet. Rec., *93*, 226-227.

Blair, L. S., Malatesta, P. F., Jacob, L., and Ewanciw, D. V. (1982): Efficacy of thiacetarsamide in experimentally infected dogs at 2 months, 4 months, 6 months, or 12 months postinfection with *Dirofilaria immitis*. Proc. 27th Ann. Meet. Am. Assoc. Vet. Parasitol., 14-15.

Blair, L. S., Malatesta, P. F., and Ewanciw, D. V. (1983): Dose response study of ivermectin against *Dirofilaria immitis* microfilariae in dogs with naturally acquired infections. Am. J. Vet. Res., *44*, 475-477.

Boray, J. C., Strong, M. B., Allison, J. R., von Orelli, M., Sarasin, G., and Gfeller, W. (1979): Nitroscanate, a new broad spectrum anthelmintic against nematodes and cestodes of dogs and cats. Austr. Vet. J., *55*, 45-53.

Buckner, R. G., and Ewing, S. A. (1977): Trichomoniasis. *In* Current Veterinary Therapy VI, Philadelphia, W. B. Saunders Co., p. 970.

Chhabra, R. C., and Singh, K. S. (1972): Diagnosis, treatment and control of spirocercosis in dogs. Ind. J. Anim. Sci., *42*, 203–207.

Chung, N. Y., Miyahara, A. Y., and Chung, G. (1977): The prevalence of feline liver flukes in the City and County of Honolulu. J. Am. Anim. Hosp. Assoc., *13*, 258-262.

Congdon, L. L., and Ames, E. R. (1973): Thiabendazole for control of *Toxocara canis* in the dog. Am. J. Vet. Res., *34*, 417-418.

Darke, P. G. G. (1976): Use of levamisole in the treatment of parasitic tracheobronchitis in the dog. Vet. Rec. *99*, 293-294.

Dey-Hazra, A. (1976): The efficacy of Droncit (praziquantel) against tapeworm infections in dog and cat. Vet. Med. Rev., No. 2, 134-141.

Dietrich, L. E. (1962): Treatment of canine lungworm infection with thiacetarsamide. J. Am. Vet. Med. Assoc., *140*, 572-573.

Dorrington, J. E. (1963): *Filaroides osleri:* The success of thiacetarsamide sodium therapy. J. S. Afr. Vet. Med. Assoc., *34*, 435-438.

Dorrington, J. E. (1968): Studies on *Filaroides osleri* infestation in dogs. Onderstepoort J. Vet. Res., *35*, 225-286.

Dubey, J. P., Miller, T. B., and Sharma, S. P. (1979): Fenbendazole for treatment of *Paragonimus kellicotti* infection in dogs. J. Am. Vet. Med. Assoc., *174*, 835-837.

Duncombe, V. M., Bolin, T. D., Davis, A. E., and Kelly, J. D. (1977a): The effect of iron and protein deficiency and dexamethasone on the efficacy or benzimidazole anthelmintics. WAAVP 8th Internat. Conf., Sydney, Australia.

Duncombe, V. M., Bolin, T. D., Davis, A. E., and Kelly, J. D. (1977b): *Nippostrongylus brasiliensis* infection in the rat: effect of iron and protein deficiency and dexamethasone on the efficacy of benzimidazole anthelmintics. Gut, *18*, 892-896.

Düwel, D., and Strasser, H. (1978): Versuche zur Geburt helminthenfreier Hundewelpen durch Fenbendazolbehandlung. Dtsch. Tierärztl. Wschr., *85*, 239-241.

Eckerlin, R. P., and Leigh, W. H. (1962): *Platynosomum fastosum* Kossack, 1910 (Trematoda: Dicrocoeliidae) in South Florida. J. Parasitol., *48* (Suppl.), 49.

Eckert, J., von Brand, T., and Voge, M. (1969): Asexual multiplication of *Mesocestoides corti* (Cestoda) in the intestines of dogs and skunks. J. Parasitol., *55* (2), 241-249.

Erb, H. N., and Georgi, J. R. (1982): Control of *Filaroides hirthi* in commercially reared Beagle dogs. Lab. Anim. Sci., *32* (4), 394-396.

Evans, J. W., and Green, P. E. (1978): Preliminary evaluation of four anthelmintics against the cat liver fluke *Platynosomum concinnum*. Austr. Vet. J., *54*, 454-455.

Faulk, R. H., and Schwirck, S. (1978): Effect of Tresaderm (thiabendazole, dexamethazone, neomycin) against otoacariasis: a clinical trial. Vet. Med. and Small Anim. Clin., *73*, 307-308.

Folz, S. D., Geng, S., Nowakowski, L. H., and Conklin, J. R. (1978): Evaluation of a new treatment for canine scabies and demodicosis. J. Vet. Pharmacol. and Therap., *1*, 199-204.

Forbes, L. S. (1966): The efficiency of bunamidine hydrochloride against young *Echinococcus granulosus* infection in dogs. Vet. Rec., *79*, 306-307.

Frenkel, J. K., and Dubey, J. P. (1972): Toxoplasmosis and its prevention in cats and man. J. Infect. Dis., *12*, 664-673.

Galliard, H. (1951a): Recherches sur l'infestation expérimentale à *Strongyloides stercoralis* au Tonkin VIII-X. Ann. Parasitol., *26* (1-2), 68-84.

Galliard, H. (1951b): Recherches sur l'infestation expérimentale à *Strongyloides stercoralis* au Tonkin. XII. Ann. Parasitol., *26* (3), 201-227.

Gemmell, M. A., and Shearer, G. C. (1968): Bunamidine hydrochloride. Its efficiency against *Echinococcus granulosus*. Vet. Rec., *82*, 252-256.

Gemmell, M. A., Johnstone, P. D., and Oudemans, G. (1975): the effect of mebendazole on *Echinococcus granulosus* and *Taenia hydatigena* infections in dogs. Res. Vet. Sci., *19*, 229-230.

Georgi, J. R., and Sprinkle, C. L. (1974): A case of human strongyloidosis apparently contracted from asymptomatic colony dogs. Am. J. Trop. Med. Hyg. *23* (5), 899-901.

Georgi, J. R., Slauson, D. O., and Theodorides, V. J. (1978): Anthelmintic activity of albendazole against *Filaroides hirthi* lungworms in dogs. Am. J. Vet. Res., *39* (5), 803-806.

Griesemer, R. A., and Gibson, J. P. (1963): The establishment of an ascarid-free beagle dog colony. J. Am. Vet. Med. Assoc., *143* (9), 965-967.

Horak, I. G. (1976): The control of ticks, fleas, and lice on dogs by means of a Sendran-impregnated collar. J. S. Afr. Vet. Assoc., *47,* 17-18.

Jones, T. C. (1979): Toxoplasmosis. In Cecil Textbook of Medicine: Paul B. Beeson, Walsh McDermott, and James B. Wyngaarden, editors. Philadelphia, W. B. Saunders Co., p. 594-598.

Kalkofen, V. P. (1971): Effect of dichlorvos on eggs and larvae of *Ancylostoma caninum*. Am. J. Trop. Med. Hyg., *20,* 436-440.

Kelly, J. D. (1977): *Canine Parasitology*. New South Wales, Australia, Post-Graduate Foundation in Veterinary Science.

King, A. B. (1976): Bunamidine hydrochloride in dogs. J. Am. Vet. Med. Assoc., *169,* 854-856.

Kotake, M. (1929a): An experimental study on passing through the mammary gland of ascaris and hookworm larvae. Osaka Igakkai Zasshi, *28,* 1251.

Kotake, M. (1929b): Hookworm larvae in the mammary gland. Osaka, Igakkai Zasshi, *28,* 2493-2518.

Kume, S. (1970): Pathogenesis of allergic shock from the use of diethylcarbamazine. In Canine Heartworm Disease. R. E. Bradley, ed., Gainesville, University of Florida, pp. 7-20.

Kume, S., Ohishi, I., and Kobayashi, S. (1962a): A new approach to prophylactic therapy against the developing stages of *Dirofilaria immitis* before reaching the canine heart. Vet. Clinics of North Amer., *8* (2), 353-378.

Kume, S., Ohishi, I., and Kobayashi, S. (1962b): Prophylactic therapy against the developing stages of *Dirofilaria immitis*. Am. J. Vet. Res., *23,* 1257-1260.

Kume, S., Ohishi, I., and Kobayashi, S. (1964): Extended studies on prophylactic therapy against the developing stages of *Dirofilaria immitis* in the dog. Am. J. Vet. Res., *25* 1527-1530.

Kume, S., Ohishi, I, and Kobayashi, S. (1967): Prophylactic therapy against the developing stages of *Dirofilaria immitis*: Supplemental studies. Am. J. Vet. Res., *28* (125), 975-978.

Levine, B. G., and Diamond, S. S. (1967): Clinical experience with medical treatment for canine heartworms. Practicing Vet., *39,* 136-140.

Lewis, G. E., and Huxsoll, D. L. (1977): Canine babesiosis. In Current Veterinary Therapy VI, Philadelphia, W. B. Saunders Co. p. 1330.

Lienert, E. (1962): Hexachlorophene (G-11) is extremely efficient in cats and dogs naturally infected with the liver fluke *Opisthorchis tenuicollis* (Rudolphi, 1819) Stiles and Hassall, 1896. Wien. Tierärztl. Monatschr., *49,* 353-359.

Little, M. D. (1978): Dormant *Ancylostoma caninum* larvae in muscle as a source of subsequent patent infection in the dog. Abstract 75, 53rd Annual Meeting, Am. Soc. Parasitology at Chicago, Ill.

Manson, E. R., and Malynicz, G. L. (1969): The use of cythioate in the treatment of demodectic mange in the dog. Austr. Vet. J., *45,* 533-534.

McCoy, O. R. (1930): The influence of temperature, hydrogen-ion concentration and oxygen tension on the development of the eggs and larvae of the dog hookworm, *Ancylostoma caninum*. Am. J. Hyg., *11,* 413-448.

McGaughey, C. A. (1950): Preliminary note on the treatment of spirocercosis in dogs with piperazine compound, acaricide (Lederle). Vet. Rec., *62,* 814–815.

Miller, J. E., Baker, N. F., and Colburn, E. L., Jr. (1977): Insecticidal activity of propoxur and carbaryl-impregnated flea collars against *Ctenocephalides felis*. Am. J. Vet. Res., *38,* 923-925.

Reedy, L. (1977): Ectoparasites. In Current Veterinary Therapy VI, Philadelphia, W. B. Saunders Co., p. 547.

Roberson, E. (1977): Antiprotozoal Drugs. In Veterinary Pharmacology and Therapeutics; L. Meyer Jones, Nicholas H. Booth, and Leslie E. McDonald, editors. Ames, The Iowa State University Press, p. 1095.

Rommel, M., Grelck, H., and Hörchner, F. (1976): Zür Wirksamkeit von Praziquantel gegen Bandwürmer in experimentell infizierten Hunden und Katzen. Ber. Münch. Tierärztl. Wochencshr., *89,* 255-257.

Ruff, M. D., Fowler, J. L., Fernau, R. C., and Matsuda, K. (1973): Action of certain antiprotozoal compounds against *Babesia gibsoni* in dogs. Am. J. Vet. Res., *34,* 641-645.

Sakamoto, T. (1977): The anthelmintic effect of Droncit on adult tapeworms of *Hydatigera taeniaeformis, Mesocestoides corti, Echinococcus multilocularis, Diphyllobothrium erinacei*, and *D. latum*. Vet. Med. Rev., No. 1, 64-74.

Seneviratna, P., Fernando, S. T., and Dhanapala, S. B. (1966): Disophenol treatment of spirocercosis in dogs. J. Am. Vet. Med. Assoc., 148, 269–274.

Sprent, J. F. A. (1956): The life history and development of *Toxocara cati* (Schrank, 1788) in the domestic cat. Parasitology, *46* (1-2), 54-58.

Sprent, J. F. A. (1961): Post-parturient infection of the bitch with *Toxocara canis*. J. Parasitol., *47,* 284.

Stockdale, P. H. G., and Smart, M. E. (1975): Treatment of crenosomiasis in dogs. Res. Vet. Sci., *18,* 178-181.

Stone, W. M., and Girardeau, M. H. (1966): *Ancylostoma caninum* larvae present in the colostrum of a bitch. Vet. Rec., *79* (24), 773-774.

Stone, W. M., and Girardeau, M. H. (1968): Transmammary passage of *Ancylostoma caninum* larvae in dogs. J. Parasitol., *54,* 426-429.

Stoye, M. (1973): Untersuchungen über die Möglichkeit pränataler und galaktogener Infectionen mit *Ancylostoma caninum* Ercolani, 1859 (Ancylostomidae) beim Hund. Zentralbl. Vet. Med. Series B, *20* (1), 1-39.

Swerczek, T. W., Nielson, S. W., and Helmbolt, C. F. (1971): Transmammary passage on *Toxocara cati* in the cat. Am. J. Vet. Res., *32* (1), 89-92.

Thomas, H., and Gönnert, R. (1978): The efficacy of praziquantel against cestodes in cats, dogs, and sheep. Res. Vet. Sci., *24,* 20-25.

Todd, K. S., Howland, T. P., and Woerpel, R. W. (1978): Activity of uredephos, niclosamide, bunamidine hydrochloride, and arecoline hydrobromide against *Mesocestoides corti* in experimentally infected dogs. Am. J. Vet. Res., *39,* 315-316.

Trejos, A., Szyfres, B., and Marchevsky, N. (1975): Comparative value of arecoline hydrobromide and bunamidine hydrochloride for the treatment of *Echinococcus granulosus* in dogs. Res. Vet. Sci., *19,* 212-213.

Williams, J. F., and Keahey, K. K. (1976): Sudden death associated with treatment of three dogs with bunamidine hydrochloride. J. Am. Vet. Med. Assoc., *168,* 689-691.

Yakstis, J. J., Egerton, J. R., Campbell, W. C., and Cuckler, A. C. (1968): Use of thiabendazole-medicated feed for prophylaxis of four common roundworm infections in dogs. J. Parasitol., *54,* 359-367.

8

PARASITES OF RUMINANTS

CONTROL OF ARTHROPODS

Arthropod Control on Beef and Dry Dairy Cattle

FACE FLY AND HOUSE FLY

The control of face flies and house flies on beef cattle and dry dairy cattle and around animal premises is a very difficult task. Control of these flies may be achieved by regular application of insecticides to animals and fly-breeding sites. Dichlorvos in mineral oil may be smeared daily on the faces of cattle for face fly control. Chlorpyrifos, coumaphos, malathion, or tetrachlorvinphos may be applied to cattle as a free-flowing dust two or three times a week or self-applied by means of self-treatment dust bags. CIOVAP, dioxathion, pyrethrin, or pyrethroid sprays may also be used. Sugar fly bait containing methomyl and muscalure (a fly attractant) is sprinkled around barns and other animal premises. Pyrethroid-containing eartags and similar devices that can be attached to animals allow a continuous, controlled release of insecticides to aid in the control of flies attacking cattle. Tetrachlorvinphos, a larvicidal organophosphate, prevents the growth of larvae of coprophilic flies in the manure of cattle fed this compound.

HORN FLY, STABLE FLY, HORSE FLIES, DEER FLIES, BLACK FLIES, AND MOSQUITOES

These flies, having piercing mouthparts, can theoretically be controlled with systemic and topical insecticides. CIOVAP spray, crotoxyphos, chlorpyrifos, coumaphos, dioxathion, famphur, malathion, trichlorfon, phosmet, methoxychlor, or tetrachlorvinphos are applied either by spray or with self-treatment dust bags or backrubbers. Tetrachlorvinphos and methoprene may be fed to cattle to prevent the development of horn flies that breed in manure. Synergized pyrethrins ap-

plied daily as a spray afford good control of all biting flies.

SCREWWORMS

Coumaphos, lindane, and dioxathion are widely employed in the treatment of cutaneous myiasis. These insecticidal agents may be applied to the cattle by dipping, but most commonly they are sprayed or smeared directly on the maggot-infested lesions.

CATTLE GRUBS

Hypoderma infection is best treated with systemic organophosphate insecticides. Coumaphos, fenthion, crufomate, phosmet, and trichlorphon are widely used as sprays, pour-ons, or spot-ons to kill the larvae in the early stages of their migration; ivermectin is also highly effective. The "safe periods" for applying these insecticides vary for different localities because of differences in fly activity. The insecticides must be applied immediately after adult *Hypoderma* activity ceases for the season. Host-parasite reactions manifested clinically by bloat, salivation, ataxia, and posterior paralysis, may occur when cattle are treated with larvicidal insecticides while *H. lineatum* larvae are in the esophagus or while *H. bovis* larvae are in the spinal canal. The host-parasite reaction was once thought to be an anaphylactoid reaction caused by antibodies produced by cattle in response to *Hypoderma* larvae. However, new experimental evidence indicates that this reaction is caused by a toxin liberated from the dead *Hypoderma* larvae. Injecton of phenylbutazone at a dosage rate of 20 mg. per kg. body weight 20 minutes before injection of larval toxin protected calves against both systemic shock and local inflammatory reactions (Eyre *et al.*, 1981). The host-parasite reaction is best treated with sympathomimetic drugs (e.g., adrenalin) and steroids to alleviate local inflammatory reactions. Atropine, the antidote for cholinesterase inhibiting agents, is contraindicated; host-parasite reaction is not a manifestation of organophosphate toxicity even though it is precipitated by organophosphate medication.

LICE

Coumaphos, crufomate, chlorpyrifos, famphur, fenthion, lindane, phosmet, trichlorfon, crotoxyphos, malathion, methoxychlor, and tetrachlorvinphos as sprays, dips, or pour-ons, provide excellent control of lice.

TICKS

Coumaphos, dioxathion, tetrachlorvinphos, malathion, lindane, or methoxychlor is effective against nonresistant ticks when applied as spray, dip, or dust. Insecticidal dusts or emulsion concentrates may be instilled into the ear canal from a squeeze bottle or oil can to eliminate spinose ear ticks (*Otobius megnini*).

MITES

Sarcoptic, chorioptic, and psoroptic mites are susceptible to sprays or dips containing lime sulfur, crotoxyphos, phosmet, and tetrachlorvinphos. Sarcoptic and psoroptic manges are reportable diseases in many states and treatment is supervised by animal health authorities. Chorioptic mange usually responds to standard louse treatments.

Arthropod Control on Lactating Dairy Cows

The application of insecticides to lactating cows producing milk for human consumption demands extreme caution, for there must not be any pesticide in the milk. READ THE LABEL BEFORE USING ANY PESTICIDE. It is against the law to use a pesticide in any manner not specified on the label, and violations with respect to dairy cows are particularly serious.

BITING FLIES AND MUSCA SPP.

Crotoxyphos, CIOVAP, dichlorvos, synergized pyrethrins, coumaphos, tetrachlorvinphos, malathion, and methoxychlor are used as sprays, and sprinkle-on dusts as well as in dust bags and backrubbers. Tetrachlorvinphos is also fed to cattle to control larvae of the horn fly and face fly in manure.

LICE

Crotoxyphos, tetrachlorvinphos, CIOVAP, synergized pyrethrins, methoxychlor, coumaphos, and malathion are applied to lactating dairy cows as sprays, in dust bags, in backrubbers, and as sprinkle-on dusts. Two applications should provide good control.

TICKS

Crotoxyphos, coumaphos, dichlorvos, and CIOVAP are applied as sprays or in backrubbers for the control of ticks. There are no restrictions when used as recommended.

CATTLE GRUBS

Mature dairy cattle have usually developed sufficient immunity to prevent the development of more than a few cattle grubs even in years when the backs of first calf heifers may be covered with warbles. Organophosphates may not be applied to lactating dairy cattle.

MANGE MITES

Crotoxyphos or lime sulfur suspension as spray or dip provides good control of chorioptic mange mites on lactating dairy cows. Sarcoptic and psoroptic mange should be reported to state disease control authorities and treatment carried out under their supervision.

Arthropod Control on Sheep and Goats

SHEEP KED

Coumaphos, diazinon, dioxathion, lindane, malathion, methoxychlor, and toxaphene as dips or sprays provide excellent control of *Melophagus ovinus* when applied after shearing. In small flocks, diazinon can be applied most conveniently with a garden sprinkling can. Use of lindane and toxaphene is illegal in some states of the U.S.A.

FLYSTRIKE

Coumaphos, diazinon, and dioxathion are recommended as sprays, dips, or local applications to affected areas in cases of cutaneous myiasis. All soiled wool and wool underrun by maggots should first be clipped away. The extent of measures taken to prevent flystrike in sheep should be proportional to the degree of risk. Clipping the wool of the breech and area around the prepuce greatly reduces the amount of moisture and filth that can be retained in those regions of the fleece. Amputation of the tail of lambs represents about the minimum of effort that ought to be expended on flystrike control but there are some parts of the world where lambs manage to grow up with their tails intact. In the Mules operation, widely practiced in Australia, redundant folds of skin from the posterior aspects of the thighs and the tail head are removed with a pair of sharp "dagging" shears. When the resultant wounds heal, the skin of the breech is drawn taut, thus extending the relatively hairless area immediately surrounding the anus and vulva and thereby reducing the moisture- and filth-carrying capacity of the breech. This operation, carried out in a minute or so without surgical preparation, anesthesia, or aftercare, seems brutal until one has had an opportunity to compare its effects on the patient with those inflicted by *Lucilia cuprina*.

LICE

CIOVAP, coumaphos, chlorpyrifos, diazinon, dioxathion, lindane, malathion, and methoxychlor provide good control of lice when applied as sprays or dips. The use of lindane and toxaphene is illegal in some states.

MANGE MITES

Sheep infested with *Psoroptes* should be treated twice with an approved dip at an interval of 10 to 14 days. Psoroptic scabies in sheep is a reportable disease and treatment is usually conducted under the supervision of animal health authorities. Lime sulfur, lindane, and toxaphene are effective but use of the latter two chemicals is prohibited in some states.

TICKS

Coumaphos, dichlorvos, dioxathion, malathion, ronnel, and toxaphene may be used as dips and sprays in the control of ticks. *Otobius megnini* ear ticks are treated with insecticidal dusts or emulsion concentrates instilled into the ear canal from squeeze bottles or oil can.

NASAL BOTS

The larva of *Oestrus ovis* is very susceptible to rafoxanide administered orally at the rate of 7.5 mg. per kg.; rafoxanide is not yet licensed in the United States, however. Crufomate, dichlorvos, or fenthion may be sprayed directly into the nostrils for the control of nasal bots.

Control of Flies on Animal Premises

Regular spraying of animal sheds, stables, and kennels with residual insecticides should provide good control of flies and other flying insects provided that reasonable effort is expended to minimize the extent of breeding sites available to these insects. Space sprays, insecticidal baits, and insecticidal resin strips offer additional control

Fenthion, diazinon, dimethoate, tetrachlorvinphos, and dichlorvos all offer excellent residual activity against house flies, face flies, horn flies, stable flies, and mosquitoes for from one to four weeks after application. Spraying resting and breeding areas is often effective.

Dichlorvos, naled, and pyrethrins are used as space sprays for feedlots and sheds. These insecticides may be misted over the backs of animals every three to seven days.

Fly baits containing dichlorvos and naled may be sprayed or sprinkled on fly-roosting areas. The sugar fly bait New Improved Golden Malrin contains methomyl and muscalure, a fly-attracting pheromone. The bait is sprinkled around barns. Muscalure attracts and keeps the flies around the bait, thus resulting in an increased kill by the insecticide.

Insect control in dairy barns and in milk rooms may be achieved with dichlorvos resin strips, baits, foggers, and sprays. Tetrachlorvinphos and the combination product CIOVAP are also used. Coumaphos is used as a spray or in dust bags. It may be applied after milking.

PROTOZOAN INFECTIONS

Toxoplasmosis and Sarcocystosis

The life histories of *Toxoplasma gondii* and *Sarcocystis* spp. are outlined in Chapter 3, and the currently known host relationships of *Sarcocystis* are listed in Table 3-1.

Toxoplasma gondii parasitizes all tissues of

all domestic animals, but clinical toxoplasmosis in ruminants is most often manifested as abortion and neonatal death caused by placentitis. Sheep and cattle acquire *T. gondii* infection by ingesting sporulated oocysts shed in the feces of cats. Cats do not belong in mangers. The presence of *T. gondii* cysts in edible carcass tissues is probably very important in the epidemiology of human toxoplasmosis. Thorough cooking overcomes this hazard.

Sarcocystosis has only recently been recognized as a clinical disease of cattle (Frelier *et al.*, 1977). Cattle become infected when they ingest sporocysts of *Sarcocystis cruzi* from dog feces. Two schizogonic generations occur in the vascular endothelium, and a third leads to the formation of the typical sarcocysts in skeletal muscle. The dog in turn is infected when it consumes uncooked infected beef, so the cycle can be interrupted either by cooking beef scraps to be fed to dogs or by preventing canine fecal contamination of cattle feedstuffs. Dogs don't belong in mangers. The prevalence and economic importance of bovine sarcocystosis remains to be assessed; objective diagnosis depends on finding schizonts in the vascular endothelium.

Coccidiosis

For pathogenesis and clinical manifestations of coccidiosis, see Chapter 3; for differential diagnosis based on oocyst morphology, see Chapter 12. In controlling coccidiosis, heavy reliance is placed on chemicals and, where coccidiosis is a problem, the chemicals are nearly indispensable. The objective of anticoccidial prophylaxis is to afford sufficient protection to the exposed ruminant to allow it to develop immunity without getting sick in the process. The chemicals reduce the magnitude of challenge and thereby prevent the disease coccidiosis; they do not prevent the infection coccidiasis. But don't expect the chemical to perform miracles. Too much contamination with oocyst-laden manure, and too much crowding, exposure, and fatigue, combined with too little feed, are the sort of conditions that can't be overcome by the best chemical.

Amprolium is recommended orally at a dosage level of 10 mg. per kg. for the treatment of active infections with *Eimeria bovis* and *E. zuernii*. A dosage level of 5 mg. per kg. daily for 21 days is used as an aid in the prevention of coccidiosis caused by *E. bovis* and *E. zuernii* during periods of exposure to oocysts.

Decoquinate is recommended as an aid in the prevention of coccidiosis caused by *E. bovis* and *E. zuernii* in ruminating calves and older cattle. Decoquinate is fed at a dosage level of 0.5 mg. per kg. for at least 28 days during periods of risk of exposure to oocysts.

Monensin at a dosage level of 0.25 mg. per kg. daily for 31 days provided excellent control of *E. bovis* in experimentally infected calves (Fitzgerald and Mansfield, 1973).

HELMINTH INFECTIONS

Trematodes

Life histories and pathogenesis of trematode parasites of ruminants are discussed in Chapter 4; for information about diagnosis, see Chapters 12 and 13. Ruminant fluke infections are usually associated with semi-aquatic landscapes because the obligatory intermediate hosts are aquatic or amphibious snails. The mode of infection is either ingestion of metacercariae encysted on vegetation (Fasciolidae and Paramphistomatidae) or penetration of the skin by cercariae (Schistosomatidae). *Dicrocoelium dendriticum* provides an important exception to this general rule by using a terrestrial snail as first intermediate host and an ant as second intermediate host. In the case of *D. dendriticum*, the ruminant becomes infected by accidentally ingesting ants while grazing.

CONTROL

Theoretically, aquatic snails can be controlled by draining swamps or by broadcasting molluscicides on the snail-infested waters but the continued existence of flukes where they have always been indicates that snail control measures are impracticable in many cases. Areas connected by streams with other snail-infested regions are generally not amenable to snail control measures. Periodic anthelmintic medication may help to reduce contamination of pastures with fluke eggs.

ANTHELMINTIC MEDICATION

Albendazole at 7.5 to 15 mg. per kg. provides control against both *Fasciola hepatica* and *Dicrocoelium dendriticum* in cattle and sheep. At present, albendazole is available only in a few states where *F. hepatica* poses a serious economic problem. Special dispensation is required to treat sheep elsewhere in the U.S.A. with albendazole. Other effective flukicides—diamphenethide, nitroxynil, oxyclozanide, rafoxanide, and triclabendazole—are not available in the U.S.A.

Cestodes

CONTROL

Adult Cestodes

The tapeworms of cattle, sheep, and goats all belong to the family Anoplocephalidae. The life histories of only a few anoplocephalids have been documented but those that have involve an arthropod intermediate host in which the infective cysticercoid develops. Infection purportedly results from the incidental ingestion of these infected arthropods by the grazing animal. Pasture renovation is recommended to destroy the surface layer of humus and thus the habitat of oribatid mites, which are the intermediate host of at least some of these cestodes, but there seems to be little experimental basis to support this recommendation. Fortunately, adult tapeworms are relatively nonpathogenic. Those species that inhabit the bile ducts cause condemnation of the liver at slaughter and lead in this way to considerable economic loss. However, the most common reason for a veterinarian's wish to find a drug to remove adult tapeworms from ruminants seems to be related to the difficulty of persuading the average client that those big, white worms are relatively harmless; it's easier to worm the stock than to convince the stockman.

Taeniid Larvae

Hydatid disease and its control were discussed in Chapter 5 in relationship to the human health hazard posed by *Echinococcus* tapeworm infections in dogs. Consideration of other important taeniid larval infections that are acquired by the ingestion of eggs in carnivoran or human feces follows.

Cysticercus tenuicollis, the larva of the canine taeniid tapeworm *Taenia hydatigena*, migrates through the liver tissue and encysts on the peritoneal membranes of cattle, sheep, swine, and certain wild ungulates. Massive invasions, such as occur when entire tapeworm segments are ingested, result in acute traumatic hepatitis, and even small numbers of migrating metacestodes are as capable as

Fasciola hepatica maritas of precipitating "black disease" in the presence of *Clostridium novyi*. However, frank disease is relatively rarely caused by *C. tenuicollis*, and the principal economic loss results from condemnation of infected livers by meat inspection authorities.

Cysticercus ovis, the larva of a second canine taeniid tapeworm *Taenia ovis*, infects the cardiac and skeletal muscles of sheep and represents the most important pathological lesion found in imported Australian mutton by American inspectors; $1,540,000 worth of boneless mutton (12.5 per cent of the total shipment) had to be sold as pet food or shipped back to Australia (Arundel, 1972).

Cysticercus bovis, the larva of the "unarmed" human tapeworm *Taeniarhynchus saginatus* (*Taenia saginata*), encysts in the striated muscles of cattle, especially the heart and muscles of mastication. Taeniid eggs survive the rigors of the septic tank as well as many contemporary sewage treatment processes, and because defecating out-of-doors is unavoidable when hunting or camping out, it is easy to see how cattle pastures become contaminated with *T. saginatus* eggs. The cysticerci that develop when these eggs are ingested by cattle are relatively inconspicuous and are easily overlooked by the lover of rare or raw ("cannibal sandwich") beef. Consequently, *T. saginatus* is a common parasite of Americans and would be far more common but for the vigilance of our meat inspectors. Condemnation of carcass meats for the presence of *T. saginatus* cysticeri results in great economic loss. Sometimes, this loss is concentrated in a particular lot of cattle and borne by a single producer. Under such circumstances, the economic loss caused by *T. saginatus* ceases to be an abstract figure and becomes of immediate concern not only to the unlucky producer but to his veterinarian too. The problem is that some person, most likely a local, has a tapeworm and that person has defecated in or near the cattle feed. People are generally uncooperative under such circumstances and the culprit is rarely identified.

Coenurus cerebralis, the larva of a canine taeniid tapeworm *Multiceps multiceps*, invades the cranial cavity of sheep, goats, and sometimes cattle. As the cyst grows over a period of six or eight months, neurological signs of progressive space occupation slowly develop. There may be blindness, incoordination, walking in circles, and pressing the head against walls, tree trunks, and the like.

Finally, the animal lies down and dies. The most common diseases that might be confused with cerebral coenurosis are bacterial encephalitis (listeriosis) and parelaphostrongylosis. Intracranial surgery is the only cure for cerebral coenurosis but lies beyond economic reality for sheep unless the shepherd is very skillful with his jackknife. The location of the larva within the skull makes some people wonder how the scolices ever reach a dog's stomach, but they must not realize that a good stout dog can crush a sheep's skull with one bite! As in the case of *Taenia hydatigena* and *T. ovis*, control can only be based on excluding dogs and other canids from sheep pastures. Unfortunately, this is often next to impossible.

ANTHELMINTIC MEDICATION

Adult Cestodes

Moniezia. In the United States, fenbendazole has been approved as a cattle anthelmintic at 5 mg. per kg., but the label bears no indication of efficacy against *Moniezia*. Overseas, fenbendazole is marketed for *Moniezia* control at a higher dosage rate, 7.5 mg. per kg., and niclosamide, resorantel, albendazole, cambendazole, oxfendazole, and mebendazole (only in sheep) are also recommended for control of tapeworms in cattle, sheep, and goats.

Thysanosoma actinoides infections were treated experimentally with 10 gm. of dichlorophene per animal (Ryff *et al.*, 1950). Bithionol at 220 mg. per kg. (Allen *et al.*, 1962), niclosamide at 100 mg. per kg. (Graber, 1969), and cambendazole at 100 mg. per kg. (Allen, 1973) were reported effective under laboratory conditions. These drugs are either not available or not approved for medication of ruminants in the U.S.A.

Avitellina (exotic) infections in sheep were successfully treated with a single dose of 15 mg. per kg. of bithionol (Guilhon and Graber, 1964). Vibe and colleagues (1972) found 100 mg. per kg. niclosamide to be very efficacious against *Thysaniezia* (exotic) and *Avitellina*.

Stilesia (exotic) infections are very difficult to treat. Tin arsenate at a dose of 350 mg. per kg. administered orally (Castel *et al.*, 1960) and dichlorophene at a rate of 250 mg. per kg. (Guilhon and Graber, 1960) were completely effective against *S. globipunctata*, but both were inactive against *S. hepatica* in sheep. The new drug praziquantel at a dosage rate of 2.5 mg. per kg. was extremely

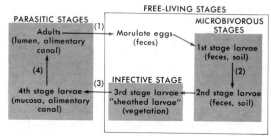

Figure 8–1. A typical strongylid life history. Stages 1 through 4 are explained in the text.

effective against *Moniezia* in sheep but doses of 8 to 15 mg. per kg. were required for the treatment of *Avitellina centripunctata, S. globipunctata,* and *S. hepatica* (Bankov, 1975, 1976; Thomas and Gönnert, 1978).

Nematodes

The Ecology of Strongylids

The typical strongylid life history as outlined in Figure 8-1 is generally applicable to members of the superfamilies Trichostrongyloidea, Strongyloidea, and Ancylostomatoidea. Important embellishments on this scheme, such as the skin penetration of hookworm infective larvae or the atypical larval development of *Dictyocaulus*, do not significantly alter the qualitative ecological and epidemiological relationships portrayed:

1. The rate of environmental contamination with eggs is in direct proportion to the degree of infection of the host population with adult worms.

2. Development and survival of the infective stage depend on the prevailing conditions of temperature and moisture. Optimum requirements vary distinctly among worm species.

3. Host resistance varies as a function of age, vigor, genetic constitution, presence or absence of an already established infection, and, in some instances, acquired immunity.

4. The maturation of the fourth stage larvae may be held temporarily in abeyance by as yet poorly understood influences. Populations of arrested larvae may be harbored for months before some unknown stimulus restarts their final development.

ADULT WORM POPULATIONS

Although some infective larvae may survive for weeks or months under suitable environmental conditions, it is the carrier host that often perpetuates strongylid infections from year to year. The infection may be maintained as a small population of adult worms, as a latent population of histotrophic larvae, or as both. Strongylids, like cold viruses and daffodils, display marked seasonal variations. The worm population is normally regulated in a way that spares the host and perpetuates the parasite, and only when this regulation breaks down do outbreaks of disease occur.

During their first season at pasture, calves, lambs, and kids acquire strongylid burdens rapidly by ingesting third stage larvae as they graze. If the vegetation is heavily contaminated with pathogenic species (e.g., *Ostertagia ostertagi* or *Haemonchus contortus*), disease and deaths may occur among these young and "inexperienced" hosts. The accumulation of infection is manifested by a corresponding increase in fecal egg output and by further contamination of the pasture. Provided sufficient warmth and moisture for larval development, the number of infective stages on vegetation will tend to increase exponentially, at least during the early part of the grazing season. However, the hosts now begin to develop resistance to further infection. The principal component of this developing resistance is a peculiar phenomenon called *premunition:* "a state of resistance to infection which is established after an acute infection has become chronic and which lasts as long as the infecting organisms remain in the body" (*Dorland's Illustrated Medical Dictionary*). The mechanism of premunition is unknown, but the phenomenon can be readily demonstrated by a variety of simple experiments. For example, if we decide to impose a severe *Haemonchus contortus* burden on a sheep that is already harboring a moderate population of these parasites, we must first remove the already established population by anthelmintic medication. Otherwise, part or all of the dose of larvae that we administer experimentally will fail to take. As premunition and other forms of host resistance develop, individual strongylid burdens reach a peak and then begin to decline. Normally, the calf, lamb, or kid enters its first winter with a substantially reduced population of adult strongylids.

What becomes of the infective larvae that the now premunized host continues to ingest as it grazes? There are three possibilities. Such larvae may be rejected, may replace established adult worms, or may become arrested in their development as fourth stage larvae, but the total number of adult worms tends to remain at a plateau. The *arrested* larvae (also referred to as *latent, inhibited,* or *hypobiotic* larvae) remain in the alimentary mucous membrane until some stimulus related to the coming of spring, or to the reproductive cycle of the host, or to both, restarts their development. For example, after lambing in spring, there is a large increase in the output of strongylid eggs in the feces of adult sheep. This "spring rise" in fecal egg counts is related principally to the maturation of the larvae that have overwintered as arrested fourth stages in the alimentary mucosae of adult sheep. On an individual basis, "spring rise" is most marked in ewes about six to nine weeks after lambing and, for this reason, is also called "postparturient rise" (Crofton, 1954). "The production of a large number of eggs about two months after parturition ensures that infective stages will be available in large numbers at a time when the sheep population is not only enlarged by lambing but also has a high proportion of susceptible individuals which have not been exposed to infection previously" (Crofton, 1963).

In summary, calves, lambs, and kids tend to carry large parasite burdens, whereas adult cattle, sheep, and goats usually have only light infections. One peak of strongylid reproductive activity is observed during the grazing season; this occurs both in mature and growing ruminants but tends to be more marked and pathogenic in the latter. A second peak occurs in mature females a few weeks after parturition and is marked by the "postparturient rise" in egg output. This increase is most marked in ewes lambing in spring, at which season a modest "spring rise" is also observed in wethers and barren ewes.

The *biotic potential* or reproductive capacity of strongylids depends jointly on the rate of production of fertile eggs and on the *generation time*, i.e., the time required for these eggs to develop into egg-producing adults. The normal degree of realization of the biotic potential tends to maintain stable worm populations that display marked periodicity but neither explode nor fade away to extinction. Normally, the probability of any individual strongylid egg reaching reproductive age is only one in thousands, so the worms must compensate by producing enormous numbers of eggs. *Haemonchus* is the most fecund, with *Oesophagostomum, Chabertia, Bunostomum, Ostertagia, Cooperia, Trichostrongylus,* and *Nematodirus* following in roughly that order. The species with low per individual reproduction rates tend to compensate either by maintaining larger adult populations (*Trichostrongylus* and *Cooperia*) or by producing eggs that are more resistant to inclemencies of the external environment (*Nematodirus*).

DEVELOPMENT AND SURVIVAL OF THE INFECTIVE STAGE

Most strongylids are capable of developing and maintaining significant populations of infective larvae over considerable ranges of temperature and moisture. Minimum conditions are of interest because they dictate the point at which the environment ceases to harbor significant infection, and optimum conditions are of interest because it is during periods favorable for the development and survival of preparasitic stages that outbreaks of clinical strongylosis usually occur.

No strongylid life history can be completed in totally arid environments, and parasitism with strongylids is correspondingly rare in desert regions. Even under apparently dry conditions, however, microhabitats may exist that contain enough moisture to allow survival if not development of eggs and larvae.

The temperature necessary for development varies with the species, and in each case the rate of development varies with the temperature. With the very significant exceptions of *Nematodirus filicollis, N. battus,* and *Ostertagia* spp., which appear to be well adapted to cold climates, the egg and larva populations of most strongylids suffer marked reductions or even disappear from northern pastures during winter. Such pastures become recontaminated in spring. *Nematodirus* infective larvae develop and remain viable in the egg shell over winter in about as harsh climates as it is profitable to practice cattle, sheep, or goat husbandry. *Ostertagia* overwinters both as infective larvae on pasture and as arrested larvae in the host population; the pasture larvae begin to die off as warmer and dryer conditions supervene.

HOST RESISTANCE

Age. A general increase in resistance to strongylid infection with age is well marked in cattle, slightly less so in sheep, and least in goats. Age resistance may break down in the face of overwhelming challenge or as a secondary result of malnutrition or disease. Old ewes may succumb to strongylidosis

when their teeth fail them, and limited milk production by ewes predisposes their nursling lambs (Whitlock, 1951). Examination of the teeth and udders of ewes should be part of any investigation of parasitic disease in sheep.

Phenotype. Whitlock (1955a, 1958) reported an inherited resistance to trichostrongylidosis in sheep. The progeny of a ram called Violet harbored smaller populations of worms and suffered less reduction in hematocrit than did the progeny of other lambs. Unfortunately, one dark and stormy night the electric transmission lines fell on Violet and blew him to glory. Years later, when he retired and turned over his Zeiss Photomicroscope to me, Dr. Whitlock had a brass plate engraved in Violet's memory and mounted on the microscope.

Premunition. The presence of a stable population of adult strongylids in the alimentary canal tends to inhibit further infection or, at least, further maturation of larvae. Removal of this stable adult population by anthelmintic medication vacates an ecological niche that is promptly filled through maturation of arrested larvae, uninterrupted development of recently ingested infective larvae, or both. For this reason, a ruminant with a *subclinical* strongylid infection should not be treated with anthelmintics unless an uncontaminated environment can be provided after treatment. The loss of premunition resulting from removal of the stable, established infection will permit rapid reinfection, perhaps with a heavier parasite load than before.

The following seeming paradox lends a measure of symmetry to this argument. If sheep are removed during peak exposure from a *Haemonchus contortus*–infested pasture to a parasite-free environment, they will develop more serious infections than if they are left on the pasture. Interrupting the flow of larvae apparently throws the regulation out of balance in some way. The inhibition of larval development by adult worms is manifested as premunition; it appears that the larvae in turn exercise a measure of control over the adults. At any rate, the practical advice to be gleaned from this is as follows: Be sure to administer an anthelmintic to *H. contortus*–infected sheep before transferring them to an uncontaminated environment, at least during the parasites' normal period of rapid population growth.

Self-cure. There are few examples of the kind of immunity that persists to protect the host against reinfection after the initial strongylid population is gone. Stoll (1929) reported an experiment ". . . in which two helminth-free lambs, upon fenced-in pasturage permitting natural repeated infection, during the summer developed, following an initial dose of *Haemonchus contortus* larvae, first an accumulation of parasites, and then a self-cure which expelled the worms and protected the animals thereafter against any significant amount of further infestation with this stomach worm." Thus was born the celebrated phenomenon called "self-cure."

Stewart (1950) observed seven periods of "self-cure" within 18 months in a flock of grazing sheep, demonstrated that an identical response could be elicited by giving large doses of infective *H. contortus* larvae, and concluded that "self-cure" taking place after periods of rain could be attributed to the intake of large numbers of *H. contortus* infective larvae. He subsequently related the rejection of the previously established adult worm population to an acute hypersensitivity reaction in the alimentary mucous membrane.

An oedematous change was evident in the mucous membrane of the abomasum or small intestine, depending upon the site of attachment of the adults, on the day on which a rise of blood histamine occurred after the administration of larvae. The intake of *H. contortus* larvae produced this change only in the abomasum of a sheep which had been infested with *H. contortus* and only in the small intestine of a sheep which had been infested with *Trichostrongylus* spp. (Stewart, 1953).

The lack of permanent protection against reinfection observed by Stewart does not necessarily invalidate Stoll's observations, but examples of functional acquired sterile immunity are rare where *H. contortus* is concerned. We had no difficulty in reinfecting lambs of the New York State Veterinary College flock with *H. contortus cayugensis* after their naturally acquired worm burdens had been removed by anthelmintic therapy, and similar results are commonly observed in other parts of the world with other subspecies of this parasite.

There is at least one definite practical consequence of "self-cure." Sheep or goats may die in the throes of evicting their worms and confuse the diagnosis by being found "uninfected" at necropsy when the clinical signs and history correctly pointed to haemonchosis. Profound anemia in grazing sheep or goats is haemonchosis unless positive evidence of another cause (e.g., acute radiation sickness) can be produced. The absence of *H. contortus* worms from the abomasum of an anemic sheep or goat in no way rules out the diagnosis of haemonchosis.

ACTIVE IMMUNITY

A durable sterile immunity is conferred in cattle by infection with the lung nematode *Dictyocaulus viviparus* and considerable success has been achieved with artificial immunization using irradiated larval vaccines (see the review by Poynter, 1963). The practical application of vaccines is, of course limited to areas of endemic dictyocaulosis, and although *D. viviparus* infection is cosmopolitan in distribution, clinical parasitic disease tends to be sporadic. Clinical dictyocaulosis is common in the British Isles, and that is where the vaccine has found ready and effective application.

DELAYED MATURATION OF LARVAE

Arrested development of larvae not only helps perpetuate certain strongylids from one year to the next but spares the host during the period of winter (or dry season) stress when energy invested in the reproduction of worms with free-living larvae would be a losing proposition biologically. Normally, these larvae mature the following spring. However, outbreaks of severe strongylidosis may result from the unseasonal maturation of arrested larvae during winter and early spring. It is important to recognize the parasitic etiology of such outbreaks in spite of their unseasonal incidence.

MANAGEMENT OF CLINICAL STRONGYLIDOSES

GENERAL CARE OF CLINICALLY ILL ANIMALS

The first step in dealing with an outbreak of strongylidosis in a herd of cattle, sheep, or goats is to identify the source of infection and to separate the animals from it. For purpose of observation and nursing, it is usually more convenient to confine the herd in a barn or drylot, and restriction of activity may help prevent losses precipitated by exertion. Never hurry acutely ill haemonchosis patients; they may drop dead at your feet. Segregate all animals showing anemia, diarrhea, weakness, or depression to facilitate therapy and to prevent their being bullied to death by their stronger fellows, but do not separate nurslings from their dams unless the owner is willing and able to cosset them.

ANTHELMINTIC MEDICATION

Administration of an anthelmintic may hasten the death of very sick animals and the owner should be forewarned of the possibility of further losses precipitated by drenching. However, the benefit of an effective anthelmintic drench in primary haemonchosis is usually dramatic. Strongylid nematodes continue to infect our cattle, sheep, and goats in spite of the plethora of safe and efficacious anthelmintic drugs. The use of anthelmintic drugs should be based upon thorough knowledge of the biology of the worms and of the climatic conditions of the area. One may treat the entire herd at regular "strategic" intervals in the hope of preventing the build-up of infective larvae in the pastures and thus prevent outbreaks of clinical strongylosis. Where contamination is particularly severe, "strategic" treatments preceding parturition and turnout to pasture, at midsummer and in fall, may need to be supplemented by "tactical" treatments at times when infection pressure may be particularly severe, as, for example, after a period of moist, warm weather particularly favorable for larval development.

Strongylids of the Alimentary Canal

The preferred drugs for ruminants in the United States are fenbendazole, ivermectin, levamisole, morantel, and thiabendazole. Coumaphos, crufomate, haloxon, and phenothiazine are also useful. All of these drugs are available in a variety of pharmaceutical forms to suit all types of farm and feedlot management systems.

Fall or early winter treatment should ideally be carried out with such anthelmintic drugs as albendazole, fenbendazole, and oxfendazole, which are active against the immature, arrested parasitic stages of Ostertagia (Duncan et al., 1976; Williams et al., 1977; Armour et al., 1978). Of these, only fenbendazole has been cleared for use in ruminants in the United States to date. The recommended dose of 5 mg. per kg. is insufficient for the removal of arrested larvae and the dose should be increased to 7.5 mg. per kg. for this purpose.

A number of reports have indicated that thiabendazole is not as effective against Hae-monchus contortus and Trichostrongylus colubriformis as it was when first introduced. The thiabendazole-resistant strains of H. contortus show cross-resistance to many other benzimidazole anthelmintics (Drudge et al., 1964; Smeal et al., 1968; Hotson et al., 1970; Theodorides et al., 1970; Kates et al., 1971; Colglazier et al., 1972, 1975; Berger, 1975; Hogarth-Scott et al., 1976; Kelly et al., 1977).

Morantel tartrate- and levamisole-resistant Ostertagia circumcincta and Trichostrongylus colubriformis have also been reported (Le Jambre et al., 1977, 1978a,b; Santiago et al., 1977, 1978). A levamisole-resistant O. circumcincta isolate was very susceptible to albendazole and oxfendazole (Le Jambre, 1979).

Lungworms

Clinical outbreaks of dictyocaulosis are treated with fenbendazole, ivermectin, or levamisole. Outside the United States, a wider selection of anthelmintic drugs is available (e.g., albendazole, cambendazole, febantel, and oxfendazole). These are highly efficacious against both adult and immature stages of Dictyocaulus. Species of Protostrongylus and Cystocaulus responded well to 15 mg. tetramisole per kg., but there was no effect on Muellerius capillaris and Neostrongylus linearis (Ramisz et al., 1975).

Eyeworms

The preferred drug for the treatment of Thelazia spp. infection in cattle is tetramisole. The drug is administered subcutaneously at the rate of 12.5 to 15 mg. per kg. A single dose produced rapid clinical recovery. Levamisole at a dosage rate of 5 mg. per kg. administered subcutaneously or 1 per cent aqueous solution as an eye lotion was also effective (Corba et al., 1969; Aruo, 1974; Vassiliades et al., 1975).

Medication of "Subclinical Parasitism" of Adult Dairy Cattle. Routine anthelmintic medication of adult dairy cattle is widely advertised to be profitable in terms of increased milk production. In general, however, antiparasitic measures can more profitably be applied to yearlings and two-year-olds; these are the cattle that tend to suffer significantly from parasitism. Parasitized replacements grow more slowly and often fail to reach their full growth potential. Such performance results in real financial loss that the producer may well be completely unaware of.

Subclinical Parasitism of Sheep. The effects of moderate parasitism in lambs were investigated by administering 5,000, 10,000, or 20,000 infective *Trichostrongylus colubriformis* larvae and comparing weight gains and feed efficiency of these artificially infected lambs with the performance of uninfected controls. Although about one half of the larvae administered became adult worms and group average fecal egg counts of 536 to 2,236 eggs per gram were observed, these levels of infection apparently caused no significant differences in average daily gain or feed efficiency (Bergstrom *et al.*, 1975).

PREVENTION AND CONTROL

Much has been written about prevention and control of strongylidoses and every scheme has its proponents and detractors, but there is no unique formula that applies in all situations.

Parasitism should be considered as a year-round game between the livestock, the strongylids, and the stockman. Certain moves at propitious times are capable of biasing the game in the stockman's favor, but these moves must not violate the rules of the game or the results may be disappointing or even disastrous. The ultimate criterion for success in any control effort is the net profit that accrues, not the number of worms fatally poisoned. The purchase of a livestock scale, as suggested by Whitlock (1955b), and adequate production records provide objective measures of success.

Control efforts may be classified under selective breeding for resistant stock, rotational grazing, and anthelmintic medication. The first of these has been employed the longest. Long before worms were recognized as disease agents, shepherds selected productive livestock for breeding, and worms claimed the lives of weaklings (against the shepherd's wishes perhaps, but to his eventual benefit; see Whitlock, 1966). There exist, in many parts of the world and under certain systems of husbandry, cattle, sheep, and goats that are capable of thriving without help from science and technology. These animals have parasites and handle them effectively as a population. Individual animals occasionally die from parasitism just as individuals occasionally get killed by predators, hung up in fences, or drowned in watering places, but the effect of minor losses such as these on the general population is minimal. On the other hand, there are also parts of the world and systems of husbandry in which the economic production of food and fiber requires intelligent intervention to suppress strongylid populations. Host resistance continues to be of paramount importance here even though conscious selection of resistant stock is seldom part of the breeding program. This is so because resistant hosts contribute less to the growth of the parasite populations than do more susceptible animals, and their presence thus tends to benefit the flock as a whole.

In theory, rotational grazing seeks to prevent or limit the intake of infective larvae by permitting animals to graze on a particular area of pasture no longer than a week so that eggs passed in their feces do not have time to develop into infective larvae, and then not allowing the animals to return until all of the larvae have died off. The considerable investment in fence construction required by rotational grazing schemes usually discourages strict observance of the rules, so the theoretical ideal is seldom realized in practice. However, any practicable rotation scheme undoubtedly increases the productivity of the pasture and may prolong the parasite generation, if only slightly (Levine and Clark, 1961).

Modern anthelmintics are efficient and comparatively nontoxic. There are places in the world where efficient livestock production is virtually impossible without them, and they are of undoubted benefit in increasing productivity wherever significant parasite losses occur. But there are limitations, hazards, and expenses that we cannot afford to ignore. No anthelmintic can overcome excessive exposure to infection just as no amount of bailing can overcome too large a leak. Crofton (1958) concluded that periodic treatment with interim reinfection merely "delayed attainment of the full parasite potential." He suggested concentrating treatments early in the pasture season to obtain maximum delay in the parasite population increase because an adult worm in spring is a potential forebear of a whole series of generations that season.

Probably the most important type of host resistance is premunition. The development of premunition in a grazing flock tends to truncate the growth curve of the parasite population by preventing the maturation of new waves of larvae and thus, in effect, prolongs the generation time. Although interference with the development of premunition is obviously to be avoided, periodic anthelmintic medication may have precisely this effect.

REFERENCES

Allen, R. W. (1973): Preliminary evaluation of levamisole, parbendazole and cambendazole as thysanosomicides in sheep. Am. J. Vet. Res., *34*, 61-63.

Allen, R. W., Enzie, F. D., and Samson, K. S. (1962): The effects of bithionol and other compounds on the fringed tapeworm, *Thysanosoma actinoides*, of sheep. Am. J. Vet. Res., *23*, 236-240.

Armour, J. Duncan, J. L., and Reid, J. F. S. (1978): Activity of oxfendazole against inhibited larvae of *Ostertagia ostertagi* and *Cooperia oncophora*. Vet. Rec., *102*, 263-264.

Aruo, S. K. (1974): The use of "Nilverm" (tetramisole) in the control of clinical signs of *Thelazia rhodesii* (eyeworm) infections in cattle. Bull. Epizoot. Dis. Afr., *22*, 275-277.

Arundel, J. H. (1972): Cysticercosis in sheep and cattle. Australian Meat Research Committee Review No. 4, 28 pp.

Bankov, D. (1975): Efficacy of praziquantel against *Stilesia globipunctata* and other cestodes in sheep. International Conference Pathophysiology of Parasitic Infections. Thessaloniki. p. 46.

Bankov, D. (1976): Opiti za diagnostika i terapiya na stileziozata po ovtsete. Vet. Nauki, *13*, 28-36.

Berger, J. (1975): The resistance of a field strain of *Haemonchus contortus* to five benzimidazole anthelmintics in current use. J. S. Afr. Vet. Assoc., *46*, 369-372.

Bergstrom, R. C., Maki, L. R., and Kercher, C. J. (1975): Average daily gain and feed efficiency of lambs with low level trichostrongylid burdens. J. Anim. Sci., *41* (2), 513-516.

Castel, P., Graber, M., Gras, C., and Chhay-Hancheng. (1960): Action de l'arseniate d'etain sur divers cestodes du mouton. Rev. Elev., *13*, 57-74.

Colglazier, M. L., Kates, K. C., and Enzie, F. D. (1972): Activity of cambendazole and morantel tartrate against two species of *Trichostrongylus* and two thiabendazole-resistant isolates of *Haemonchus contortus* in sheep. Proc. Helminth. Soc. Wash., *39*, 28-32.

Colglazier, M. L., Kates, K. C., and Enzie, F. D. (1975): Cross-resistance to other anthelmintics in an experimentally produced cambendazole-resistant strain of *Haemonchus contortus* in lambs. J. Parasitol., *61*, 778-779.

Corba, J., Scales, B., and Froyd, G. (1969): The effect of DL-tetramisole on *Thelazia rhodesii* (eye-worm) in cattle. Trop. Anim. Health Prod., *1*, 19-22.

Crofton, H. D. (1954): Nematode parasite populations in sheep on lowland farms. I. Worm egg counts in ewes. Parasitology, *44*, (3/4), 465-477.

Crofton, H. D. (1958): Nematode parasite populations in sheep on lowland farms. IV. The effects of anthelmintic treatment. Parasitology, *48*, 235-242.

Crofton, H. D. (1963): Nematode parasite populations in sheep and on pasture. Farnham Royal, Bucks, England. Commonwealth Agricultural Bureaux.

Drudge, J. H., Szanto, J., Wyant, Z. N., and Elam, G. (1964): Field studies on parasite control in sheep: Comparison of thiabendazole, ruelene, and phenothiazine. Am. J. Vet. Res., *25*, 1512-1518.

Duncan, J. L., Armour, J., Bairden, K., Jennings, F. W., and Urquhart, G. M. (1976): The successful removal of inhibited fourth stage *Ostertagia ostertagi* larvae by fenbendazole. Vet. Rec., *98*, 342.

Eyre, P., Boulard, C., and Deline, T. (1981): Local and systemic reactions in cattle to *Hypoderma lineatum* larval toxin: Protection by phenylbutazone. Am. J. Vet. Res., *42*, 25-28.

Fitzgerald, P. R., and Mansfield, M. E. (1973): Efficacy on monensin against bovine coccidiosis in young Holstein-Friesian calves. J. Protozool., *20*, 121-126.

Frelier, P. Mayhew, I. G., Fayer, R., and Lunde, M. N. (1977): Sarcocystosis: a clinical outbeak in dairy calves. Science, *195*, 1341-1342.

Graber, M. (1969): A propos du pouvoir anthelmintique du *N* -(2'-chloro-4' nitrophenyl-5 chlorosalicylamide chez le mouton. Rev. Elev. Med. Vet. Pays Trop., *22*, 217-228.

Guilhon, J., and Graber, M. (1960): Recherches sur l'activité du G4 à l'égard des principaux cestodes parasites du mouton. Rev. Elev., *13*, 297-304.

Guilhon, J., and Graber, M. (1964): Action du thio bis (hydroxydichlorophenyle) sur les cestodes des ruminants. Bull. Acad. Vet. Fr., *37*, 493-497.

Hogarth-Scott, R. S., Kelly, J. D., Whitlock, H. V., Ng, B. K. Y., Thompson, H. G., James, R. E., and Mears, F. A. (1976): The anthelmintic efficacy of fenbendazole against thiabendazole-resistant strains of *Haemonchus contortus* and *Trichostrongylus colubriformis* in sheep. Res. Vet. Sci., *21*, 232-237.

Hotson, I. K., Campbell, N. J., and Smeal, M. G. (1970): Anthelmintic resistance in *Trichostrongylus colubriformis*. Austr. Vet. J., *46*, 356-360.

Kates, K. C., Colglazier, M. L., Enzie, F. D., Lindahl, I. L., and Samuelson, G. (1971): Comparative activity of thiabendazole, levamisole, and parbendazole against natural infections of helminths in sheep. J. Parasitol., *57*, 356-362.

Kelly, J. D., Hall, C. A., Whitlock, H. V., Thompson, H. G., Campbell, N. J., and Martin, I. C. (1977): The effect of route of administration on the anthelmintic efficacy of benzimidazole anthelmintics in sheep infected with strains of *Haemonchus contortus* and *Trichostrongylus colubriformis* resistant or susceptible to thiabendazole. Res. Vet. Sci., *22*, 161-168.

Le Jambre, L. F., Southcott, W. H., and Dash, K. M. (1977): Resistance of selected lines of *Ostertagia circumcincta* to thiabendazole, morantel tartrate, and levamisole. Int. J. Parasitol., *7*, 473-479.

Le Jambre, L. F., Southcott, W. H., and Dash, K. M. (1978a): Development of a simultaneous resistance in *Ostertagia circumcincta* to thiabendazole, morantel tartrate, and levamisole. Int. J. Parasitol., *8*, 443-447.

Le Jambre, L. F., Southcott, W. H., and Dash, K. M. (1978b): Effectiveness of broad spectrum anthelmintics against selected strains of *Trichostrongylus colubriformis*. Austr. Vet. J., *54*, 570-574.

Le Jambre, L. F. (1979): Effectiveness of anthelmintic treatments against levamisole-resistant *Ostertagia*. Austr. Vet. J., *55*, 65-67.

Levine, N. D., and Clark, D. T. (1961): The relation of weekly pasture rotation to acquisition of gastrointestinal nematodes by sheep. Ill. Vet., *4* (4), 42-50.

Poynter, D. (1963): Parasitic bronchitis. Adv. Parasitol., *1*, 179-212.

Ramisz, A., Urban, E., and Piechocki, B. (1975): Badania nad przydatnoscia tetramizolu (Nilverm) do zwalczania inwazji nicieni z rodziny g Protostrongylidae u owiec. Med. Weter., *31*, 677-679.

Ryff, J. F., Browne, J. O., Stoddard, H. L., and Honess, R. F. (1950): Removal of the fringed tapeworm from sheep. J. Am. Vet. Med. Assoc., *117*, 471-473.

Santiago, M. A. M., Costa, V. C., and Benevenga, S. F. (1977): *Trichostrongylus colubriformis* resistante ao levamisole. Rev. Centro Ciencias Rurais, *7*, 421-422.

Santiago, M. A. M., Costa, V. C., and Benevenga, S. F. (1978): Antividade anti-helmintica do dl-tetramisole e do thibendazole uma estirpe do *Trichostrongylus colubriformis* resistente ao levamisole. Rev. Centro Cienias Rurais, *8*, 257-261.

Smeal, M. G., Gough, P. A., Jackson, A. R., and Hotson, I. K. (1968): The occurrence of *Haemonchus contortus* resistant to thiabendazole. Austr. Vet. J., *44*, 108-109.

Stewart, D. F. (1950): Studies on the resistance of sheep to infestation with *Haemonchus contortus* and *Trichostrongylus* spp. and on the immunological reactions of sheep exposed to infestation. IV. The antibody response to natural infestation in grazing sheep and the "self-cure" phenomenon. Austr. J. Agr. Res., *1*, 427-439.

Stewart, D. F. (1953): Studies on the resistance of sheep to infestation with *Haemonchus contortus* and *Trichostrongylus* spp. and on the immunological reactions of sheep exposed to infestation. V. The nature of the "self-cure" phenomenon. Austr. J. Agr. Res., *4*, 100-117.

Stoll, N. R. (1929): Studies with the strongyloid nematode *Haemonchus contortus*. I. Acquired resistance of hosts under natural reinfection conditions out-of-doors. Am. J. Hyg., *10*, 384-418.

Theodorides, V. J., Scott, G. C., and Laderman, M. (1970): Strains of *Haemonchus contortus* resistant against benzimidazole anthelmintics. Am. J. Vet. Res., *31*, 859-863.

Thomas, H., and Gönnert, R. (1978): The efficacy of praziquantel against cestodes in cats, dogs and sheep. Res. Sci., *24*, 20-25.

Vassiliades, G., Bouffet, P., Friot, D., and Toure, S. M. (1975): Traitement de la thelaziose oculaire bovine au Senegal. Rev. Elev. Med. Vet. Pays Trop., *28*, 315-317.

Vibe, P. P., Sultankulov, T. D., and Petrov, V. S. (1972): Ispytanie fenesala, Oksida, bitionola i bitirazina pri avitellinoze i tizaniezoze ovets. Byull. Vses. Inst. Gel'mintol. No. 9, 18-19.

Whitlock, J. H. (1951): The relationship of the available natural milk supply to the production of the trichostrongylidoses in sheep. Cornell Vet., *41* (3), 299-311.

Whitlock, J. H. (1955a): Trichostrongylidosis in sheep and cattle. Proc. Am. Vet. Med. Assoc., 92nd Annual Meeting, 123-131.

Whitlock, J. H. (1955b): A study of the inheritance of resistance to trichostrongylidosis in sheep. Cornell Vet., *45* (3), 422-439.

Whitlock, J. H. (1958): The inheritance of resistance to trichostrongylidosis in sheep. I. Demonstration of the validity of the phenomenon. Cornell Vet., *48* (2), 127-133.

Whitlock, J. H. (1966): Biology of a nematode. *In* Biology of Parasites, Soulsby, E. J. L., ed. New York, Academic Press.

Williams, J. C., Knox, J. W., Sheehan, D., and Fuselier, R. H. (1977): Efficacy of albendazole against inhibited early fourth stage larvae of *Ostertagia ostertagi*. Vet. Rec., *101*, 484-486.

9

PARASITES OF HORSES

ARTHROPODS

Identification and life histories of parasitic arthropods, the injuries they inflict, and the diseases they transmit are considered in Chapters 1 and 2. For further details on insecticides, see Chapter 11.

FLIES

Gasterophilus

The life histories of all *Gasterophilus* species are generally similar but differ in some important details. Adult *Gasterophilus* flies have vestigial mouthparts and cannot feed; they live only long enough to mate and deposit their eggs on the haircoat of a horse. Larvae that hatch from these eggs enter the horse's mouth by tactics peculiar to the species of fly and burrow into the oral tissues. After several weeks, they reenter the lumen, are swallowed, and remain attached to the walls of the stomach and intestine for almost a year. At last they release their grip and pass out with the feces to pupate in the soil. Adult botflies emerge from the pupal cases in three to nine weeks, depending on the ambient temperature. Botfly activity continues through summer and fall but ceases completely when cold weather sets in.

Treatment for stomach bots is traditionally delayed until a month after the first frost to allow the recently acquired larvae to complete their sojourns in the oral tissues and to reach the stomach, where they are more accessible to insecticidal attack. This strategy is based on the assumption that uptake of infection ceases with the advent of cold weather. In the case of *Gasterophilus intestinalis,* however, the eggs glued to the hairs of the forelegs remain infective long after frost has put an end to the adult flies. These eggs must be destroyed if enduring results are to be achieved by antibot medication. These eggs may be removed from the haircoat with a special fine-toothed comb available from saddlery shops, but the process is rather slow and laborious. If more than a very few horses are involved, the larvae can be lured out of their egg cases by copious sponging with water at 40° to 48°C. (104° to 118°F). The sudden rise in ambient temperature provides the adequate stimulus for hatching; addition of 0.06 per cent coumaphos, 0.12 per cent malathion, or 0.03 per cent lindane assures rapid destruction of these larvae as they emerge. The eggs of *G. nasalis* and *G. hemorrhoidalis* have all hatched by the time cold weather arrives and do not require special attention at debotting time. *Gastrophilus* control can be achieved with dichlorvos, trichlorfon, and carbon disulfide administered by stomach tube. Ivermectin is highly effective against both stomach bots and the earlier stages migrating in the tissues of the mouth when administered as a paste at 0.2 mg. per kg.

Biting Flies

Biting flies (stable flies, mosquitoes, horse and deer flies, and occasional horn flies) attack horses on warm days throughout the summer. Regular application of insecticidal preparations (i.e., pyrethrins, synergized pyrethrins, pyrethroids, coumaphos, stirofos, dichlorvos, and lindane) is indicated.

Efforts to control *Stomoxys calcitrans* should include elimination of breeding sites and application of insecticides to areas where they habitually rest. Repellents in the form of sprays or smears may afford relief for several hours. Discourage black fly attack by smearing petroleum jelly to the inner surface of the pinna of the horse's ears. Horse flies and deer flies are most difficult to kill or repel; the best solution is often to stable the horses during the hours of peak fly activity.

Face Flies and House Flies

These nonbiting flies feed on secretions around the eyes, nostrils, and mouth and on blood that continues to ooze from wounds made by horse flies; they annoy horses to distraction on warm, sunny days. Life histories of these flies and transmission by them of infectious agents is considered in Chapter 1. Face fly control may be attempted by application of stirofos, coumaphos, or pyrethrins to the entire horse, and elimination or insecticidal treatment of breeding sites (i.e., cow manure) when feasible. Face flies do not pursue their victims indoors, so stabling horses during hours of peak fly activity often proves to be the best solution.

Control of house flies is based on elimination of breeding sites (manure and decaying organic matter) and regular application of insecticides. Dichlorvos, naled, stirofos, fenthion, Ravap, and permethrin may be sprayed on horses. Pyrethrin sprays may be applied to the entire horse two to four times a week. Residual sprays (dimethoate) applied to walls of animal quarters every two weeks throughout the summer are quite effective in reducing fly populations. Baits may be set out wherever flies congregate. Vapona resin strips may be hung from the ceiling of closed barns.

LICE

Lice are found on horses principally during winter and spring (Fig. 9–1). Two spray applications of coumaphos, malathion, or lindane two weeks apart should provide adequate control. In cold weather, dusting horses with a mixture of rotenone and synergized pyrethrins is a less stressful procedure.

TICKS

Disease transmission and injuries inflicted by ticks is discussed in Chapter 2. In horses particularly, tick-attachment sites may become markedly irritated and lead to an itch-scratch cycle marked by serious self-mutilation. Coumaphos is effective as a spray or dust when applied to the entire horse. Malathion is easily sponged or sprayed on horses as a 0.12 per cent aqueous solution. Always wear rubber gloves and wash skin thoroughly after handling organophosphate and carbamate insecticides. Lindane smear may be applied to the external ear canal for the removal of *Otobius megnini*.

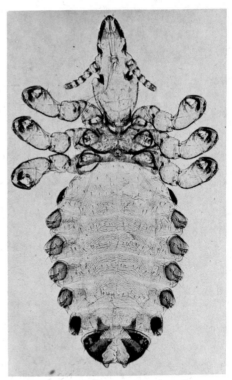

Figure 9–1. *Haematopinus asini* (x25).

MANGE MITES

Severe irritation caused by mange mites may lead to serious self-mutilation by affected horses. Two applications of lindane one week apart are effective. Mange is contagious and sometimes communicable. Isolate mangy horses and sterilize all water buckets, brushes, curry combs, and the like. Stalls should be thoroughly disinfected or left vacant for two to three weeks.

PROTOZOANS

BABESIOSIS

Babesia caballi and *B. equi* are susceptible to many antiprotozoal drugs, but in the United States, only imidocarb dipropionate is approved for use in horses. Imidocarb dipropionate is administered subcutaneously at 2 mg. per kg. repeated once after 24 hours for the treatment of *B. caballi*, and at 4 mg. per kg. repeated at 72 hour intervals for *B. equi*.

COCCIDIOSIS

Eimeria leuckarti and *Klossiella equi* appear to be nonpathogenic, which is fine because no treatment is available for either infection.

HELMINTHS

Life Histories

STRONGYLIDS

Strongylus vulgaris

The Infective Stage. The extrahost development of *S. vulgaris* is typical of strongylids in general (Fig. 8-1). Development to the infective stage requires adequate moisture and temperatures in the range 8 to 39°C.; the time required is inversely related to temperature (e.g., about 8 to 10 days at 18°C., 16 to 20 days at 12°C.). In arid regions, scattering the droppings with a tractor and harrow reduces strongyle larva populations by breaking up the manure and causing it to dry out before the larvae have reached the desiccation-resistant third stage. However, in more humid regions, the interior of even scattered manure remains sufficiently moist long enough for development to the third stage. Once *S. vulgaris* larvae have arrived at the third stage, they are very resistant to cold and desiccation and can survive on pasture through a northern winter or in stored dry hay for many months. The longevity of *S. vulgaris* third stage larvae depends mainly on the food reserves in their intestinal cells; the greater the activity of the larvae, the more rapidly these reserves become exhausted. However, it is imprudent to depend on *S. vulgaris* to wear itself out no matter how warm and humid the weather may be. Any pasture that has held a horse within a year can be assumed to be contaminated with *S. vulgaris* infective larvae.

The Intra-Arterial Migrations of Strongylus vulgaris. About 56 species of the family Strongylidae parasitize the cecum and colon of the horse (Lichtenfels, 1975), and as many as 15 or 20 different species are commonly found in a single host. The most important of these, because of its destructive migrations in the mesenteric and other arteries, is the "bloodworm," *Strongylus vulgaris*. In 1870, Otto Bollinger hypothesized that occlusion of the intestinal arteries by verminous thrombi and emboli could account for the majority of equine colic cases, both fatal and nonfatal. Since then, the etiological relationship between *S. vulgaris* and colic has been extensively debated and somewhat investigated, although not to an extent commensurate with its scientific and practical importance.

The meticulous experimental observations and well-thought-out conclusions of Enigk (1950, 1951a) provide the basis for the following outline. For the reader interested in greater detail than can be presented here, I have published an English translation of Enigk's papers (Georgi, 1973), and all serious students of equine medicine and pathology should study the review by Ogbourne and Duncan (1977).

When ingested by a horse, the infective third stage larvae of *S. vulgaris* cast off their sheaths in the lumen of the small intestine and enter the wall of the cecum and ventral colon. Here the larvae penetrate to the submucosa, where they undergo the third molt, which is completed by the seventh to eight day after infection. Leaving their third stage cuticles surrounded by round cells, the fourth stage larvae penetrate nearby small arterioles that lack an internal elastic lamina and wander in the intima of these vessels and progressively larger branches of the cranial mesenteric artery.

Enigk observed that *S. vulgaris* cannot penetrate the internal elastic lamina, which thus confines the larvae to the intima and helps keep them on their proper course. Thus constrained, the rapidly migrating larvae reach the colic and cecal arteries by the eighth to the fourteenth day after infection and the cranial mesenteric artery by the eleventh to the twenty-first day (Enigk, 1950; Duncan and Pirie, 1972). Some of the larvae push on into the aorta and its branches, where they may cause important pathological changes. However, larvae proceeding beyond the cranial mesenteric artery are probably lost to their species because of the improbability of their finding their way back to the cecum and ventral colon to breed.

After two to four months of migrating in the intima, the fourth stage larvae that have not gone astray or become trapped deep in thrombi are carried away by the bloodstream to the small arteries in the subserosa of the intestinal wall. The larvae, now grown large, occlude these small arteries, whose walls then become inflamed and, in due course, destroyed. The larvae thus liberated from the arterial tree then enter the surrounding tissue and become encapsulated in pea- to bean-sized nodules wherein the final molt occurs. Some larvae complete the final molt even before returning to the intestinal wall (see Fig. 13-19). According to Duncan and Pirie (1972), most of the larvae found in the cranial mesenteric lesions at four months postinfection have molted to the fifth stage, although the fourth stage cuticle is still retained as a sheath. This sheath is cast off before these immature adults return to the intestinal wall. Finally, the immature adults enter the lumen of the cecum and ventral colon, mature, and commence reproductive activity at about six months after infection. One rarely finds more than 100 or 200 adult *S. vulgaris* worms in a horse, and their egg production usually constitutes 10 per cent or less of the total strongylid output.

Pathophysiology of Verminous Arteritis. The migrations of fourth stage *S. vulgaris* larvae cause arteritis, thrombosis, and embolism of the cranial mesenteric artery and its branches. Although these arterial lesions exist to some degree in almost every horse, and principal branches are frequently completely occluded by them, fatal infarction of the bowel wall is relatively infrequent. This seeming paradox suggests a Darwinian interpretation. Of all domestic animals, the horse has by far the most elaborate system of anastomoses in the arterial supply to the large intestine; the colic vessels are particularly well supplied with the means for rapidly establishing effective collateral circulation (Dobberstein and Hartmann, 1932). In an evolutionary context, this may be interpreted as evidence that *S. vulgaris,* which has no direct counterpart in other domestic animals, has probably been occluding horses' intestinal arteries and thus exerting selection pressure for ages.

However, in spite of this exceptional adaptation, obstruction of the intestinal arteries does occasionally lead to fatal infarction of the bowel. Even temporary curtailment of blood flow pending establishment of collateral circulation may account for a high proportion of clinical colic cases from which the patient recovers. Further, the fatal intestinal displacements often interpreted at necropsy examination to be the cause of colic sysmptoms are more likely to be the result of abnormalities of intestinal tone and motility brought about by verminous thromboembolism and of the horse's violent efforts to obtain relief.

Resolution of Verminous Arteritis. After the larvae have migrated back to the intestinal lumen, the arterial lesions heal (Duncan and Pirie, 1975; Pauli *et al.*, 1975). These lesions also heal dramatically after destruction of the larvae by albendazole medication. Development and resolution of verminous arteritis can be studied radiographically in young foals by injecting contrast medium

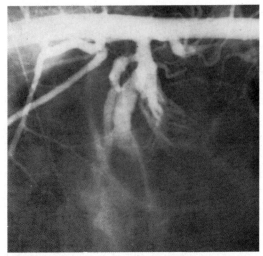

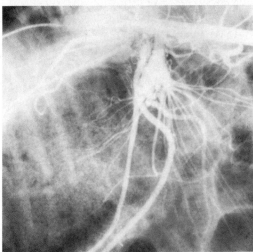

Figure 9–2. Resolution of equine verminous arteritis following larvicidal therapy with albendazole as visualized by contrast arteriography. The upper radiograph was taken one month after infection with 500 *Strongylus vulgaris* larvae, and albendazole therapy was started immediately afterward. The lower radiograph was taken one month after albendazole therapy. See text for explanation.

through a catheter that has been introduced into the aorta by way of a peripheral artery (Slocombe *et al.*, 1977). Two such radiographs compose Figure 9-2. The upper radiograph of a two month old pony foal was taken one month after 500 *S. vulgaris* larvae were administered via nasogastric tube. The cranial mesenteric and ileocecal arteries are enlarged, and blood flow through the colic artries is greatly diminished, as evidenced by the lack of contrast medium flowing through them. The lower radiograph of the same foal was taken one month after albendazole therapy; now the stem arteries have returned to nearly normal size, and the contrast medium clearly outlines the colic arteries, indicating a greatly increased flow through those vessels (Rendano et al., 1979).

Anthelmintic Therapy Directed Against Migrating S. vulgaris Larvae. Albendazole administered by nasogastric tube at 25 mg. per kg. three times a day for five days yielded dramatic larvicidal effect against fourth and immature fifth stage *S. vulgaris* in the cranial mesenteric arterial system (Rendano et al., 1979). In subsequent studies, high efficiency was obtained in treating artificially and naturally infected ponies at a lower dosage level, i.e., 50 mg. per kg. twice a day for two days (Georgi et al., 1980). Unfortunately, albendazole is not available for treating horses in the United States. Thiabendazole, administered on two successive days at a dosage rate of 440 mg. per kg. each day was found to be active against 7 to 18 day old larvae of *S. vulgaris,* but very slight activity was noted against older larvae (Drudge and Lyons, 1970). Fenbendazole administered orally to naturally infected ponies at 60 mg. per kg. reduced the number of *S. vulgaris* in the anterior mesenteric arterial system at necropsy (Duncan et al., 1977). When administered at 10 mg. per kg. for five days or at 50 mg. per kg. for three days at eight weeks after artificial infection with infective larvae of *Strongylus vulgaris,* fenbendazole was nearly 100 per cent efficient (Slocombe et al., 1983). Intramuscular injection of ivermectin at 0.2 mg. per kg. eliminated nearly all of the fourth stage larvae from the cranial mesenteric artery and its tributaries (Slocombe et al., 1982).

Strongylus edentatus and Strongylus equinus

Adult *Strongylus edentatus* and *S. equinus* are about twice as large as *S. vulgaris,* probably twice as bloodthirsty, and considerably more difficult to remove with anthelmintic drugs, but their larvae are not as pathogenic. The migration routes followed by larvae of *S. edentatus* and *S. equinus* have been elucidated by Wetzel (1940), Wetzel and Kersten (1956), and McCraw and Slocombe (1974, 1978).

Strongylus edentatus. The third stage larvae of *S. edentatus* burrow into the wall of the large intestine and reach the liver via the portal veins. Enclosed in nodules in the hepatic parenchyma, they molt to the fourth stage in about two weeks. The fourth stage larvae then wander about in the hepatic tis-

sue for about two months, growing larger as they go. Leaving the liver by way of the hepatic ligaments, the larvae wander for months in the parietal retroperitoneal tissues and eventually make their way to the base of the cecum and thence to the bowel lumen. The prepatent period is usually cited as 11 months but may be as short as 6 months (McCraw and Slocombe, 1978).

Strongylus equinus. The third stage larvae of *S. equinus,* like those of *S. vulgaris,* undergo their third molt in nodules in the wall of the cecum and colon. About 11 days after infection, the newly molted fourth stage larvae leave their intestinal nodules, cross the peritoneal space, and enter the right half of the liver, which, in the living horse, lies in contact with the cecum. These larvae wander about in the hepatic tissue for two months or longer before emerging and entering the pancreas or abdominal cavity, in which locations they complete their development to the fifth stage. The fourth molt occurs about four months after infection. Finally, these adult worms peretrate the wall of the large intestine and reenter the lumen to mate. The prepatent period of *S. equinus* is nine months.

Triodontophorus and the Small Strongylids

Triodontophorus spp. and the forty-odd species of cyathostomes do not migrate far beyond the mucous membrane of the colon and therefore the pathogenic effects of their larvae are considerably less dramatic than those inflicted by larvae of *Strongylus* spp. However, the cyathostomes are always the most abundant parasites in the large intestine of the horse, their eggs usually represent 80 per cent or more of the total strongyle egg output, and they are occasionally responsible for cases of persistent, severe diarrhea. Several of the more common species have developed resistance to benzimidazole anthelmintics, as explained later on in this chapter.

ASCARID

The Infective Stage. The thick outer proteinaceous layer of the *Parascaris equorum* egg shell (see Fig. 12-32) is very sticky and enables the eggs to adhere to stall walls, mangers, water buckets, mares' teats, and other objects. Infective larvae develop within these eggs in a week or two and remain within the protective shell until it is swallowed by a horse. The epidemiology of *P. equorum* infection therefore differs considerably from that of strongylids, with their free-swimming infective larvae, and, in fact, rather resembles that of the pinworm *Oxyuris equi*, discussed below. Unfortunately, most chemical disinfectants available in North America have no appreciable effect on ascarid eggs. Therefore, effective stall sanitation for the control of ascarids consists of weekly removal of all manure and bedding and thorough cleaning of all surfaces with a high pressure cleaner or steam jenny. Most horsemen find such a program excessively laborious and rely instead on anthelmintics to suppress production and environmental contamination with the eggs of *P. equorum*. But because of the extraordinary longevity and hardihood of ascarid eggs, contamination, however gradual, tends to be cumulative, and thorough cleaning at least of the foaling stall and of the mare's udder and teats before foaling is well worth the effort.

Migrations of Parascaris equorum Within the Host. When the infective egg of *Parascaris equorum* is swallowed by a foal, the larva hatches, burrows into the wall of the small intestine, and is carried to the liver by the portal vein. After migrating about in the hepatic tissues, the larva enters a hepatic vein and is carried by the caudal vena cava, heart, and pulmonary artery to the lung, where it enters an alveolus. After completing a molt in the lungs, the larva ascends in the expectorant mucus of the tracheobronchial tree and returns by way of the lumen of the esophagus and stomach to the intestine, where it completes a final molt and matures. The first waves of invading larvae inflict mainly mechanical injury; one observes little more than petechial hemorrhages. However, as the host becomes sensitized to *Parascaris* antigens, the tissues respond to the presence of larvae with infiltrations of eosinophilic leukocytes and other inflammatory cells. The damage done to the liver and lungs eventually heals, but the chronic reduction in functional capacity suffered during what is normally a period of rapid growth leaves its mark on the yearling; it will never be what it could have been.

STRONGYLOIDES

The Infective Stage. *Strongyloides westeri*, like other members of the genus, develops rapidly in passed feces to the infective filariform stage, which usually enters the host by penetrating its skin or oral mucous membranes.

Transmammary Infection. The remarkable fact about *Strongyloides westeri* is that the adult worms are encountered principally in suckling and weaning foals; the dam of an infected foal sheds no *S. westeri* eggs even though she is the source of infection. Infection is transmitted from the dam to the foal by way of the mammary gland (Lyons *et al.*, 1969, 1973), and the foals begin to shed eggs in their feces at 10 days to two weeks after birth. Diarrhea rather frequently afflicts foals between the ninth and thirteenth day of life, thus occurring coincidentally with the first postparturient estrus of the mare. Enigk and colleagues (1974) presented convincing evidence that this so-called "foal heat diarrhea" is caused by *S. westeri* and is not related to any alteration in the chemical composition of the mare's milk. Heavy infections in foals persist for 10 weeks; lighter infections may last two or three times as long. Occasionally, very light infections are observed in yearlings and older horses. These may represent percutaneous infections in hosts that were not exposed as sucklings (Enigk *et al.*, 1974).

PINWORMS

The Infective Stage. The infective larva of *Oxyuris equi* develops within the eggshell four or five days after the gravid female worm has cemented it to the skin of the anus or perineum. Masses of cement gradually dry, crack, and detach from the skin in flakes containing thousands of infective eggs. These flakes adhere to mangers, water buckets, and walls, thus contaminating the environment of the stable. Paper towels or disposable cloths are to be preferred for cleansing the perineum of horses because any nondisposable object, such as a sponge or towel, will inevitably become heavily contaminated with *O. equi* eggs. Then when the sponge or towel is applied to a horse's muzzle after a workout or used to "clean" the bit, the future brightens up for *O. equi*. The prepatent period is five months.

TAPEWORMS

The Infective Stage. *Anoplocephala* spp. cysticercoids develop in oribatid mites that live in the humus layer of the soil. Oribatid mites are most numerous on permanent pastures but rare on cultivated fields. Plowing and reseeding pastures may therefore make life somewhat difficult for these intermediate hosts but probably cannot be relied on as measures to control *Anoplocephala* spp.

Anoplocephala perfoliata tends to attach to the mucous membrane in clusters near the ileocecal valve. This clustering results in ulceration of the mucous membrane and inflammation with thickening and induration of the deeper layers of the intestinal wall. These pathological changes probably account for some cases of persistent diarrhea and may predispose to intussusception of the ileum into the cecum or rupture of the bowel wall in the vicinity of the ileocecal valve. Diagnosis of *A. perfoliata* infection is based on distinguishing the eggs from those of *A. magna* and *Paranoplocephala mammilana* (see Fig. 12-31).

Development of Strongyle, Ascarid, and Strongyloides Infections in Foals

Ann F. Russell (1948) studied the sequential changes in the composition of worm populations in 26 foals from seven different Thoroughbred studs. She performed fecal egg counts and identified infective larvae developing in fecal cultures from samples collected from these foals every week from the age of four weeks to at least six months of age and, in a few cases, to more than one year of age.

In Figure 9-3, egg counts are plotted against age for *Strongyloides westeri*, for *Parascaris equorum*, and for the family Strongylidae collectively. Note that *S. westeri* infection

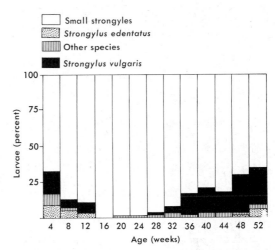

Figure 9–4. Percentage of larvae of different species of strongyles in fecal cultures. Data obtained from monthly observations of 26 foals. Adapted from Russell, 1948. From The Horse by J. Warren Evans, Anthony Borton, Harold F. Hintz, and L. Dale Van Vleck. W. H. Freeman and Company. Copyright 1977.

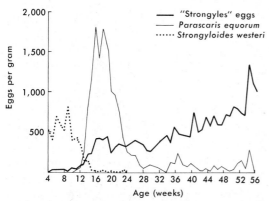

Figure 9–3. Average number of eggs of *Parascaris equorum*, "strongyles," and *Strongyloides westeri* counted per gram of manure. Data obtained from weekly observations of 26 foals. Adapted from Russell, 1948. From The Horse by J. Warren Evans, Anthony Borton, Harold F. Hintz, and L. Dale Van Vleck. W. H. Freeman and Company. Copyright 1977.

reached a maximum early in life, then rapidly dropped to a low level, and finally disappeared at about five months of age; this accords perfectly with what we now know about the mammary transmission of *S. westeri*.

Parascaris equorum eggs first appeared at about 12 weeks of age, after which egg counts rose steeply to a peak and then rapidly fell but, instead of disappearing completely, persisted at a low level indefinitely. The 12 week delay in appearance of *P. equorum* eggs corresponds closely to the prepatent period of this parasite, and we may deduce from this that the infection was acquired soon after birth. Thus, anthelmintic medication of the pregnant mare, careful bathing of her udder and teats, and thorough cleaning of the foaling box are logical measures for the prevention of significant infection of foals with *P. equorum*. The persistence of infection at a low level in horses of all ages and the extraordinary resistance of the egg to the rigors of the external environment make *P. equorum* a difficult parasite to control.

The third and most important curve shown in Figure 9-3 represents a gradual increase in the composite strongyle egg counts during the first year of life. In order to interpret this curve, it is necessary to take into account the relative abundances of *Strongylus vulgaris*, *S. edentatus*, and the "small strongylids" as determined by fecal culture and identification of the infective larvae; these findings are portrayed in Figure 9-4. This figure shows that the eggs of the small strongylids always predominated, representing, at various ages, between 80 and 100 per cent of the total strongyle eggs shed in the feces of these foals. This is to be expected in view of the 6 to 11 month prepatent periods of *Strongylus* spp. and the general predominance of cyathostomes in horses. It is curious, therefore, that small numbers of *S. vulgaris* and *S. edentatus* eggs appear in fecal samples of foals up to 12 weeks of age. Russell (1948) observed this phenomenon in every one of her 26 foals and interpreted it as evidence of *coprophagia*. This ingestion of feces by foals is probably related to the normal process of "seeding" the cecum and colon with beneficial microorganisms essential for the digestion of cellulose, but it also presents a clear opportunity for invasion by parasites.

As Figures 9-3 and 9-4 show, strongylid egg output increases steadily and *S. vulgaris* and *S. edentatus* eggs appear on schedule at 6 months and 11 months, respectively. This clearly indicates that strongylid infection begins shortly after birth of the foal and proceeds without interruption thereafter. Because young foals are much more susceptible to the pathogenic effects of these parasites than are older horses, it follows that the greatest efforts should be directed toward preventing excessive exposure, especially during the first months of life.

Anthelmintic Medication and Control

The equine practitioner now has a large number of safe and effective broad spectrum anthelmintics to choose from. On breeding farms, all horses over two months old should be dewormed every four to eight weeks (Drudge and Lyons, 1965). The principal objective of this program is to prevent contamination of the environment with strongyle eggs; that is why it is essential that all horses on the premises be treated. Piperazines are effective against both ascarids and cyathostomes and are thus the logical choice for worming foals up to six months of age. Thereafter, drugs effective against *Strongylus* spp. should be substituted.

Based upon epidemiological evidence, the most essential of all strategic treatments is that administered in spring, around foaling time. It is during this period that the adult worm population is greatly augmented through maturation of arrested and migrating larvae. The fecundity of thse worms is also increased, and larger numbers of larvae reach the infective stage, thus posing a threat to young, susceptible horses. Elimination of these egg laying worms in spring thus renders the pastures safer for grazing horses (Duncan, 1974).

Adult *Strongylus vulgaris*, *S. edentatus*, *S. equinus*, cyathostomes, *Oxyuris*, and *Parascaris* are susceptible to cambendazole, dichlorvos, febantel, fenbendazole, ivermectin, levamisole with piperazine, mebendazole, oxfendazole, oxibendazole, pyrantel pamoate, and thiabendazole alone or with piperazine. Administration of dichlorvos, piperazine–carbon disulfide complex with phenothiazine, trichlorfon, carbon disulfide, or ivermectin in fall and early spring affords control of ascarids and stomach bots. Cambendazole, oxibendazole, and thiabendazole are effective against *Strongyloides westeri*. Mirck and Van Meurs (1982) reported that ivermectin was effective against *S. westeri*.

Anthelmintic Resistance. Phenothiazine, thiabendazole, cambendazole, mebendazole, fenbendazole, oxfendazole, and febantel are no longer as effective against small strongylids as they were when first introduced (Drudge and Elam, 1961; Drudge and Lyons, 1965; Drudge et al., 1977, 1979; Slocombe et al., 1977; Hagan, 1979). Drudge and colleagues (1979) identified five species (*Cyathostomum catinatum*, *C. coronatum*, *Cylicocyclus nassatus*, *Cylicostephanus goldi*, and *C. longibursatus*) that exhibited cross resistance to cambendazole, fenbendazole, mebendazole, oxfendazole, and thiabendazole. However, all of these worms were highly susceptible to 10 mg. per kg. of oxibendazole, a 2-amino substituted benzimidazole. Resistant populations may also be controlled with dichlorvos, pyrantel pamoate, or ivermectin, or by administering a benzimidazole with piperazine. The selection of resistant populations of these five cyathostome species to benzimidazole anthelmintics has been rather rapid. Duncan (1982) suggests that in any worm control program one should alternate drugs of different chemical structure every six to twelve months to reduce the likelihood of development of resistant worm populations, but there is no experimental evidence to support this recommendation. The benzimidazole anthelmintics continue to retain excellent potency against the large strongylids and other nematode parasites of horses.

Because resistance is the inevitable result

of frequent, regular anthelmintic medication, a better course might be to worm only those horses with significant fecal egg counts (e.g., 100 eggs per gram). The objective, after all, is to reduce the rate of contamination of the environment with eggs. This approach is discussed in greater detail in Chapter 12.

The stomach worms *Draschia* and *Habronema* are very refractory to many modern broad spectrum anthelmintics. Carbon disulfide, when administered with large amounts of 2 per cent sodium bicarbonate, afforded excellent efficacy against *Draschia* and *Habronema* (Wright et al., 1931). Ivermectin is also highly effective against these stomach worms.

Anoplocephala perfoliata was reported by Kelly and Bain (1975) to be very susceptible to 15 mg. per kg. micronized mebendazole but Slocombe found this drug to be without effect at dosage levels below 35 mg. per kg. Slocombe (1979) found pyrantel at 13.2 to 19.8 mg. base per kg. highly effective. Niclosamide at 200 mg. per kg. eliminated nearly 99 per cent of the tapeworm burden from infected horses (Safaev, 1972) but has uniformly failed against *Anoplocephala* spp. in our experience.

Onchocerca. For those who remain convinced that killing *Onchocerca* spp. microfilariae is of benefit to the equine host, the following treatment may be tried. Diethylcarbamazine is fed to horses at 4 mg. per kg. for four days and the entire course repeated one week later. Continuous administration of diethylcarbamazine during the *Culicoides* fly season should provide good protection against *Onchocerca* (McMullan, 1972). Ivermectin administered intramuscularly at 0.2 mg. per kg. is highly effective against microfilariae of *Onchocerca* but many treated horses develop subcutaneous edema. When one considers that dead microfilariae engender a greater inflammatory reaction than live microfilariae, it really doesn't make much sense to go about poisoning them.

Cutaneous and Conjunctival Habronemiasis. Ronnel, in doses of 100 mg. per kg. administered every two weeks until the lesions are healed, has been reported to be effective when combined with local treatment (Wheat, 1961). Intralesional injection of 2 to 3 ml. of 10 per cent solution of fenthion promotes healing of habronemic granulomas (Rossoff, 1974). The gritty masses on conjuctival membranes must be excised to prevent injury to the cornea. Ivermectin appears to be emerging as the treatment of choice for cutaneous habronemiasis (Herd and Donham, 1981).

REFERENCES

Bollinger, O. (1870): Die Kolik der Pferde und das Wurmaneurysma der Eingeweidearterien. Eine pathologische und Klinische Untersuchung. Beitr. Vergleich. Path. u. Path. Anat. Hausth. München, Heft I.

Dobberstein, J., and Hartmann, H. (1932): Über die Anastomosenbildung im Bereich der Blind- und Grimmdarmarterien des Pferdes und ihre Bedeutung für die Entstehung der embolischen Kolik. Berl. Tierärztl. Wochenschr., 48, 399-402.

Drudge, J. H., and Elam, G. (1961): Preliminary observations on the resistance of horse strongyles to phenothiazine. J. Parasitol., 47 (Suppl.), 38-39.

Drudge, J. H., and Lyons, E. T. (1965): Newer developments in helminth control and Strongylus vulgaris research. Proc. 11th Ann. Meeting A.A.E.P., Miami Beach, Florida, pp. 381-389.

Drudge, J. H., and Lyons, E. T. (1970): The chemotherapy of migrating strongyle larvae. International Conf. Eq. Infect. Diseases, Paris, 1969, Proceedings, pp. 310-322.

Drudge, J. H., Lyons, E. T., and Tolliver, S. C. (1977): Resistance of equine strongyles to thiabendazole: Critical tests of two strains. Vet. Med. Small Anim. Clin., 72, 433-435, 437-438.

Drudge, J. H., Lyons, E. T., and Tolliver, S. C. (1979): Benzimidazole resistance of equine strongyles–critical tests of six compounds against population B. Am. J. Vet. Res., 40, 590-594.

Duncan, J. L. (1974): Field studies on the epidemiology of mixed strongyle infection in the horse. Vet. Rec., 94, 337-345.

Duncan, J. L., and Pirie, H. M. (1972): The life cycle of Strongylus vulgaris in the horse. Res. Vet. Sci., 13, 374-379.

Duncan, J. L., and Pirie, H. M. (1975): The pathogenesis of single experimental infections with Strongylus vulgaris in foals. Res. Vet. Sci., 18, 82-93.

Duncan, J. L., McBeath, D. G., Best, J. M. J., and Preston, N. K. (1977): The efficacy of fenbendazole in the control of immature strongyle infections in ponies. Equine Vet. J., 9, 146-149.

Duncan, J. L. (1982): Internal parasites of horses: Treatment and Control. In Practice, 4, 183-188.

Enigk, K. (1950): Zür Entwicklung von Strongylus vulgaris (Nematodes) in Wirtstier. Z. Tropenmed. Parasitol., 2, 287-306.

Enigk, K. (1951a): Weitere Untersuchungen zür Biologie von Strongylus vulgaris (Nematodes) in Wirtstier. Z. Tropenmed. Parasitol., 2, 523-535.

Enigk, K., Dey-Hazra, A., and Batke, J. (1974): Zür klinischen Bedeutung und Behandlung des galaktogen erworbenen Strongyloides Befalls der Fohlen. Dtsch. Tierärztl. Wochenschr., 81, 605-607.

Georgi, J. R. (1973): The Kikuchi-Enigk model of Strongylus vulgaris migrations in the horse. Cornell Vet., 63, 220-263.

Georgi, J. R., Rendano, V. T., King, J. M., Bianchi, D. G., and Theodorides, V. J. (1980): Equine verminous arteritis; efficiency and speed of larvicidal activity as influenced by dosage of albendazole. Cornell Vet., 70, 147-152.

Hagan, C. J. (1979): More on febantel and trichlorfon. Vet. Med. Small Anim. Clin., *74*, 6.

Herd, R. P., and Donham, J. C. (1981): Efficacy of ivermectin against cutaneous *Draschia* and *Habronema* infection (summer sores) in horses. Am. J. Vet. Res., *42*, 1953-1955.

Kelly, J. D., and Bain, S. A. (1975): Critical test evaluation of micronized mebendazole against *Anoplocephala perfoliata* in the horse. N. Z. Vet. J., *23*, 229-232.

Lichtenfels, J. R. (1975): Helminths of Domestic Equids. Special Issue: Proc. Helminth. Soc. Wash., *42*, 92 pp.

Lyons, E. T., Drudge, J. H., and Tolliver, S. (1969): Parasites from the mare's milk. Blood Horse, *95*, 2270-2271.

Lyons, E. T., Drudge, J. H., and Tolliver, S. (1973): On the life cyle of *Strongyloides westeri* in the equine. J. Parasitol., *59*, 780-787.

McCraw, B. M., and Slocombe, J. O. D. (1974): Early development of and pathology associated with *Strongylus edentatus*. Can. J. Comp. Med., *38*, 124-138.

McCraw, B. M., and Slocombe, J. O. D. (1978): *Strongylus edentatus*: development and lesions from ten weeks postinfection to patency. Can. J. Comp. Med., *42*, 340-356.

McMullan, W. C., (1972): Onchocercal filariasis. Southwestern Vet., *25*, 179-191.

Mirck, M. H., and Van Meurs, G. K. (1982): The efficacy of ivermectin against *Strongyloides westeri* in foals. The Veterinary Quarterly, *4*, 89-91.

Ogbourne, C. P., and Duncan, J. L. (1977): *Strongylus vulgaris* in the horse: its biology and veterinary importance. CIH Misc. Pub. No. 4, CAB, Farnham Royal, Slough, England, 40 pp.

Pauli, B., Althaus, S., and Von Tscharner, C. (1975): Über die Organisation von Thromben nach Arterienverletzungen durch wandernde 4. Larvenstadien von *Strongylus vulgaris* beim Pferd (licht- und elektronmikroscopische Untersuchungen). Beitr. Pathol., *155*, 357-378.

Rendano, V. T., Georgi, J. R., White, K. K., Sack, W. O., King, J. M., Theodorides, V. J., and Bianchi, D. G. (1979): Equine verminous arteritis. An arteriographic evaluation of the larvicidal activity of albendazole. Equine Vet. J., *11*, 223-231.

Rossoff, I. S. (1974): Handbook of Veterinary Drugs. New York, Springer Publishing Co., p 215.

Russell, A. F. (1948): The development of helminthiasis in thoroughbred foals. J. Comp. Pathol., *58*, 107-127.

Safaev, Ya. S. (1972): Efficacy of fenasal (niclosamide) against *Anoplocephala* infections in horses. Veterinariia (Moskow) *49* (1) sect. *5*, 68-69.

Slocombe, J. O. D., Rendano, V. T., Owen, R. ap R., Pennock, P. W., and McCraw, B. M. (1977): Arteriography in ponies with *Strongylus vulgaris* arteritis. Can. J. Comp. Med., *41* (2), 137-145.

Slocombe, J. O. D. (1979): Prevalence and treatment of tapeworms in horses. Can. Vet. J. *20*, 136-140.

Slocombe, J. O. D., McCraw, B. M., Pennock, P. W., and Vasey, J. (1982): Effectiveness of ivermectin against later 4th-stage *Strongylus vulgaris* in ponies. Am. J. Vet. Res., *43*, 1525-1529.

Slocombe, J. O. D., McCraw, B. M., Pennock, P. W., and Baird, J. D. (1983): Effectiveness of fenbendazole against later 4th-stage *Strongylus vulgaris* in ponies. Am. J. Vet. Res., *44*, 2285-2289.

Wetzel, R. (1940): Zür Entwicklung des grossen Palisadenwurmes (*Strongylus equinus*) im Pferde. Arch. für Wissench. Tierheilk., *76*, 81-118.

Wetzel, R., and Kersten, W. (1956): Die Leberphase der Entwicklung von *Strongylus edentatus*. Wien. Tierztl. Monatsch., *43*, 664-673.

Wheat, J. D. (1961): Treatment of equine summer sores with a systemic insecticide. Vet. Med., *56*, 477-478.

Wright, W. H., Bozicevich, J., and Underwood, P. C. (1931): Critical experiments with carbon bisulphide in the treatment of habronemiasis. J. Roy. Army Vet. Corps, *2*, 66-70.

10

PARASITES OF SWINE

ARTHROPODS

Control of External Parasites

LICE

CIOVAP, coumaphos, dioxathion, ivermectin, malathion, methoxychlor, tetrachlorovinphos, and fenthion provide good control of lice when applied as sprays or poured on the topline from shoulders to hips. Ivermectin, also effective against mange mites, is not as yet approved for swine. It is good practice when treating swine to also apply insecticide to the bedding of the holding pens. Usually two applications are adequate.

MITES

Mange mites are susceptible to crotoxyphos and malathion sprays applied twice at an interval of two weeks. Ivermectin is highly effective in treating sarcoptic mange.

HELMINTHS

Ascaris suum

The pathological effects of adult *Ascaris suum* infections in the small intestine are less dramatic than those of the larval migrations but they are undoubtedly significant. There may be diarrhea, but the most important effect is interference with proper nutrition and normal growth. Heavily infected pigs fail to make economically profitable gains. Occasional bizarre accidents such as occlusion of the bile duct or perforation of the bowel wall result from the tendency of ascarids to wander.

Diagnosis of clinical ascarosis frequently depends on clinical and necropsy findings because the main pathological events occur during the prepatent stage. Clinical signs of severe respiratory distress in a group of growing pigs and the discovery of extensive petechial and ecchymotic pulmonary hemorrhages and edema contribute to a diagnosis of acute ascarosis. Pieces of lung tissue should be minced and placed in a Baermann apparatus to demonstrate the migrating larvae. Less acute cases are marked by respiratory distress, varying degrees of malnutrition, and lesions of interstitial pneumonia. Chronic ascarosis is marked by stunting, emaciation, a copious outpouring of *Ascaris suum* eggs in the feces, and lesions of chronic interstitial pneumonia and hepatic fibrosis; such pigs are hopeless from an economic point of view.

Anthelmintic Medication. *Ascaris suum,* the economically most important nematode of swine, continues to menace the swine industry in spite of its susceptibility to piperazines, hygromycin B, dichlorvos, fenbendazole, levamisole, and pyrantel tartrate. It is obvious that drugs alone are not successful in controlling this ubiquitous parasite. However, treating and cleaning sows with soap and warm water two weeks before moving them to the farrowing crates will materially reduce the contamination to which the piglets will be exposed. Treating again at weaning with continuing attention to the hygienic conditions of the premises should keep the growing pigs reasonably free of *A. suum.* Continuous provision of feeds containing pyrantel tartrate prevents the migration and establishment of *A. suum.* Pyrantel tartrate is the only approved drug that kills the infective larva immediately after it hatches in the small intestine. Continuous administration of thiabendazole prevents the migration of larvae through the lungs but not through the liver.

In summary, control efforts should be directed at preventing infection of pigs during the first few weeks of life. Anthelmintic medication of the sow prior to farrowing, careful sanitation at farrowing time, and avoidance of exposure of young pigs to contaminated soils all serve to limit early infection.

Strongyloides ransomi

The tiny parthenogenetic *Strongyloides ransomi* female lies deeply embedded in the mucous membrane of the small intestine. The eggs shed in the feces contain first stage rhabditiform larvae that develop into infective third stage filariform larvae in two or three days, or slightly longer if a generation of free-living adults is included in the cycle. Infection occurs by penetration of the skin or oral mucosae by filariform larvae. These may follow a tracheal migration route to maturation in about six days or a somatic migration route to accumulate as arrested larvae in the adipose tissues, especially those of the mammary area. Tracheal migration and maturation is the usual outcome in piglets and occurs to some extent in older pigs. Mature gilts tend instead to store *S. ransomi* larvae in their adipose tissues and to shed them later in the colostrum and milk. The third stage larvae shed in the colostrum and milk are said to be "advanced" as compared with the third stage larvae that originally infected the gilt because they are slightly larger and their genital primordia are longer, wider, and more conspicuous, and because they mature in suckling pigs in only two to four days instead of six days.

Transmammary infection is the key to the epidemiology of *S. ransomi* infection. Piglets separated at birth from their dam and reared artificially were free of *S. ransomi* infection, whereas piglets allowed to nurse began to shed eggs in their feces two to four days after birth (Moncol and Batte, 1966). This initial transmammary infection thus serves to contaminate the environment of the sow and litter, thereby augmenting the mature worm burdens of the piglets and rebuilding the sow's tissue store of arrested larvae for subsequent litters (Moncol, 1975).

Strongyloidosis of piglets is an acute enteritis with bloody diarrhea (dysentery), rapid emaciation, anorexia, anemia, and stunting. There may be death losses but, from an economic standpoint, these may be an significant than the retarded growth of the survivors.

Anthelmintic Medication. Strongyloides ransomi can be treated in neonatal pigs with levamisole resinate or thiabendazole.

Trichuris suis

Trichuris suis threads the narrow esophageal portion of its body in and out of the mucous membrane of the cecum and, in severe infections, the colon too. The eggs appear in the feces in the one-cell stage, and the infective first stage larvae develop within them in about two months at summer temperatures. These eggs will remain infective for several years in soil and hatch only when they are ingested by a pig. All molts occur in or on the alimentary mucous membrane, and the whipworms mature and begin laying eggs about six weeks after infection.

Very severe infections of young swine with *T. suis* cause catarrhal enteritis with clinical signs of diarrhea, dehydration, anorexia, and retardation of growth (Batte *et al.*, 1977). Control of *T. suis* infection depends on separating swine from the source of infective eggs, which usually is contaminated soil or filthy housing.

Anthelmintic Medication. Trichuris suis is susceptible to hygromycin B and dichlorvos.

Hyostrongylus rubidus

Hyostrongylus rubidus is a typical trichostrongyloid nematode somewhat resembling *Ostertagia* in its habits. The adult worms parasitize the stomach and produce typical strongyle eggs that cannot be reliably distinguished from those of *Oesophagostomum* spp. infecting swine. Ensheathed third stage larvae develop within a week under optimum conditions; these are infective when swallowed by swine. Like *Ostertagia, H. rubidus* invades the gastric glands where the third and fourth molts take place. *Hyostrongylus rubidus* evokes a catarrhal, sometimes diphtheritic, gastritis with ulceration and secretion of a tenacious mucus. Clinical signs include anemia and inappetence with occasional melena as evidence of gastric hemorrhage. Hyostrongylosis is mainly a disease of adult pigs at pasture.

Anthelmintic Medication. Hyostrongylus rubidus (and *Ascarops strongylina*) are susceptible to dichlorvos.

Oesophagostomum spp.

The most important effect of *Oesophagostomum* spp. is the formation of nodules in the gut wall by developing third stage larvae. The fourth stage larvae emerge from these nodules as early as two weeks after infection, or they remain for several months. Nodule formation may be accompanied by catarrhal enteritis, spoils sausage casings, and probably interferes with maximum growth of young swine. A rise in egg output by sows peaks at six or seven weeks after farrowing and then drops off rapidly. This could be an important epidemiological factor in situations favorable for the development of infective larvae.

Anthelmintic Medication. Oesophagostomum spp. are susceptible to dichlorvos, fenbendazole, levamisole resinate, and pyrantel tartrate.

Macracanthorhynchus hirudinaceus

The thorny-headed worm of swine is a parasite of the small intestine, where it attaches itself to the wall by its proboscis (see Fig. 6-66). The body is flattened and transversely wrinkled, which causes this parasite to be mistaken for a tapeworm occasionally. The large eggs have three concentric ellipsoidal shells and contain an *acanthor* larva when shed in the host's feces (see Fig. 12-34). Development to the *cystacanth* stage infective for pigs occurs in May beetles, dung beetles, or water beetles in about three months. Pigs acquire *M. hirudinaceus* infection when rooting for beetle grubs, but the infected adult beetle is also a source of cystacanths. The prepatent period is two or three months.

Anthelmintic Medication. There is no effective treatment for *M. hirudinaceus* infection. Benzimidazole anthelmintics may be tried.

Stephanurus dentatus

The adult kidney worm of swine *Stephanurus dentatus* occurs in cysts in the perirenal fat, the renal pelvis, the walls of the ureters, and the adjacent tissues of swine. The life history may be direct or may involve earthworms as facultative intermediate hosts, infection occurring by ingestion or skin penetration of third stage larvae or by ingestion of infected earthworms. Once in the body of the pig, the larvae enter the liver and spend four to nine months wandering destructively there. Some are trapped by an encapsulating tissue reaction, but the rest migrate to the retroperitoneal tissues surrounding the kidneys and ureters. Eggs appear in the urine 9 to 16 months after infection and persist for three years or longer. Piglets may become infected *in utero* (Batte *et al.*, 1960, 1966).

Stephanurus dentatus larvae migrate abortively in other hosts (e.g., cattle) and frequently lose their way in pigs. Not only liver and kidney, but also choice loin chops are frequently condemned because of these destructive larvae. Migration of *S. dentatus* larvae in the spinal cord may cause posterior paralysis, but otherwise the clinical signs of infection are not distinctive. Extensive liver damage may lead to emaciation and death.

A control program has been suggested that takes ingenious advantage of the exceptionally long prepatent period of *S. edentatus* (Stewart and Tromba, 1957). Gilts only are used for breeding and are marketed immediately after weaning their first litter. Using this system, the prevalence of infection on a cooperating farm was reduced from 93 per cent to nil within two years. Unfortunately, the "gilt-only" method has not been widely adopted, and *S. dentatus* continues to be a major problem of swine husbandry in the southeastern United States (Marti *et al.*, 1977).

Anthelmintic Medication. Levamisole and fenbendazole are the approved anthelmintics for the treatment of *Stephanurus dentatus* infections. Albendazole, ivermectin, and fenbendazole are very active against both adult and immature *S. dentatus* but none of these is approved for use in swine in the U.S.A.

Trichinella spiralis

The life history and human health implications of *Trichinella spiralis* infection are discussed in Chapter 6.

Anthelmintic Medication. The enteric and tissue stages are susceptible to thiabendazole (Campbell and Cuckler, 1962a, 1962b, 1964, 1966; Hennekeuser *et al.*, 1969).

Metastrongylus spp.

Anthelmintic Medication. Levamisole resinate is the only approved anthelmintic with activity against swine lungworms.

Cysticercus spp.

Cysticercus tenuicollis, the larva of the dog tapeworm *Taenia hydatigena*, migrates through the liver tissue before settling down on the peritoneal membranes. Severe invasions involve considerable trauma and reactive inflammation, and sometimes result in adhesions of the liver to the diaphragm and various other organs. It seems likely that such involvement would interfere with normal development of the pig and it certainly leads to rejection of the liver at slaughter. Dogs do not belong in pig feeders.

Cysticercus cellulosae, the larva of the human tapeworm *Taenia solium*, is not as common as *C. tenuicollis*, but it represents a significant hazard to human health. People become infected with *Taenia solium* by ingesting the cysticerci in undercooked pork. After the tapeworm matures, the person's feces contain a steady supply of eggs, which may be conveyed to the mouth at any time by a lapse in personal hygiene. When the eggs reach the stomach, the oncospheres hatch out, enter the gut wall, and wander far and wide in the body, slowly developing into cysticerci. Apparently the *milieu intérieure* of man resembles that of swine closely enough to satisfy the development requirements of *Cysticercus cellulosae*. However, humans are not quite as satisfactory intermediate hosts as swine, so the cysticerci tend to take up aberrant locations such as the eye, brain, and spinal cord. Occasional cases of human cysticercosis and coenurosis are also caused by larvae of canine taeniids.

REFERENCES

Batte, E. G., Harkema, R., and Osborne, J. C. (1960): Observations on the life cycle and pathogenicity of the swine kidney worm (*Stephanurus dentatus*). J. Am. Vet. Med. Assoc., *136*, 622-625.

Batte. E. G., Moncol, D. J., and Barber, C. W. (1966): Prenatal infection with the swine kidney worm (*Stephanurus dentatus*) and associated lesions. J. Am. Vet. Med. Assoc., *149*, 758-765.

Batte, E. G., McLamb, R. D., Muse, K. E., Tally, S. D., and Vestal, T. J. (1977): Pathophysiology of swine trichuriasis. Am. J. Vet. Res., *38*, 1075-1079.

Campbell, W. C., and Cuckler, A. C. (1962a): Thiabendazole treatment of the invasive phase of experimental trichinosis in swine. Ann. Trop. Med. Parasitol., *56*, 500-505.

Campbell, W. C., and Cuckler, A. C. (1962b): Effect of thiabendazole upon experimental trichinosis in swine. Proc. Soc. Exper. Biol., *110*, 124-128.

Campbell, W. C., and Cuckler, A. C. (1964): Effect of thiabendazole upon the enteral and parenteral phases of trichinosis in mice. J. Parasitol., *50*, 481-488.

Campbell, W. C., and Cuckler, A. C. (1966): Further studies on the effect of thiabendazole on trichinosis in swine, with notes on the biology of the infection. J. Parasitol., *52*, 260-279.

Hennekeuser, H. H., Pabst, K., Poeplau, W., and Gerok, W. (1969): Thiabendazole for the treatment of trichinosis in humans. Tex. Rep. on Biol. and Med., *27* (Suppl. 2), 581-596.

Marti, O. G., Fincher, G. T., and Stewart, T. B. (1977): Effect of cambendazole on swine kidneyworm *Stephanurus dentatus*. Vet. Parasitol., *3*, 89-93.

Moncol, D. J. (1975): Supplement to the life history of *Strongyloides ransomi* Schwartz and Alicata, 1930 (Nematoda: Strongyloididae) of pigs. Proc., Helminth. Soc. Wash., *42*, 86-92.

Moncol, D. J., and Batte, E. G. (1966): Transcolostral infection of newborn pigs with *Strongyloides ransomi*. Vet. Med. Small Anim. Clin., *61*, 583-586.

Stewart, T. B., and Tromba, F. G. (1957): The control of the swine kidney worm, *Stephanurus dentatus*, through management. J. Parasitol., *43* (Suppl.), 19-20.

CHAPTER

11

ANTIPARASITIC DRUGS

Vassilios J. Theodorides

A parasiticide is a poison that is more toxic to parasites than to their hosts. The degree of discrimination is sometimes small, sometimes considerable, but never complete, so that application of parasiticides always entails some hazard to the host. As a matter of fact, it is always easier to explain the deleterious effects that parasiticides frequently exert on the host than to explain how they kill parasites.

In his quest for an agent that would kill the spirochete of syphilis, Paul Ehrlich investigated a series of organic compounds and found what he was looking for in "Compound 606," the six hundred and sixth compound investigated. Compared with modern efforts, which often involve screening many thousands of compounds, success came early to Paul Ehrlich. Manufacturers spend vast fortunes in their search for new drugs. Their investments must usually be recovered between the time approval is awarded for public sale of a particular product (this may take 9 or 10 years) and the time their patent rights run out. After that, free competition tends to reduce the profit that can be realized from the products that still happen to be in popular demand.

Stages in the development of a typical insecticide or anthelmintic proceed approximately as follows: First, as mentioned earlier, many thousands of compounds must usually be screened before one is found that shows promise. The screening procedure, in the case of an anthelmintic, could require the demonstration of *in vivo* activity against some convenient parasite (e.g., *Nematospiroides dubius*, *Nippostrongylus brasiliensis*, *Syphacia obvelata*, or *Hymenolepis nana* of laboratory rodents; *Ascaridia galli* or *Heterakis gallinarum* of chickens). A preliminary estimate of mammalian toxicity, the LD_{50} (median lethal dose), is also obtained from experiments on rats or mice.

The activity screening tests and preliminary toxicity studies greatly reduce the list of suitable candidates but are of little value in predicting the effect of a particular drug either on a particular species of domestic animal or on its customary assemblage of parasites. Responses of various species and strains to poisons (except to the so-called indifferent narcotics and general protoplasmic poisons) are usually quite selective, often idiosyncratic. Thus, ascarids are very sensitive to piperazines, whereas hookworms are quite refractory; most breeds of cattle and dogs tolerate judicious applications of organophosphorus insecticides, whereas Brahman cattle and greyhound and whippet dogs are very likely to be fatally intoxicated by such treatment. The necessary information can only be obtained through experiments on domestic animals and the parasites for which the anthelmintic is intended.

When a manufacturing firm files a New Drug Application with the Food and Drug Administration (FDA), it must submit specimens of the product and all chemicals used in its manufacture along with complete information on its chemistry, process of manufacture, and quantitative assay methods. Protocols and results of all experiments conducted on the pharmacolgical activity and mammalian toxicity of the compound and copies of all relevant published reports must also be submitted. Drugs intended for animals that are used for human food must be accompanied by data on tissue residues and the route and rate of excretion of the parent compound and its metabolites. The amount and the structure of the longest residing tissue residues must also be determined and, if the substance has similarities to known carcinogenic chemicals, a lifetime (three year) toxicity experiment is then required in rats and mice. The Environmental Protection Agency (EPA) requires an environmental impact analysis of the new compound. Phytotoxicity and the effects of the drug on fish and other lower animals must also be vigorously studied. Before a new anthelmintic or any new parasiticide can be approved, well controlled experiments must be carried out involving slaughter of the test animals and determinations of residual worm burdens after treatment. Confirmation experiments must be conducted by several independent laboratories as a series of *field tests* in different geographic regions of the United States.

The package label is required by law to bear all the necessary cautions and to notify the user about all adverse reactions that have been discovered. Six months after a product enters the market and at regular intervals thereafter, the manufacturer is required to report to FDA any adverse reactions that have come to light and to add appropriate notices to the label or withdraw the product from the marketplace. As a result, the label (or package insert) has become one of the most objective and current sources of information on parasiticides.

According to Webster's New Collegiate Dictionary (seventh edition), a *proprietary* is a "drug that is protected by secrecy, patent, or copyright against free competition as to name, product, composition, or process of manufacture." Proprietaries always receive a proprietary name and a generic name. For example, YOMESAN is Chemagro Corporation's name for niclosamide, and EQUIZOLE, THIBENZOLE, AND OMNIZOLE are Merck's names for various preparations of thiabendazole. The generic name is for scientific communication and the proprietary name is for advertising (which usually entrenches the proprietary name in the vernacular of the professions). In the pharmaceutical industry, the word "proprietary" is applied in a more restricted sense to products intended for sale to the general public "over the counter" to distinguish them from the "ethical" products that are restricted for sale to veterinarians. Many manufacturers and distributors market identical products under both "proprietary" and "ethical" labels.

The relative safety and ease of administration of many modern parasiticides render them quite suitable for lay use. The physical act of introducing the drug into the gullet has, in many cases, ceased to require professional attention. Rather than regret the lost exercise or further encourage such mummeries as the "ethical" *vs.* "proprietary" nonsense, veterinarians should concentrate their efforts on the nine tenths of the field that remains: applying their knowledge of parasite biology to devising and practicing effective measures for parasite control.

Resistance to Parasiticides. Regular application of antiparasitic drugs to populations of parasites inevitably results in the development of resistant parasite populations through selection of resistant phenotypes. Eventually, the once effective drug ceases to work and must be replaced by another. Unfortunately, the replacement may also fail against the resistant strain, especially if it is a chemical congener of the original. This has happened often enough to serve us warning. We are going to have to develop better ways of controlling parasites than crudely and blindly lashing away at them with one chemical after another.

The literature on parasiticidal drugs is enormous. In the interests of both economy and readability, we have found it necessary to omit specific reference citations from the text of this chapter. A list of references at the end of this chapter includes the important sources for the material presented here, however. Specific treatments presented in Chapters 7 through 10 are documented at the ends of those chapters.

INSECTICIDES

The Federal Environmental Pesticide Control Act (FEPCA) of 1972 is administered by the Environmental Protection Agency (EPA) and controls the distribution, sale, and *use* of pesticides within each state as well as between states. This act even specifies what penalties may by imposed for the *misuse* of pesticides. State governments may establish even stricter standards than those set by FEPCA. For example, at the time of this writing, preparations of lindane and toxaphene are manufactured and sold within the United States for application to livestock other than dairy cattle, but the use of these chemicals as pesticides on domestic animals including pets is prohibited in many states. Curiously, preparations of lindane are available on prescription in some of these very same states for use in human pediculosis and sarcoptic mange. Users of pesticides thus bear a legal responsibility in the United States for knowing which chemicals they are currently permitted to use and for using these chemicals only in strict accordance with the indications and directions on the package labels. Current information on pesticides should be sought from the pesticide coordinator, extension entomologist with livestock responsibility, or extension veterinarian appointed by the state agricultural extension services and land grant colleges. These people are prepared to provide authoritative and detailed information on insecticides. They may periodically publish recommendations covering a great variety of insecticide applications. Veterinarians should ask to be placed on the mailing list for such publications and should seek expert advice whenever doubt arises with respect to the proper and lawful use of insecticides.

The diversity of structure, biological activity, and toxicity among insecticides is exceeded only by the number and variety of insects, mites, and ticks that we are trying to control. The label of every insecticide container must be read carefully and understood before the contents are applied to the animal. *The label is the most up-to-date and authoritative source of information available.*

Botanicals

The botanical insecticides are derived from plant materials. Ground plant parts (flowers, leaves, stems, roots) or their extracts may be formulated as a variety of application forms. Essential oils from plants are often used as insect attractants or repellents. Botanical insecticides, particularly pyrethrins, have excellent toxic effects against a variety of crop and animal insect pests, very short persistence in the environment, and relatively low toxicity to animals. Pyrethroids are synthetic pyrethrumlike compounds with superior kill and knockdown activity. Rotenone is the insecticidal component of the roots of several plants.

PYRETHRINS

The flower head of the pyrethrum plant *Chrysanthemum cinerariaefolium* contains six closely related insecticidal substances that are known as *pyrethrins*. Pyrethrinlike compounds produced synthetically in the laboratory are called *pyrethroids*. Pyrethrins and pyrethroids are rapidly degradable in the presence of moisture, air, and light, and are also rapidly biodegradable. Pyrethrins are very soluble in kerosene but insoluble in water. The oral LD_{50} of pyrethrum for rats is 200 to 1500 mg. per kg., depending on the purity of the product, and the dermal LD_{50}

for rats is greater than 1800 mg. per kg. Pyrethrins may produce some inhalation problems in rats, but regular aerosol applications should not produce any adverse reactions in domestic animals. Pyrethrins are toxic to fish and aerosols should not be used near fish tanks, but regular usage has had very little impact on game fish and other wildlife. Pyrethrins rapidly knock down, paralyze, and kill arthropods by disrupting sodium and potassium ion transport in nerve membranes. Residues of pyrethrins are sometimes repellent. Pyrethrins are frequently combined with a synergist such as piperonyl butoxide or N-octyl bicycloheptene dicarboximide.

Many commercially available insecticides formulated as aerosols, fogs, and mists contain either pyrethrins alone or a mixture of pyrethrins and a synergist (e.g., AURIMITE, BUZZOFF, CERUMITE, D-FLEA, DIRYL, FLAIR, F.L.T. POWDER, FLEABAN, FLICK, K.F.L. SHAMPOO, LIQUA-SECT, LIQUAI-DATE, HAVA-CIDE, HEATHCLIFF'S FLEA AND TICK SPRAY FOR CATS, MYCODEX PET SHAMPOO, NOVALCIDE, PARA BOMB-M, PARA-GO, PARA S-1, PET PEST SPRAY, PYRESEPT SHAMPOO, SEBBATIX, SECT-A-SPRAY, SPECTRO, THERADEX, THERA-GROOM, TICK KILL, VET-KEM PET SPRAY, and ZERO-MITE).

Pyrethrin aerosols, smokes, fogs, sprays, and powders control face flies, horse flies, house flies, stable flies, mosquitoes, fleas, lice, and ticks. Enclosed areas may be sprayed with an electric thermal fog dispenser. Pyrethrins are registered for application without limitations to beef and lactating dairy cattle and in dairy barns and milk houses. Pyrethrins are not persistent insecticides. Therefore, regular and repeated application is necessary. Resistance to pyrethrins has been reported in house flies and in some cattle ticks.

WARNING. Pyrethrins should not be applied to kittens less than four weeks old or to suckling puppies. In case of poisoning, antihistamines may be of some antidotal value; nervous manifestations can be controlled with phenobarbital, and diarrhea with atropine.

PYRETHROIDS

Pyrethroids are synthetic pyrethrumlike substances. These new chemicals are more potent and possess greater knockdown effect than do the plant pyrethrins. Pyrethroids are biodegradable but sufficiently stable when exposed to air and light so that weekly or biweekly applications provide excellent control of insects. They have a greater insecticidal effect when the temperature is lowered; in chemist's language, they have a negative temperature coefficient. Pyrethroids initially stimulate and then depress nerve cell function and eventually cause paralysis. The fast knockdown of flying insects is the result of rapid muscular paralysis. Pyrethroids have low mammalian toxicity but they are toxic to fish. Allethrin, tetramethrin, resmethrin, fenvalerate, flumethrin, permethrin, cypermethrin, and decamethrin are some of the pyrethroids used in the United States and abroad.

Allethrin

Allethrin, a first generation pyrethroid, is a mixture of several optical isomers. It is a clear, amber-colored, viscous liquid insoluble in water and soluble in alcohol, carbon tetrachloride, and kerosene. It is incompatible with alkalis. Allethrin has low mammalian toxicity; the LD_{50} for rats is greater than 920 mg. per kg. Allethrin is formulated in aerosols, oil sprays, and dusts with and without the common pyrethrum synergists. It is used mainly in the control of flies and mosquitoes in houses and as sprays for farm buildings and farm animals including dairy animals. Synergized allethrin sprays are safe to use on dogs and cats. FELETHRIN is available for the control of fleas and ticks. No restrictions exist for the use of allethrin on milk- and meat-producing animals.

Permethrin

Permethrin, a third generation pyrethroid, is an extremely active insecticide with rapid knockdown effect against a variety of insects. It occurs as a colorless, crystalline solid and as a pale yellow, viscous liquid soluble in most organic solvents and slightly soluble in water. The acute oral LD_{50} for rats is greater than 4000 mg. per kg., but permethrin is very toxic to fish. Permethrin is photostable, effective residues lasting four to seven days on crop foliage. Permethrin is registered as a residual animal quarters treatment (dairy barns, feedlots, stables, poultry houses, swine and other animal housing) for the control of house flies, stable flies, and other manure breeding flies. ECTIBAN tape and ECTIBAN wettable powder are the commercially available formulations.

Fenvalerate

Fenvalerate is a clear, yellow, viscous liquid with a mild odor. It is soluble in kerosene and xylene but insoluble in water, and is very photostable. The acute oral LD_{50} for rats is 451 mg. per kg., the acute dermal LD_{50} in rabbits is 2,500 mg. per kg., but fenvalerate is highly toxic to fish. Fenvalerate is formulated for long residual insecticidal activity. ECTRIN is used in dairy and beef cattle eartags for control of horn flies, face flies, Gulf Coast ticks, and spinose ear ticks, and as an aid in the reduction of stable fly and house fly populations around livestock quarters.

Resmethrin

Resmethrin is a waxy, off-white to tan solid with chrysanthemate odor. It is moderately soluble in kerosene but insoluble in water; it is not synergized to any appreciable extent by pyrethrum synergists. Of great significance is resmethrin's low mammalian toxicity; the acute oral LD_{50} for rats is 4,240 mg. per kg. Resmethrin shows excellent knockdown effect and is cleared for use in aerosols and pet shampoo (DURAKYL shampoo) for the control of fleas on dogs and cats. DURAKYL pet yard and kennel spray is applied weekly to dog and cat quarters for control of fleas. Resmethrin sprays are also used to control flying and crawling insects in enclosed areas.

ROTENONE

Rotenone is the insecticidal component of derris root, cubé root, and many leguminous shrubs that acts as an inhibitor of mitochondrial respiratory enzymes. It is insoluble in water but very soluble in alcohols, acetone, carbon tetrachloride, chloroform, and many other organic solvents. Rotenone decomposes on exposure to light and air. The oral LD_{50} for rats is 133 mg. per kg., and for white mice, 350 mg. per kg., but it is very toxic to fish. Rotenone, alone or synergized, is the main insecticidal ingredient in such products as BENZYLHEX, CANEX, CANOLENE, GOODWINOL, MITONE, AND PARAGO. Rotenone may be applied to cats, dogs, horses, and cattle in dust, ointment, or liquid form for the control of a variety of arthropod parasitisms including localized demodicosis in dogs.

WARNING. Kittens less than four weeks old and suckling puppies should not be treated with rotenone products. Rotenone is toxic to swine, fish, and snakes, may be carcinogenic in rats, and should not be applied to these animals. Cats and dogs may vomit after licking rotenone from their coats.

Carbamates and Organophosphates

Carbamates and organophosphates are the most commonly used insecticides. One should be aware of their toxic effects on animals. These insecticides exert their toxic action by inhibiting an important enzyme of the nervous system, namely acetylcholinesterase. The carbamate and organophosphate insecticides bind and inactivate acetylcholinesterase with the result that acetylcholine accumulates at the neural synapse. The accumulation of acetylcholine produces signs of acute poisoning which are principally the result of acetylcholine's *muscarinic* effects on parasympathetic postganglionics (miosis, lacrimation, salivation, vomiting, diarrhea, frequent urination, dyspnea, bradycardia, and hypotension) and its nicotinic effects at the neuromuscular junctions (rapid involuntary muscle twitching and scattered fasciculations followed by severe weakness and paralysis). Death is usually due to respiratory failure. Acetylcholine is broken down in healthy animals by the enzyme acetylcholinesterase but phosphorylation or carbamylation of this enzyme blocks this activity. Phosphorylation of cholinesterase is a reversible reaction but separation of the enzyme from the phosphate ligand is very slow. Recovery from carbamate poisoning, on the other hand, is relatively rapid. Many organophosphorus insecticides show a chronic neurotoxicity with degeneration of long axons in the spinal cord and peripheral nerves (e.g., sciatic nerve). Atropine administered parenterally is the preferred antidote for carbamate and organophosphate poisoning. Organophosphate poisoning may also be reversed with PROTOPAM (pralidoxime chloride) *but this drug is contraindicated in carbamate poisoning.* The principal action of pralidoxime chloride is to reactivate actylcholinesterase, which in turn destroys the accumulated acetylcholine so that the synapses and neuromuscular junctions can once again function normally. Pralidoxime chloride also slows *aging* of phosphorylated cholinesterase, which process is characterized by a progressive refractoriness to reactivation. Pralidoxime chloride is relatively short-acting, so repeated dosing may

be required. Artificial respiration may be required in severe cases of carbamate and organophosphate poisoning.

Carbamates and particularly organophosphates should not be used in conjunction with other cholinesterase inhibitors, other insecticides, or phenothiazine because the effect of these chemicals on cholinesterase reserves is cumulative. Organophosphates should not be applied to greyhound and whippet dogs or to certain breeds of cattle (Chianina, Charolais, Gelbvieh, Simmental, Brahman); these breeds suffer *idiosyncratic* reactions to this class of compound.

Application of organophosphates to cattle infested with *Hypoderma* larvae may lead to *host-parasite reaction* (page 160).

Carbamates

CARBARYL

Carbaryl (SEVIN) is a white, crystalline solid sparingly soluble in water but freely soluble in most nonpolar organic solvents. Carbaryl is rapidly hydrolyzed in alkaline media, but has good residual insecticidal effect as it is ordinarily used. The half-life of carbaryl is seven to nine days in soil and one to five days in fresh water. The mammalian toxicity of carbaryl is low; the oral LD_{50} for female rats is 500 mg. per kg. Carbaryl is highly toxic to honeybees, however.

Carbaryl and other carbamate insecticides kill insects by inhibiting the activity of acetylcholinesterase in the ganglia. The poisoned insects display hyperactivity, ataxia, convulsions, and paralysis, and finally die.

Dogs and Cats. Carbaryl alone or in combination with pyrethrins, rotenone, synergists, and methoxychlor is used to control fleas, lice, and ticks. Products containing carbaryl include: DIRYL POWDER, E-Z DIP, F-L-T BOMB, F-L-T POWDER, MYCODEX SHAMPOO, NORSECT AEROSOL, PARA DIP, PARA-GO, PARA POWDER, PARA S-1 AEROSOL, PET SPRAY, SECT-A-SPRAY, SPECTRO-SPRAY, AND VET KEM flea and tick powder and collars. Adult dogs and cats infested with fleas, lice, or ticks may be dipped or washed with products containing 0.5 to 1 per cent carbaryl. A free-flowing dust formulation containing 2 to 5 per cent carbaryl may also be used. The dust is sprinkled over the animal and then is rubbed thoroughly into the coat. The flea and tick collar is claimed to provide protection for up to four months. For quick action, aerosol application is recommended. Unfortunately, fleas and ticks in many areas have developed resistance to carbaryl.

Premises. Kennels, dog houses, and other sleeping quarters may be sprayed or dusted with carbaryl formulations. For continuous protection, regular application every seven days is recommended.

WARNING. Do not use other cholinesterase-inhibiting chemicals together with products containing carbaryl. Puppies and kittens under four weeks should not be treated with carbaryl preparations. Read the label for other specific product restrictions, If animals show signs of poisoning, administer atropine.

METHOMYL

Methomyl is a crystalline solid with a slight sulfurous odor, soluble in water and ethanol, and very soluble in methanol. Methomyl is very toxic to mammals. The oral LD_{50} for rats is 17 mg. per kg.

Methomyl has demonstrated a broad spectrum of activity against a wide range of insects infesting vegetables and field crops. It has a very rapid action. Flies are killed when they come into contact with or ingest methomyl. Methomyl is the insecticidal ingredient in the IMPROVED SUGAR GOLDEN MARLIN FLY BAIT. This product also contains a fly-attractant pheromone (MUSCALURE).

WARNING. Methomyl is toxic to fish and honeybees. Methomyl should be kept away from domestic animals. In case of poisoning, administer atropine.

PROPOXUR

Propoxur (BAYGON, SENDRAN), a substituted phenyl *N*-methylcarbamate, is a white to tan, crystalline solid, practically insoluble in water but soluble in methanol and many other polar organic solvents, and only slightly soluble in cold hydrocarbons. Propoxur decomposes in alkaline media. Propoxur has quick knockdown action and affords residual effect for four to six weeks. It is toxic to birds and honeybees but can be used safely on and around domestic mammals. The oral LD_{50} for rats is 100 mg. per kg.

Dogs and Cats. Propoxur is the active ingredient in many pet shampoos, aerosols, and flea and tick collars. The shampoos and aerosols provide quick kill of fleas and ticks,

and the collars may provide protection for up to five months. The ZODIAC TICK COLLAR contains propoxur in a slow-release form and it is claimed that this collar works even when it is wet. Propoxur wettable powder (PRO DIP 50) is dissolved in water and applied with a sponge for the control of fleas and ticks.

WARNING. Propoxur, like all carbamate and organophosphate insecticides, inhibits the activity of acetylcholinesterase. Atropine is the antidote for carbamate poisoning.

Organophosphates

CHLORFENVINPHOS

Chlorfenvinphos (SUPONA) is an amber liquid sparingly soluble in water at pH 4 to 7, soluble in alkaline aqueous media with rapid decomposition, and very soluble in most organic solvents. Chlorfenvinphos is very toxic to rats, with an oral LD_{50} of 10 to 40 mg. per kg., but it is much less toxic to other animals. The oral LD_{50} for mice is 117 to 200 mg. per kg. and for dogs, 12 grams per kg. Chlorfenvinphos persists in soil for a long time and therefore may be used for the control of soil insects.

Chlorfenvinphos is formulated as a 24.5 per cent emulsifiable concentrate (DERMATON DIP), which is diluted before use to 0.1 per cent (4 ml. emulsifiable concentrate per liter). For control of fleas and ticks on dogs, the diluted insecticide is applied either by dipping or by sponging over the entire body every week or two. DERMATON is also an effective premises spray for use in yards, kennels, and dog runs.

WARNING. Do not use on cats. Gloves must be worn during the application of DERMATON. For standard precautions to be followed in dealing with organophosphorus insecticides, see page 191.

CHLORPYRIFOS

Chlorpyrifos (DURSBAN) is a white, crystalline solid, highly soluble in most organic solvents and insoluble in water. It is moderately persistent in the environment and is useful for the control of mosquito and fly larvae, fire ants, and termites. The acute oral LD_{50} in rats is 163 mg. per kg. and the acute dermal LD_{50} in rabbits is 2000 mg. per kg.

Chlorpyrifos sprays and dips (SECTA-A-CHLOR, MARMADUKE SPRAY, DIP) are indicated for the control of fleas and ticks on dogs only. It is claimed that one application will kill fleas and protect against reinfestation for up to one month. For more effective control of fleas one should also spray bedding and resting areas. It is suggested that pregnant bitches and pups under 10 weeks of age should not be treated with chlorpyrifos.

DURSBAN 44 INSECTICIDE is indicated for the control of lice and horn flies on beef cattle. Apply the required dose to one spot on the topline between the shoulder blades. Do not re-treat for 30 days.

WARNING. Do not treat veal calves, dairy cattle of any age, cows within 21 days before or 14 days after calving, or slaughter cattle within 14 days of slaughter. For standard precautions to be followed in dealing with organophosphorus insecticides, see page 191.

COUMAPHOS

Coumaphos is a crystalline powder insoluble in water but extremely soluble in aromatic hydrocarbons. It is of relatively low toxicity for mammals. Mice are very sensitive, however; their oral LD_{50} is 55 mg. per kg., whereas the oral LD_{50} for rats is 90 to 110 mg. per kg. Coumaphos hydrolyzes slowly under alkaline conditions, but rapid degradation occurs in the liver of cattle. Coumaphos is used in a variety of formulations on animals and premises for the control of a wide range of parasitic arthropods. Coumaphos is also registered as 2 and 11.2 per cent feed premixes and as 0.32 per cent feed crumbles (BAYMIX) for the control of susceptible gastrointestinal nematodes of cattle.

Cattle. Coumaphos controls cattle grubs with a single application of a ready-to-use 4 per cent formulation (CO-RAL). This is applied in fall as soon as possible after *Hypoderma* fly activity ceases.

For the control of cattle lice, horn flies, and ticks, coumaphos is applied as a 1 to 5 per cent dust with self-treatment dust bags, as 1 per cent in oil with backrubbers, and as sprays prepared by diluting 11.6, 24, or 25 per cent emulsifiable concentrates with water. For the control of screwworms, apply the 1 to 5 per cent ready-to-use dust or 10 per cent spray foam around the wound. Coumaphos may be used on beef and lactating dairy cattle without limitations for slaughter or use of milk for food.

Sheep and Goats. Coumaphos 0.25 to 5 per cent sprays, dips, or dust applications are effective against fleeceworms, screwworms, lice, keds, ticks, and chorioptic mites.

Swine. Coumaphos 0.25 to 3 per cent spray or 1 to 5 per cent ready-to-use dust is applied to pigs for the control of lice and screwworm infestations. Swine bedding may also be treated with 1 per cent dust.

WARNING. The label must be read carefully before applying any of the many preparations of coumaphos. When concentrated pour-on or dip is applied to cattle, milk should not be used for 14 days after treatment. Coumaphos should not be applied to cattle within 14 days of slaughter, and goats and sheep should not be treated within 15 days of slaughter. Coumaphos should not be applied to lactating dairy goats or to dry dairy goats within 14 days of freshening. For standard precautions to be followed in dealing with organophosphorus insecticides, see page 191.

CROTOXYPHOS

Crotoxyphos (CIODRIN) is a light straw-colored liquid, slightly soluble in water and aliphatic hydrocarbons, but soluble in acetone, chloroform, ethanol, and highly chlorinated hydrocarbons. Its half-life in alkaline aqueous solutions is 35 hours; in acidic media it hydrolyzes somewhat more slowly. CIODRIN is a contact and stomach insecticide, effective against flies, lice, ticks, and mites on beef and lactating dairy cattle, swine, goats, sheep, and horses. The oral LD_{50} for rats is 125 mg. per kg. and the acute dermal LD_{50} for rabbits is 385 mg. per kg. CIODRIN is marketed as a 14.4 per cent emulsifiable concentrate (CIODRIN) and as an emulsifiable mixture (CIOVAP) of 10 per cent crotoxyphos and 2.5 per cent dichlorvos.

Cattle. The products containing crotoxyphos are diluted to 0.25 to 1 per cent in water or oil and applied to beef and lactating dairy cattle with a sprayer or backrubber for the control of face flies, horn flies, stable flies, house flies, mosquitoes, ticks, and chorioptic mites.

Sheep and Goats. CIODRIN and CIOVAP are applied with a sprayer at the rate of 1 gallon of 1 per cent aqueous solution per animal for the control of lice and ticks. Treatment may be repeated every seven days if necessary.

Swine. CIODRIN and CIOVAP are sprayed on swine at the rate of 1 gallon of a 0.25 per cent aqueous solution or 1 to 2 quarts of a 0.5 per cent aqueous solution per head for the control of flies and lice. Applications may be repeated after seven days.

WARNING. For standard precautions to be followed in dealing with organophosphorus insecticides, see page 191.

CRUFOMATE

Crufomate is an odorless, white, crystalline powder. The commercial product (RUELENE) is a yellow, viscous oil. Crufomate is soluble in most organic solvents; its solubility in water is about 0.15 per cent. The oral LD_{50} for rats is 770 to 1000 mg. per kg.

Cattle. Crufomate is used in beef and non-lactating dairy cattle mainly for the control of *Hypoderma* grubs, horn flies, and lice. It is also sold as an anthelmintic drench for cattle, sheep, and goats. Crufomate may be applied to cattle as a pour-on, spray, or dip. As a pour-on, the diluted drug is applied by pouring it on the animal's topline at the rate of 62 mg. per kg. (0.66 ml. of 9.4 per cent aqueous solution per kg., but not more than 22 grams, i.e., 234 ml., per animal). The dip is a 0.25 per cent aqueous solution of crufomate, and the spray is a 0.375 per cent solution.

WARNING. Crufomate should not be applied to dairy cows during lactation or within three days of calving, or to cattle subjected to any kind of stress. Treatment may be repeated in 21 days. Beef cattle should not be treated within seven days of slaughter. For standard precautions to be followed in dealing with organophosphorus insecticides, see page 191.

CYTHIOATE

Cythioate is the *N*-substituted homologue of famphur. The oral LD_{50} for rats is 160 mg. per kg. and the oral LD_{50} for cats is 220 mg. per kg., even if the dose is divided over two to five days. Dogs fed 15 to 200 ppm. of cythioate daily (6 to 80 mg. per kg.) developed slight to marked inhibition of erythrocyte and plasma cholinesterase activities. Repeated oral doses with 10 times the recommended dose produced transitory tremors and weakness of the neck muscles.

Cythioate oral 1.6 per cent liquid and 30 mg. tablets (PROBAN) are indicated for the control of fleas on dogs. Cythioate is administered orally at the rate of 3.3 mg. per kg., either as 1 ml. of the solution per 4.5 kg. or one 30 mg. tablet per 9 kg., every third day.

In Europe, cythioate is also adminstered to cats at 1.5 mg. per kg. once a week for the control of fleas. Some veterinarians instill 2 drops of PROBAN liquid into each ear of the cat twice as week. Cythioate may also be useful against *Demodex, Otodectes,* lice, and ticks.

WARNING. Pregnant females or any animal under stress should not be treated with cythioate. For standard precautions to be followed in dealing with organophosphorus insecticides, see page 191.

DIAZINON

Diazinon is a colorless liquid, very soluble in ethanol, acetone, xylene, and petroleum oils and only sparingly soluble in water. The 90 per cent pure technical product is a pale to dark brown oil. Diazinon is a contact and stomach insecticide. The oral LD_{50} for rats is 300 to 400 mg. per kg.; the acute dermal LD_{50} in rabbits is 4000 mg. per kg.

Sheep. Diazinon 0.03 to 0.06 per cent in water is sprayed on sheep for the control of lice, blowfly maggots, keds, and ticks. A 2 per cent dust may also be used.

Premises. Diazinon shows long residual effect against ticks and insects. It is applied as a spray in barns and other farm buildings. A 5 per cent dust or bait formulation may be applied to cracks, crevices, and other places where insects congregate.

WARNING. Sheep treated with products containing diazinon should not be slaughtered for two weeks. This insecticide must not be applied in dairy barns and milk rooms. For standard precautions to be followed in dealing with organophosphorus insecticides, see page 191.

DICHLORVOS

Dichlorvos (VAPONA, DDVP) is a colorless to amber liquid. Its solubility in water is about 1 per cent, in kerosene 3 per cent, and greater in most organic solvents. The oral LD_{50} for rats is 56 to 80 mg. per kg. of the technical chemical; the acute dermal LD_{50} in rabbits is 107 mg. per kg. Dichlorvos has contact, systemic, and fumigant, quick knockdown insecticidal action but little residual effect. Its half-life in neutral aqueous media is about 8 hours; rapid hydrolysis is also noted in the mammalian body. In slow-release pharmaceutical forms, dichlorvos demonstrates a high degree of activity against the economically important nematodes of dogs, cats, swine, and horses (see ANTHELMINTICS).

Cattle. Dichlorvos, at a concentration of 0.5 to 1 per cent in water or oil, is sprayed on beef and lactating dairy cattle at the rate of 30 to 60 ml. per head for the control of face flies, horn flies, stable flies, houseflies, and mosquitoes. A combination of 0.25 per cent dichlorvos and 1 per cent crotoxyphos in emulsifiable form or oil base (CIOVAP) is applied by sprayer, backrubber, or electric mixer to beef and lactating dairy cattle for the control of flies, lice, ticks, and chorioptic mites. RAVAP, a combination product of dichlorvos and tetrachlorvinphos, is used for the control of flies, lice, and ticks, including the spinose ear tick in beef cattle.

Sheep and Goats. Dichlorvos and the combination product CIOVAP are applied to sheep and goats with a coarse sprayer for the control of flies, lice, ticks, and mites.

Swine. Dichlorvos and CIOVAP are used for the control of flies and lice. They are applied by spraying at the rate of 3.8 liters of 0.25 per cent solution or 0.9 to 1.9 liters of 0.5 per cent solution per head.

Dogs and Cats. Dichlorvos collars and tags are worn around the animals' neck for protection against fleas.

Horses. Dichlorvos is registered as a feed additive for the control of *Gasterophilus* larvae.

Premises. Insect control in dairy barns, feedlots, horse barns, and surrounding resting and breeding areas may be achieved with dichlorvos resin strips, baits, foggers, and regular spraying. VAPONA resin strips or bait strips are suitable for fly control in milk rooms.

WARNING. Dichlorvos collars must not be worn by Persian cats, sick cats, or greyhound or whippet dogs. Exposure to water reduces the effectiveness of dichlorvos collars. The collar must be removed before bathing animals and may be replaced when the animal's haircoat has dried completely. Applications of dichlorvos to animals may be safely repeated every 7 to 14 days. Food animals should not be treated within one day of slaughter. For standard precautions to be followed in dealing with organophosphorus insecticides, see page 191.

DIMETHOATE

Dimethoate (CYGON) is a white crystalline solid with a mercaptan odor that is very soluble in polar organic solvents such as alcohols and ketones; its solubility in water is about 4 per cent. Dimethoate is registered as a premises and space insecticide. The oral LD_{50} for rats is 150 to 300 mg. per kg.; the acute dermal LD_{50} for guinea pigs is 1000 mg. per kg. For the control of adult houseflies, dimethoate is used as a residual spray on walls of agricultural buildings and animal quarters at the concentration of 1 to 1.25 per cent and, when sprayed on breeding areas, it kills housefly larvae. The residual effect lasts up to eight weeks.

WARNING. Dimethoate should not be applied in dairy barns and milk rooms. Care must be taken to avoid contamination of feed and drinking water. For standard precautions to be followed in dealing with organophosphorus insecticides, see page 191.

DIOXATHION

Dioxathion (DELNAV) is a tan, nonvolatile liquid, practically insoluble in water but soluble in aromatic hydrocarbons, ethers, and ketones. It decomposes rapidly in alkaline media and under heat but is compatible with other insecticides. Under conditions of normal usage, dioxathion shows long residual insecticidal and acaricidal activity. Insects are killed by direct contact or by ingesting the chemical. The acute toxicity for laboratory animals varies with the purity of the material. The oral LD_{50} for rats is about 45 mg. per kg. of the technical dioxathion; the acute dermal LD_{50} for rats is 235 mg. per kg. Dioxathion is available as 10.5 per cent (KEMTOX), 20.4 per cent (CO-NAV), and 30 per cent (DEL-NAV) emulsifiable concentrates. When diluted with water, these products are suitable for application to animals by spray, dip, pour-on, or backrubber.

Cattle. Dioxathion at 0.15 per cent in water (e.g., 1 gallon of 30 per cent emulsifiable concentrate per 200 gallons of water) is applied to beef cattle by spraying or dipping for the control of face flies, horn flies, screwworms, lice and ticks. A more concentrated (0.6 per cent) aqueous solution is applied by pouring one liter on the back and shoulders of each animal. Dioxathion 1.5 per cent in oil is used in backrubbers. The animals may be sprayed every 14 days but the pour-on application should not be repeated within 30 days.

Sheep and Goats. For the control of keds, lice, myiasis maggots, and ticks, dioxathion 0.15 per cent in water (one tablespoonful of dioxathion 30 per cent emulsifiable concentrate per gallon) is applied by spray or dip. Treatment may be repeated every two weeks.

Swine. For control of lice and ticks, dioxathion 0.15 per cent in water is applied by spray or dip. Treatment may be repeated every two weeks.

Horses. For control of flies, lice, and ticks, dioxathion 0.15 per cent is applied by spray or dip.

Dogs. For control of fleas, lice, and ticks, 0.15 per cent dioxathion is applied by spray or dip. Treatment may be repeated every seven days.

Premises. For control of fleas, lice, and ticks in kennels, in dog runs, and on lawns, 0.5 per cent dioxathion is applied as a spray.

WARNING. Dioxathion should not by applied to dairy animals (or in dairy barns), to cats, foals, or Brahman cattle, or to greyhound or whippet dogs. Calves under three months of age should not be dipped. Sows should not be treated within two weeks of farrowing or nursing. Treated animals may be slaughtered without any waiting period. For standard precautions to be followed in dealing with organophosphorus insecticides, see page 191.

FAMPHUR (FAMOPHOS)

Famphur is a crystalline powder, very soluble in chlorinated hydrocarbons, insoluble in aliphatic hydrocarbons, and soluble in water at about 100 mg. per liter. The acute oral LD_{50} is 35 mg. per kg. for rats and 400 mg. per kg. for sheep; the acute dermal LD_{50} for rabbits is 2730 mg. per kg.

Famphur in 13.2 per cent liquid formulation (WARBEX, BO-ANA) is poured on the topline of cattle at the rate of 43.6 mg. per kg. (33 ml. per 100 kg. up to a maximum of 120 ml.) for the control of *Hypoderma* grubs and sucking lice. A single application should be made in fall as soon as possible after adult fly activity ceases. WARBEX dust for self-application by dust bag is used to control horn flies on cattle.

WARNING. Famphur should not be used within a few days of treatment with other cholinesterase-inhibiting chemicals and should not be used on lactating dairy cows or on dry cows within 21 days of calving; on calves less than three months old; on animals stressed from castration, dehorning, or overexcitement; or on sick or convalescent animals. Brahman bulls should not be exposed to products containing famphur. Cattle should not be slaughtered within 35 days after application of famphur. For standard precautions to be followed in dealing with organophosphorus insecticides, see page 191.

FENTHION

Fenthion (BAYTEX) is an oily liquid with a slight garlicky odor. It is very soluble in most organic solvents but sparingly soluble in water and relatively stable in acidic media, alkaline media, and heat. As a result, fenthion is a highly persistent insecticide. The oral LD_{50} for male rats is 255 to 298 mg. per kg.; the acute dermal LD_{50} for male rats is 1680 mg. per kg.

Cattle. Fenthion is applied as a ready-to-use 3 per cent pour-on (TIGUVON) along the topline of beef and nonlactating dairy cattle at the rate of 33 ml. per 100 kg. for the control of flies, lice, and *Hypoderma* grubs. Products containing higher concentrations of fenthion (LYSOFF) must be diluted immediately before use. For spot treatment, 3 ml. per 100 kg. of a 20 per cent solution of fenthion in oil (SPOTTON) may be used. Fenthion may also be sprayed on or applied by backrubbers. For the control of grubs, fenthion must be applied in fall immediately after adult fly activity ceases.

Swine. Fenthion is applied to swine as a pour-on for the control of lice.

WARNING. One application per season is adequate for the control of *Hypoderma* grubs. Cattle should not be slaughtered within 35 days following a single application. If the drug is applied a second time for the control of cattle lice, usually 35 days after the first application, the cattle should not be slaughtered within 45 days of the second application. Fenthion should not be applied to dairy cows within 28 days of calving and should not be used on lactating dairy cows, on calves less than 3 months old, or on animals under stress. Swine should not be treated within 14 days of slaughter. For standard precautions to be followed in dealing with organophosphorus insecticides, see page 191.

MALATHION

Malathion (CYTHION) is a clear to amber liquid with a garlicky odor. It is slightly soluble in water, sparingly soluble in petroleum oils, but miscible in most organic solvents, including alcohols, aromatic hydrocarbons, and vegetable oils. Malathion hydrolyzes rapidly in aqueous media below pH 5 and above pH 7; it also is quickly metabolized by mammals. Malathion is a very safe general purpose insecticide. The oral LD_{50} for rats is 1000 to 1400 mg. per kg.; the acute dermal LD_{50} for rabbits is 4100 mg. per kg.

Because of its compatibility with other insecticides, malathion is formulated with methoxychlor (VET-KEM DAIRY AND LIVE-STOCK DUST), with toxaphene (KEMAL and LINDOX M), with pyrethrins and synergists (PARA BOMB-M-1 pressurized spray), and with pyrethrins, synergists, and methoxychlor (PET PEST SPRAY aerosol). One should weigh the increased spectrum of each combination against the prolonged residual effect and possible residues in edible products when deciding whether to use a particular product.

Cattle. Malathion is indicated in beef and nonlactating dairy cattle for the control of face flies, horn flies, lice, and ticks. It is applied at concentrations of 1.25 per cent in water, 2 per cent in oil, or 5 per cent in ready-to-use dust. Application may be repeated in 10 to 14 days. For the control of horn flies on lactating dairy cattle, 3 to 4 tablespoons per head of 4 to 5 per cent malathion dust may be sprinkled on the back and neck.

Sheep and Goats. Animals infested with keds and ticks are dipped in or sprayed with 0.6 per cent malathion in water. Five per cent malathion dust may be applied by hand or power duster.

Swine. Lousy swine may be treated with 0.6 per cent malathion in water, 0.5 per cent malathion in oil, or 6 per cent malathion dust.

Horses. Malathion 0.12 per cent in water is indicated for the control of stable flies, lice, and botfly eggs.

Premises. For the control of flies around farm buildings, malathion is applied in water as a 2.5 per cent residual spray. In dairy barns and milk rooms, 1 to 1.25 per cent bait formulation is applied to fly roosting areas as a spray or by brushing. Adult, larval, and pupal fleas and *Cheyletiella* mites can be controlled by spraying premises with 0.5 per cent solution of malathion.

WARNING. Malathion dip or spray should not be applied to lactating dairy cattle or goats or to dry animals within two weeks of freshening. Malathion should not be applied to premises within five hours before milking or during milking. Calves under one month

of age should not be treated with malathion. Avoid contamination of feed, water, milk, and milking equipment. With regard to combination products in particular, be certain to follow the safety restrictions printed on the label. For standard precautions to be followed in dealing with organophosphorus insecticides, see page 191.

NALED

Naled (DIBROM), obtained by bromination of dichlorvos, is usually liquid and has an acrid odor. Crystalline naled with a low melting point (27°C) has also been prepared. Pure naled is very slightly soluble in water but readily soluble in organic solvents, except aliphatic hydrocarbons. Naled is completely hydrolyzed in water within 48 hours at room temperature. Mammalian toxicity is relatively low; the oral LD_{50} for rats is 430 mg. per kg.; the acute dermal LD_{50} for rabbits is 1100 mg. per kg.

Naled is used as a short-term residual insecticide for the control of houseflies, stable flies, mosquitoes, and gnats in livestock barns, sheds, and feedlots, but direct application to animals must be avoided. For space treatment, 1 part of the 37 per cent emulsifiable concentrate is mixed with 100 parts of water. Freshly diluted naled is applied every three to seven days at the rate of 9.3 liters per hectare (5 gallons per acre) with a mist blower directed above the animals and pens. Dry or wet baits are sprinkled on fly roosting areas. Naled should not be applied to milk rooms; avoid contaminating milk, milking equipment, water, feed, and eggs.

PHOSMET

Phosmet (PROLATE, IMIDAN) is an off-white, crystalline powder with an unpleasant odor, sparingly soluble in water but soluble in most organic solvents except aliphatic hydrocarbons. It is relatively stable in neutral and acidic media but rapidly hydrolyzed in aqueous alkaline media. The oral LD_{50} for male rats is 147 to 316 mg. per kg.; the acute dermal LD_{50} for rabbits is 3160 mg. per kg.

Cattle. Phosmet is used as a spray or pour-on (GX-118, KEMOLATE) for the control of horn flies and cattle grubs. It is applied at the rate of 66 ml. of 4 per cent mixture per 100 kg. but not exceeding 240 ml. per animal. Apply in fall as soon as possible after adult fly activity has ceased. For the control of horn flies, lice, ticks, and sarcoptic mites, one may use 5 per cent phosmet in self-treatment dust bags.

Dogs and Cats. Phosmet 11.6 per cent in aromatic petroleum solvents (PARAMITE) is registered for the control of fleas, ticks, and sarcoptic mange mites. A single application of diluted PARAMITE (16 ml. PARAMITE per liter of water) is said to be adequate for the treatment of sarcoptic mange in dogs. This regimen will also control fleas and ticks for 16 days. Phosmet did not significantly depress the erythrocyte cholinesterase of dogs when applied at 2.7 times the recommended rate. Fleas and ticks on cats may be controlled for 9 to 16 days by applying a more diluted solution (8 ml. PARAMITE per liter of water).

WARNING. Dogs or cats under 8 weeks of age should not be treated with phosmet. Treatment should not be repeated more often than every seven days. Calves under three months of age, dairy animals, and beef animals within 21 days of slaughter should not be treated. For standard precautions to be followed in dealing with organophosphorus insecticides, see page 191.

RONNEL (FENCHLORPHOS)

Ronnel is a white, crystalline powder sparingly soluble in water but very soluble in most organic solvents. Ronnel has low mammalian toxicity. The oral LD_{50} for rats is 1.25 to 1.75 grams per kg.; the acute dermal LD_{50} for rabbits is 1000 mg. per kg. Ronnel is rapidly metabolized in the rat and in cattle. Ronnel (TROLENE, ECTORAL, CATRON, AND RID-EZY) is used as an animal systemic and premises insecticide in a variety of pharmaceutical formulations (spray, dip, pour-on, dust, smear, backrubber, feed mineral block, mineral supplement in granular form, and liquid feed supplement). Manufacture of ronnel has been discontinued in the United States at the time of this writing but may again become available.

Cattle. Ronnel (TROLENE) is fed to beef and nonlactating dairy cattle for the contol or *Hypoderma* grubs, lice, and horn flies. It may be fed as a free-choice feed mineral block, as a mineral supplement in granular form, or as a liquid feed supplement containing 0.26 to 6 per cent ronnel. Ronnel is applied to cattle as a spray, dip, or pour-on, or by backrubber for the control of horn flies, lice and ticks. Screwworm infestation is treated by local application of ronnel preparations to the wounds.

Sheep. Ronnel is used on sheep as a spray, dip, or spot treatment for control of keds, lice, and myiasis larvae.

Swine. Ronnel is applied to swine by spray or dust and is also used to spray hog pens and bedding to control flies and lice.

Dogs and Cats. Ronnel is administered orally in tablet form and topically as a spray or dip for the control of lice, fleas, ticks, and *Otodectes, Sarcoptes,* and *Demodex* mites in dogs, and fleas, lice, and *Otodectes* mites in cats. Fleas and lice on dogs and cats are controlled by either dipping or sponging 0.25 per cent ronnel solution over the entire body or by administering ECTORAL tablets at the rate of 27.6 to 55 mg. per kg. on alternate days. Ticks may be controlled by dipping dogs in 1 per cent ronnel solution or by administering ECTORAL tablets at the rate of 50 mg. per kg. daily. For ear mites in dogs and cats, apply 1 per cent ronnel to the ear canals as needed. For sarcoptic mange, apply 1 per cent ronnel to the entire body three times at seven-day intervals. For treatment of canine demodectic mange, apply a fresh 1 per cent solution topically every four days and administer ECTORAL tablets daily at the rate of 55 to 77 mg. per kg. Treatment should be continued for three weeks after all mites found in skin scrapings are dead. Ronnel aerosol spray applied with a fogger provides effective control of fleas and ticks in enclosed areas.

WARNING. Ronnel is a cholinesterase inhibitor and should not be used within a few days of exposure to other cholinesterase-inhibiting drugs. Lactating dairy cows and goats should not be treated with ronnel. If treatment of dairy cows and goats is carried out, then the milk must not be used for 7 to 10 days after the last application. Animals should not be treated within 10 days of slaughter. In dogs, doses over 500 mg. of ronnel per kg. of body weight cause emesis. Adverse reactions may occur at even lower doses. For standard precautions to be followed in dealing with organophosphorus insecticides, see page 191.

TETRACHLORVINPHOS (STIROFOS)

Tetrachlorvinphos is a white, crystalline powder sparingly soluble in water and hydrocarbons but soluble in most organic solvents. Of low mammalian toxicity, the oral LD_{50} of tetrachlorvinphos for rats is 4000 to 5000 mg. per kg.; the acute dermal LD_{50} for rabbits is 2500 mg. per kg. Tetrachlorvinphos is marketed under the proprietary names RABON and GARDONA as emulsifiable concentrate, wettable powder, and dust, and as a mixture of 2.3 per cent tetrachlorvinphos and 5.7 per cent dichlorvos (RAVAP).

Cattle. For the control of face flies, horn flies, houseflies, stable flies, lice, ticks, and chorioptic mites, RABON and RAVAP may be applied manually or by dust bag as a ready-to-use 3 per cent dust, by spraying aqueous suspensions, or by backrubber application of concentrates diluted in oil. RABON prevents the growth of horn fly and face fly larvae when fed to beef and dairy cattle in complete ration, mineral supplements, or molasses blocks at the rate of 1.54 mg. per kg. per day. Regular spraying of barns is recommended for control of flies.

Swine. RABON 3 per cent ready-to-use dust or 0.5 per cent wettable powder are applied directly to swine for the control of lice. Treatment may be repeated in two weeks if necessary.

Dogs and Cats. RABON 9.5 per cent in collars (UNIPET) is used for control of fleas and ticks on dogs and cats. It is claimed that UNIPET collars remain effective for two to three months and that wetting does not reduce their effectiveness.

TRICHLORFON (METRIFONATE)

Trichlorfon is a white, crystalline powder moderately soluble in water, very soluble in chloroform and alcohols, and slightly soluble in aromatic hydrocarbons; decomposition is rapid in alkaline media. Trichlorfon has high insecticidal activity and low mammalian toxicity. Trichlorfon is hydrolyzed *in vivo* into dichlorvos, which kills insects by inhibiting the enzyme acetylcholinesterase. The oral LD_{50} for rats is 450 mg. per kg.; the dermal LD_{50} for rats is over 500 mg. per kg. Trichlorfon is marketed under many proprietary names (NEGUVON, DYREX, DYLOX, CASECT, GRUB AND LOUSE POUR-ON, and GX-120 POUR-ON) primarily for the control of *Hypoderma* grubs, horn flies, and lice in cattle.

Cattle. For control of *Hypoderma* grubs and as an aid in the control of lice and horn flies, trichlorfon is applied as a ready-to-use 8 per cent mix to the topline of beef and nonlactating dairy cattle at the rate of 33 ml. per 100 kg., not exceeding 120 ml. per animal. The animals may alternatively be sprayed with 1

per cent trichlorfon. Trichlorfon treatment should be carried out in fall as soon as possible after the end of adult fly activity.

Premises. Trichlorfon in bait blocks, dry bait, liquid bait, and syrup bait is used to control flies in dairy barns and milk rooms.

WARNING. Trichlorfon should not be applied to lactating dairy cows, to dry cows within 21 days of calving, or to sick and stressed animals. Do not treat cattle within 21 days of slaughter. Do not contaminate milk and milk-handling equipment. For standard precautions to be followed in dealing with organophosphorus insecticides, see page 191.

Chlorinated Hydrocarbons

Chlorinated hydrocarbons are now in disfavor because of their persistence in the environment. In many states, it is illegal for dairymen to use or store chlorinated hydrocarbons on their farms but the use of these chemicals is permitted in the farm residence. Chlorinated hydrocarbons produce neuromuscular hyperexcitability. Poisoning of domestic animals is treated with nervous system depressants such as phenobarbital.

LINDANE

Lindane is the gamma isomer of benzene hexachloride. It is a crystalline powder with a slight musty odor, insoluble in water and slightly soluble in alcohols, ether, benzene. and chloroform. The oral LD_{50} for rats is 100 to 130 mg. per kg. and the level of toxicity is similar for domestic animals. Lindane stimulates the mammalian central nervous system, resulting in hypertension, bradycardia, polypnea, and restlessness, followed by body tremors, salivation, grinding of the teeth, and convulsions. The animal dies of either cardiac or respiratory failure. Lindane rapidly kills insects by interfering with the normal functions of the nervous system.

Lindane is characterized by a high rate of biodegradability. It is used alone in a wide range of formulations (emulsifiable concentrates, wettable powders, oil base sprays, smokes, dusts, aerosols, and smears) for the control of lice, ticks, mites, and screwworms. Lindane is also one of the active ingredients in a number of combination products such as BENZYL BENZOATE WITH LINDANE, DEMSARDEX, FENATOX, MYCODEX SHAMPOO WITH LINDANE, THERADEX WITH LINDANE, THIONIUM SHAMPOO

WITH LINDANE, AND SECTILIN SHAMPOO.

Beef Cattle. Lindane (LINSPRAY) is indicated at a concentration of 0.03 to 0.06 per cent in water as spray or dip for the control of lice, mange mites, and ear ticks in beef cattle. Calves three to six months old should be sprayed only with dilute lindane (0.03 per cent). Lindane 3 per cent as a smear (MYZIN) or in a bomb (SW-T BOMB), is used for spot treatment of screwworm and ear tick infestations. Lindane 0.2 per cent oil is applied by backrubbers, and 1 per cent is used for manual and dust bag applications.

Sheep and Goats. Lindane is applied as spray or dip at concentrations of 0.03 to 0.06 per cent in water for the control of fleeceworms, keds, lice, psoroptic mange, and ticks. Sheep or goats may be treated with 1 per cent dust formulation. For spot treatment of screwworms, a 3 per cent smear is employed.

Swine. Lindane (0.03 to 0.08 per cent emulsion in water, 0.02 per cent in oil, 1 per cent in dust, or 3 per cent in smear) is applied to swine by spray, dip, manual dusting, backrubbers, or spot treatment for the control of lice, sarcoptic mange, and screwworms. Repeat treatment in 14 days if necessary.

Dogs. Lindane is the insecticide in many pet shampoos (MYCODEX, SECTILIN, THERADEX, AND THIONIUM) intended for the control of lice, fleas, and ticks. KWELL shampoo, cream, and lotion products for human use contain 1 per cent lindane and are very effective medications for sarcoptic mange. The application should be repeated every five to seven days for five to seven weeks. Lindane 0.03 per cent in oil, may be used for the control of ear mites. Lindane, 1 per cent in water (GAMMEX), is recommended for dipping dogs infested with fleas, lice, mites, or ticks.

Horses. Lindane 0.03 per cent is sponged or sprayed on horses for the control of face flies, stable flies, ticks (including *Otobius*), screwworms, lice, and botfly eggs.

Premises. Lindane, 1.25 per cent in water, 0.1 per cent formulated with other insecticides, 0.5 per cent in oil, or 1 per cent in dust, is applied to interior surfaces of agricultural buildings for the control of flies and other nuisance insects.

WARNING. Lindane should not be applied to cats, dairy cattle, or calves under three months old. Cattle, sheep, goats, and pigs should not be dipped within 60 days or sprayed within 30 days of slaughter. Do not apply lindane to sows from two weeks before until three weeks after farrowing. Do not treat animals in cold, stormy weather or animals that are overheated or sick. Lindane must not be used around dairy barns and milk rooms.

METHOXYCHLOR

Methoxychlor (MARLATE) is the methoxy analogue of DDT. It is a dimorphic crystalline powder, practically insoluble in water but soluble in alcohol. Although methoxychlor has prolonged residual insecticidal activity, it shows very little tendency to accumulate in animal fat depots. The oral LD_{50} for rats is 6 grams per kg. Methoxychlor is used either alone or with organophosphate insecticides and synergists (e.g., piperonyl butoxide). Like DDT, methoxychlor presumably interferes with ion movement along the axons. The poisoned insects show tremors, hyperexcitability, and paralysis.

Cattle. Methoxychlor 0.5 per cent in oil is mist sprayed at 75 ml. per animal on beef and nonlactating dairy cattle for the control of stable flies, horn flies, and lice. The application may be repeated every three weeks. Methoxychlor as dust (LINTOX), dip, and wettable powder is used on beef and dairy cattle. Lactating cows may be spot treated with dust formulations only. The oil base emulsion and the dust formulations are applied to animals with appropriate self-treatment equipment such as backrubbers and dust bags, respectively.

Sheep and Goats. Methoxychlor 1 per cent emulsion in water is applied to sheep and goats by spraying or dipping, and 50 per cent powder is applied by hand dusting for the control of keds and lice.

Swine. To control lice, methoxychlor 5 per cent in oil may be applied by rubbing devices, 1 per cent emulsion in water or 0.5 per cent in oil may be used for spraying or dipping, or 50 per cent dust may be applied by hand or mechanical duster.

Dogs and Cats. Methoxychlor in combination with pyrethrins, piperonyl butoxide, and carbaryl (PARA S-1 AEROSOL) is applied to dogs and cats for the control of fleas, lice, and ticks. It also repels mosquitoes and gnats.

Horses. Methoxychlor 0.7 per cent is sprayed or sponged on horses for the control of flies and lice.

WARNING. Methoxychlor should not be applied to cattle more frequently than once every three weeks and should not be applied within five hours of milking. Calves less than one month old and lactating goats should not be treated. During barn treatment, care must be taken not to contaminate milk, water, or feedstuffs. Do not treat overheated animals.

Formamidines

The formamidines are a promising new group of acaricidal compounds effective against cattle ticks and mange mites of sheep and dogs. Formamidines kill by inhibiting monoamine oxidase and are very effective against pests that have developed resistance to organophosphates and carbamates. In the United States, amitraz is approved for the treatment of generalized canine demodicosis.

AMITRAZ

Amitraz is a crystalline compound soluble in organic solvents and only slightly soluble in water. The acute oral LD_{50} for rats is 800 mg. per kg.; the dermal LD_{50} for rabbits is greater than 200 mg. per kg. When applied to the skin of dogs as a 0.025 per cent solution, amitraz produced transient sedation, depression of the rectal temperature, and elevation of blood glucose. Amitraz was well tolerated by dogs when administered orally at 0.25 mg. per kg. daily for 90 days but at 1 to 4 mg. per kg., hyperglycemia was consistently observed. In clinical studies, transient sedation was the most frequently observed untoward effect.

MITABAN liquid contains 19.9 per cent amitraz and is diluted to a 0.025 per cent solution for the treatment of generalized demodicosis in dogs. The contents of one 10.6 ml. vial is mixed with 2 gallons of warm water for each of three to six treatments spaced 14 days apart. It is suggested that treatment be continued until no viable mites are found in skin scrapings made at two successive treatments or until six treatments have been applied. The product information leaflet mentions that one should not use amitraz for treatment of localized demodicosis or scabies.

WARNING. The safety of amitraz has not been evaluated in pregnant bitches or in dogs younger than 4 months. Mitaban concentrate is flammable. Wear rubber gloves when preparing dilutions and applying these to dogs.

Pheromones

(2)-9-Tricosene (MUSCALURE)

MUSCALURE is a synthetic pheromone, a substance female houseflies produce to attract male houseflies. It is a clear, odorless oil, miscible in hexane. MUSCALURE may actually act as an aggregration pheromone, luring both male and female flies, rather than as a sex attractant for male flies only.

The sugar fly bait NEW IMPROVED GOLDEN MALRIN contains 0.25 per cent MUSCALURE, as attractant, and 1 per cent methomyl, as insecticide. The attractant lures and keeps the flies around the bait, thus resulting in an increased kill by the insecticide.

WARNING. Animals must not be allowed to ingest this product.

Repellents

DEET (N,N-Diethyl-m-toluamide)

DEET is an odorless liquid miscible in water, alcohol, and benzene, but practically insoluble in petroleum ether. Its oral LD_{50} for rats is 2000 mg. per kg. DEET is used as a repellent for mosquitoes, gnats, flies, fleas, ticks, and chiggers. For continuing protection, frequent applications are necessary.

DIMETHYL PHTHALATE

Dimethyl phthalate is an oily liquid with slight aromatic odor that is insoluble in water but miscible in alcohol and chloroform. It is used as a repellent for mosquitoes, flies, fleas, and chiggers. Dimethyl phthalate in cottonseed oil (RITAMIDE) may be used for the treatment of ear mite infestations in dogs and cats. We recommend that the clinician select instead one of the many acaricidal drugs for the control of ear mite infestations.

DI-N-PROPYL ISOCINCHOMERONATE

Dipropyl isochinchomeronate is a relatively safe chemical with an oral LD_{50} for rats of 5.2 to 7.2 grams per kg. The chemical is best known by its proprietary name, MGK

REPELLENT 326. It is usually formulated with other insect repellents, insecticides, or synergists. MGK REPELLENT 326 is registered for application as a spray to beef and dairy cattle, goats, sheep, swine, and agricultural premises.

WARNING. Milk, animal feeds, and drinking water should not be contaminated.

R-11

R-11 is a liquid sparingly soluble in water that is best known by its proprietary name, MGK REPELLENT 11. The oral LD_{50} for rats is 2500 mg. per kg. R-11 is used in a spray (SECT-A-SPRAY) in combination with pyrethrins, piperonyl butoxide, and carbaryl. This product is indicated for the control of fleas, lice, and ticks on dogs and cats. It is difficult to understand the reason for combining an insect repellent with such active insecticidal substances. In general, insect repellents offer very little residual protection against insects infesting dogs and cats.

Growth Regulators

METHOPRENE

Methoprene is an amber liquid sparingly soluble in water but soluble in organic solvents. It is of low toxicity to mammals. The oral LD_{50} for rats is 34.6 grams per kg. Methoprene is a growth regulator; it prevents insects from reaching maturity by arresting larval development, which in turn results in the death of the larvae.

In special slow-release formulations (ALTOSID SR-10), methoprene was found to be highly efficacious against larvae of mosquitoes, houseflies, stable flies, horn flies, and face flies. Methoprene has very little residual effect.

Cattle. ALTOSID CP-10, a premix containing 10 per cent methoprene, is incorporated into mineral blocks and feed supplements. Feeding these medicated feedstuffs to beef and dairy cattle to provide an intake of 0.5 to 1.0 mg. per kg. body weight per month results in good control of coprophilic dipteran flies, particularly horn flies. The formulated drug undergoes very little breakdown as it passes through the alimentary tract. The unmetabolized methoprene eliminated in the manure disturbs the growth of the maggots, thus preventing the development of adult horn flies.

PRECOR is a methoprene formulation for indoor control of dog and cat fleas; it acts on the flea larvae.

WARNING. Feed supplements containing methoprene should be withdrawn from cattle 14 days before slaughter.

Synergists

N-OCTYL BICYCLOHEPTENE DICARBOXAMIDE

N-octyl bicycloheptene dicarboxamide inhibits the microsomal detoxification of insecticides, thus maximizing their toxicity. It is registered for application to beef and dairy cattle, sheep, goats, horses, swine, dogs, and cats and to agricultural buildings and animal quarters for the control of annoying insects. It is often formulated with piperonyl butoxide and insecticides as aerosols, pressurized sprays, and free-flowing dusts (FLICK SHAMPOO, NORSECT, PET PEST SPRAY, PYRESEPT SHAMPOO, SERO-MITE, TICK-KILL).

PIPERONYL BUTOXIDE

Piperonyl butoxide is a pale yellowish liquid, soluble in alcohols, benzene, Freons, and other organic solvents. It is very safe for animals. The oral LD_{50} for rats is about 7.5 grams per kg. Chlorinated hydrocarbons, carbamates, organophosphates, and particularly pyrethrins and rotenone are synergized by piperonyl butoxide. The insecticidal activity of these compounds is enhanced because piperonyl butoxide inhibits degradation of the insecticide by the insect's microsomal enzymes.

AURIMITE, CERUMITE, DIRYL, D-FLEA, FLEABAN, FLAIR, FLICK, F-L-T BOMB, F-L-T POWDER, HAVA-CIDE LIQUID, K.F.L. SHAMPOO, NORSECT, PARA BOMB-M-1 SPRAY, PARA S-1 AEROSOL, PET PEST SPRAY, PYRESEPT SHAMPOO, SECT-A-SPRAY, SECTRO, THERA-GROOM SHAMPOO, TIC-CIDE, TICK-KILL, VET-KEM PET SPRAY, AND ZERO-MITE all contain piperonyl butoxide as a synergist formulated with pyrethrins, malathion, carbaryl, or methoxychlor.

Miscellaneous Insecticides

BENZYL BENZOATE

Benzyl benzoate is a colorless, crystalline, leaflet or an oily liquid with pleasant aromatic odor and sharp burning taste. It is insoluble in water and glycerol but soluble in alcohol, chloroform, ether, and oils. The oral LD_{50} for rats is 1.7 grams per kg. Toxic levels of benzyl benzoate depress the nervous system, resulting in vertigo, incoordination, coma, and death from respiratory or heart failure.

Benzyl benzoate is effective against most ectoparasites. It should only be used on dogs infested with sarcoptic, otodectic, or demodectic mites, however. Benzyl benzoate is marketed either alone (DEMODEK) or formulated with lindane (BENZYL BENZOATE WITH LINDANE and DEMSARDEX). MITONE contains benzyl benzoate and rotenone, BENZYL-HEX contains benzyl benzoate, lindane, and rotenone, and MANGE LOTION contains benzyl benzoate, lindane, rotenone, and dichlorophene. For spot treatment of localized infestations, apply daily to all lesions for at least seven days. For the treatment of generalized forms of sarcoptic and demodectic mange, first clip the hair from the entire body and bathe the dog to remove all crusty materials. MANGE LOTION is then applied while the dog is still wet. It is recommended that only one third of the body be treated with the acaricide at one time. Benzyl benzoate has no residual effect. Therefore, repeated applications are required. Demodectic mange may require prolonged therapy. Sarcoptic mange is usually cured with two applications.

WARNING. Benzyl benzoate–containing drugs should not be used on cats. If application is carried out by dipping, protect the patient's eyes with a bland ointment.

DIPHENYLAMINE

Diphenylamine (N-phenylbenzeneamine) is a crystalline solid with floral odor, insoluble in water but soluble in ethyl alcohol, propyl alcohol, benzene, ether, and glacial acetic acid. The oral LD_{50} for guinea pigs is 300 to 1000 mg. per kg.

Diphenylamine is formulated as a 5 to 30 per cent smear or lotion to be smeared with a brush on and around the wound for the control of screwworms in horses.

WARNING. Diphenylamine should not be applied to dairy or meat-producing animals, cats, dogs, or man.

SULFUR

Sulfur is a polymorphic, yellow, crystalline powder that is insoluble in water, sparingly soluble in alcohol, but very soluble in carbon disulfide. It is one of the oldest miticidal drugs and is still used for the treatment of manges, particularly on cats and lactating dairy animals. Sulfur is formulated as a free-flowing dusting powder, micronized wettable powder, microdispersed colloidal sulfur 3 per cent (SULTEX), and sulfur ointment. It is also formulated with keratolytic substances such as salicylic acid and as the lime-sulfur solution (ORTHORIX), an aqueous solution of calcium sulfide, poylsulfide, and thiosulfate.

Farm Animals. Animals infested with sarcoptic, psoroptic, or chorioptic mites are dipped or pressure sprayed with colloidal sulfur or with lime-sulfur solution diluted 1:40 with warm water. Sulfur dust may also be rubbed into the hair of infested animals. The application may be repeated in 10 to 12 days, if necessary. There are no restrictions on the application of lime-sulfur.

Dogs and Cats. Cats infested with notoedric mites are bathed first and then sprayed, dipped, or washed with lime-sulfur solution diluted 1:40 with warm water. The treatment is repeated every five days. Dogs infested with sarcoptic mites may also be treated with lime-sulfur solution.

ANTIPROTOZOALS

We have tried here to briefly characterize the biological activities of a few approved and some nonapproved but legally obtainable antiprotozoal drugs. As with any drug, the information on the label or package insert must always be read and followed before administering antiprotozoal agents.

AMPROLIUM

Amprolium is an odorless, crystalline powder that is soluble in water. A 10 per cent aqueous solution has an acidic reaction. As a coccidiostat, amprolium is fed in broiler rations at a concentration of 0.125 per cent. The coccidiostatic activity of amprolium is related to its ability to competitively antagonize the physiological role of thiamine as a coenzyme.

Cattle. For treatment of active *Eimeria bovis* and *E. zuernii* infections in cattle, amprolium (formulated as 9.6 per cent drench solution, 20 per cent soluble powder, or 1.25 per cent feed crumbles) is administered by drench or top-dressed on the feed at the approximate dosage of 10 mg. per kg. for five consecutive days. For prevention of coccidiosis caused by *E. bovis* and *E. zuernii* during periods of exposure, a dose level of 5 mg. per kg. daily for 21 days is recommended. Amprolium premix (AMPROVINE) is used for beef and dairy calves. Other species of *Eimeria* are also susceptible to amprolium, but the drug label claims efficacy only against *E. bovis* and *E. zuernii*. Cattle dosed with 50 mg. per kg. of amprolium per day did not develop adverse reactions.

Sheep and Goats. Amprolium has not yet been cleared for sheep and goats by FDA. Coccidiosis in sheep and goats can be controlled with amprolium or with potentiated amprolium with ethopobate at 55 mg. per kg. twice a day for 19 days; medication should start before the animals have been exposed to infective oocysts.

WARNING. Animals should not be medicated within 24 hours of slaughter.

DECOQUINATE

Decoquinate is an approved coccidiostatic drug for the control of *Eimeria* infections in chickens and cattle.

Cattle. Decoquinate is indicated for prevention of coccidiosis caused by *E. bovis* and *E. zuernii* in ruminating calves and older cattle. It is fed at 0.5 mg. per kg. per day for at least 28 days during periods of exposure to infective oocysts.

WARNING. Decoquinate should not be fed to breeding animals or lactating dairy cows. Complete feeds containing decoquinate should be consumed within seven days of manufacture. Bentonite should not be used in decoquinate feeds.

IMIDOCARB DIPROPIONATE

In the United States, imidocarb dipropionate (IMIZOL EQUINE) is approved for use in horses and zebras for the control of *Babesia* infections. It is administered intramuscularly in the neck region at 2 mg. per kg. repeated once after 24 hours for treatment of *Babesia caballi* infections. For *B. equi* infections, imidocarb is administered at 4 mg. per kg. repeated four times at 72 hour intervals. Imidocarb is also effective against *Babesia* and *Anaplasma* infections in cattle but has not been cleared for cattle in the United States.

WARNING. Overdosage may produce salivation, colic, diarrhea; reactions similar to organophosphorus poisoning. Imidocarb is a cholinesterase inhibitor and should not be used with other cholinesterase-inhibiting drugs. It should not be administered to horses less than one year old, to mares near term, or to horses intended for human food. Imidocarb dipropionate is sold only under permit issued by the director of the National Program Planning Staff, Veterinary Services, APHIS, USDA, to licensed veterinarians and is available from Wellcome Animal Health Division, Burroughs Wellcome Co.

METRONIDAZOLE

Metronidazole (FLAGYL) is a light yellow, crystalline powder, sparingly soluble in water and in ethanol but soluble in diluted acids. It is used in man for the treatment of *Trichomonas vaginalis*, *Giardia lamblia*, and *Entomoeba histolytica* infections. Metronidazole has not been approved by FDA for veterinary use but is available at pharmacies as FLAGYL, a product for human use.

Cattle. Metronidazole is indicated for the treatment and control of *Trichmonas foetus* infections. It is administered intravenously at 75 mg. per kg. three times at 12 hour intervals.

Dogs. Metronidazole is indicated for the treatment of giardiasis and trichomoniasis. The recommended dose is 50 mg. per kg. administered orally once a day for five consecutive days. Daily dosage of dogs with 100 mg. per kg. for 30 days was well tolerated but higher levels produced adverse reactions (tremors, muscle spasms, weakness, incoordination, and ataxia).

WARNING. Metronidazole causes pulmonary tumors in mice and increases the incidence of various neoplasms, particularly mammary tumors in female rats.

MONENSIN

Monensin is an antibiotic with coccidiostatic and growth-promoting activities. It is used in poultry and cattle. In calves experimentally inoculated with *Eimeria bovis* oocysts, monensin at 16.5 to 33 grams per metric ton of feed (resulting in an intake of at least 0.25 mg. per kg.) fed daily for 31 days, prevented the development of clinical signs of coccidiosis. In lambs, prophylactic administration of monensin at 1 mg. per kg. prevented diarrhea and reduced oocyst shedding. Therapeutic administration of monensin to naturally infected lambs at 1 mg. per kg. was useful in controlling hemorrhagic diarrhea and shedding of oocysts in the feces. Monensin has not been cleared for the treatment of coccidian infections in ruminants. Monensin is very toxic to horses.

QUINACRINE HYDROCHLORIDE

Quinacrine hydrochloride is a bright yellow, crystalline powder with a bitter taste. It is soluble at a dilution of 1:35 in water, sparingly soluble in ethanol, and insoluble in acetone, benzene, and ether. A one per cent aqueous solution has an acidic reaction. Quinacrine was used as an antimalarial, especially during World War II, but, because of its toxicity and relatively weak activity against *Plasmodium vivax*, has now been replaced by other antimalarials. ATABRINE (a product for human use) has not been approved by FDA for veterinary use but ATABRINE tablets are available from Winthrop Laboratories.

Dogs. Quinacrine is indicated for the control of *Giardia, Taenia* and *Diphyllobothrium* infections. For large breeds, quinacrine is administered orally at 200 mg. per dog three times on the first day and twice a day during the following six days. Small breeds receive 100 mg. per dog twice on the first day and once daily for the folowing six days. Puppies are dosed with 50 mg. twice a day for six days.

WARNING. A single oral dose of 300 mg. per kg. for 15 days or 110 mg. per kg. for 27 days is lethal for dogs. The most prominent sign is vomiting, the occurrence of which may be reduced by simultaneous administration of sodium bicarbonate. Quinacrine is a strong inhibitor of cholinesterase.

SULFADIMETHOXINE

Sulfadimethoxine is indicated for the control of enteritis caused by coccidia in dogs. The recommended oral dose is 55 mg. per kg. for the first day and 27.5 mg. per kg. per day for the following four days. It is good practice to continue therapy until the dog is asymptomatic for at least 48 hours. Periodic administration of sulfadimethoxine to dogs prevents the build-up of coccidian oocysts in the soil. A single oral dose of 160 mg. sulfadimethoxine per kg. was well tolerated; 3.2 grams per kg. produced only diarrhea.

SULFAGUANIDINE

Feed containing 0.2 per cent sulfaguanidine is fed continuously to sheep for the prevention of coccidiosis. It is most likely that the same regimen can be applied to the prevention of coccidiosis in goats and cattle under stress. Medicated ration should be fed continuously beginning as early as possible in the exposure period and continuing as long as protection is required.

SULFAMETHAZINE

The sodium salt of sulfamethazine may be administered in water or feed, or intravenously to cattle, sheep, and goats for the control of coccidiosis. During outbreaks, up to 0.5 per cent concentration is mixed with the feed. Alternatively, 130 mg. sulfamethazine per kg. may be administered orally on the first day and followed by 65 mg. per kg. every 12 hours for four days.

WARNING. Animals should be provided with plenty of water when they are on sulfonamide medication. Withdrawal recommendation should be followed for food-producing animals.

ANTHELMINTICS

Anthelmintics approved by the Bureau of Veterinary Medicine of the Food and Drug Administration are described here in alphabetical order according to their generic names. A few anthelmintics in common use in other countries are also described briefly.

ALBENDAZOLE

Albendazole is the thio analogue of oxibendazole, a 2-amino-substituted benzimidazole. It is a very stable, white, odorless powder that is insoluble in water and only slightly soluble in most organic solvents. The oral LD_{50} for rats is 2400 mg. per kg. In dogs and rats dosed with albendazole at levels up to 30 mg. per kg. per day for 90 days, there were no anatomical or physiological alterations attributable to the drug. No teratogenesis was observed in mice dosed with up to 30 mg. per kg. per day from day 6 to day 15 of gestation. The "no effect" level in rats was 5 mg. per kg.

Albendazole is a broad spectrum anthelmintic effective against gastrointestinal nematodes, lung nematodes, cestodes, and lung and liver trematodes. It is a registered anthelmintic in many countries but it has not as yet been cleared by FDA in the United States. When the FDA banned the use of hexochloroethane, a carcinogen, the cattle industry was left without an approved, safe, and effective anthelmintic for use in fascioliasis of cattle and sheep. Albendazole, proven safe and effective against *Fasciola hepatica* in cattle at 10 mg. per kg. and against *Fascioloides magna* in sheep at 7.5 mg. per kg., and widely used in many countries of the world, was in process for approval by FDA for use in the United States. Because of the dire need of the livestock industry, FDA allowed albendazole to be made available on the basis of an emergency Investigational New Animal Drug (INAD). Albendazole, distributed by Norden Laboratories to veterinarians only, is cleared for use only in states where fascioliasis is a serious problem in cattle and sheep. A 180 day withdrawal period was established by FDA for use of albendazole under the emergency INAD. They concluded that this lengthy withdrawal afforded an adequate margin of safety to consuming humans for any albendazole residues that might remain in the edible tissues of treated animals at the time of slaughter. This is a provisional investigational clearance. A complete approval for use in cattle has not yet been obtained as of this date.

Cattle. Albendazole (VALBAZEN) is administered orally as a drench at 7.5 mg. per kg. for the control of *Haemonchus, Ostertagia*, and *Trichostrongylus* in the abomasum, *Nematodirus, Cooperia, Trichostrongylus, Bunostomum, Oesophagostomum*, and *Moniezia* in the intestines, and *Dictyocaulus* in the lungs. Many larval forms, including the hypobiotic early fourth stage of *Ostertagia*, are very susceptible to albendazole. Ten to 15 mg. per kg. afforded consistently excellent activity against adult *Fasciola hepatica*. A single dose of 75 mg. of albendazole per kg. of body weight was well tolerated. Albendazole was embryotoxic when administered to cows at a dosage rate of 25 mg. per kg. during the first 7 to 17 days of gestation. The conception rate of cows dosed after the 21st day of gestation was comparable to controls and all cows gave birth to normal calves.

WARNING. Overseas, animals should not be treated within 14 days of slaughter; milk must not be used for human consumption until 72 hours after treatment.

Sheep. Albendazole drench (VALBAZEN) is administered orally at 3.8 mg. per kg. for the control of *Haemonchus, Ostertagia*, and *Trichostrongylus* in the abomasum, *Nematodirus, Cooperia, Marshallagia, Bunostomum, Gaigeria, Chabertia, Oesophagostomum, Moniezia*, and *Avitellina* in the intestines, and *Dictyocaulus* in the lungs. For the control of *Fasciola hepatica*, albendazole is administered at 4.75 to 7.5 mg. per kg.. The maximum tolerated dose in sheep is reported to be around 37.5 mg. per kg.

Albendazole may induce fetal skeletal abnormalities when administered at a dosage level of 11 mg. per kg. or more to ewes during the first 10 to 17 days of pregnancy. No untoward effects have been reported after its use in many thousands of sheep, however.

WARNING. Care should be taken to adhere to recommended dosages particularly when treating ewes during the first month of pregnancy. Sheep should not be treated within 10 days of slaughter.

Horses. Initial experimentation indicates that albendazole administered by stomach tube at 5 mg. per kg. was highly active against *Strongylus vulgaris, S. edentatus*, and *S. equinus*, adult small strongyles, and adult and larval stages of *Oxyuris equi*. At a dosage rate of 25 mg. per kg. three times a day for five days or 50 mg. per kg. twice a day for two days, albendazole was extremmly efficacious against the fourth stage larva of *Strongylus vulgaris* in the anterior mesenteric arterial system.

Dogs and Cats. Albendazole demonstrated excellent activity against *Ancylostoma, Toxocara, Trichuris*, and *Taenia* in dogs at a dosage level of 25 mg. per kg. administered orally or in feed for three to five days. Its activity was slight against *Dipylidium*. A single dose of 100 mg. per kg. was reported to be active against *Mesocestoides corti* in dogs. One bitch with active *Paragonimus kellicotti* infection was successfully treated with albendazole paste at 30 mg. per kg. per day for 12 days. Albendazole controlled *Paragonimus kellicotti* infections in cats at 25 mg. per kg. twice a day for 7 to 14 days. *Filaroides hirthi* infections in dogs were controlled with albendazole at 25 to 50 mg. per kg. twice daily for five days.

ARECOLINE HYDROBROMIDE

Arecoline hydrobromide is a bitter, white, crystalline solid. One gram dissolves in about 1 ml of water or in 10 ml of ethanol; it is slightly soluble in chloroform. The subcutaneous LD_{50} in dogs is about 5 mg per kg. Arecoline hydrobromide exerts its anticestodal effect by paralyzing the muscles controlling the attachment apparatus of the tapeworms and at the same time by increasing the host's intestinal motility cholinergically to aid in the expulson of the worms.

Arecoline hydrobromide in tablet form (ARECO-CAINE) is used in dogs and cats for the removal of *Taenia, Dipylidium,* and *Echinococcus* tapeworms. The drug is administered orally at 0.9 to 2.0 mg. per kg. after 12 to 18 hours of fasting. If catharsis does not occur within two or three hours (usually the animals defecate within 15 to 45 minutes), a saline or soap enema should be administered. It is suggested that the lower dose be used to avoid undesirable toxic effects such as discomfort, hypersalivation, intestinal cramping, vomiting, severe diarrhea, and depression.

WARNING. Sick, emaciated, or pregnant animals must not be treated with arecoline hydrobromide.

ARSENAMIDE SODIUM (THIACETARSAMIDE)

Arsenamide is a white, crystalline powder sparingly soluble in cold water and very soluble in warm ethanol and methanol. Arsenamide sodium 1 per cent (10 mg. per ml.) buffered solution is marketed under a variety of proprietary names (ARSENAMIDE SO-DIUM, CAPARSOLATE SODIUM, FILARIMIDE). It is administered intravenously at 2.2 mg. per kg. twice a day for two or three days for the treatment of adult *Dirofilaria immitis* infection in dogs. For dogs in poor condition, a more conservative dose, 2.2 mg. per kg. once daily for 15 days, is recommended. Blair and coworkers (1982) demonstrated that the early fifth stages and two year old adult heartworms are the most susceptible to arsenamide. Adolescent female worms are less susceptible than males are. It is now clear that an unyielding heartworm infection, an apparent drug failure, indicates the presence of maturing worms. Repeated arsenamide therapy at intervals of a few months should eventually lead to complete elimination of the worms.

BUNAMIDINE HYDROCHLORIDE

Bunamidine hydrochloride is an odorless, white, crystalline solid, soluble in methanol. The oral LD_{50} for mice is about 540 mg. of the base per kg. of body weight. Bunamidine hydrochloride (SCOLABAN) is administered orally to dogs for the removal of *Dipylidium, Taenia, Mesocestoides,* and *Echinococcus,* and to cats for the removal of *Dipylidium* and *Hydatigera taeniaeformis* tapeworms. Because the worms die and disintegrate within the host's intestinal tract, they are not often seen in the feces after treatment. Bunamidine is administered to cats and dogs at the rate of 25 to 50 mg. per kg. up to a maximum of 600 mg. The tablets should be administered whole and should not be broken, crushed, mixed with the food, or dissolved in liquid because bunamidine irritates the oral mucosa. Bunamidine should be given on an empty stomach. The presence of intestinal contents and mucus reduces anthelmintic efficacy. The animal may be fed about three hours after medication. Treatment should not be repeated within 14 days.

In the treatment of *Echinococcus* infection, a second dose should be administered in 48 hours, and a third dose four to six weeks later to remove the worms that were immature at the initial treatment.

WARNING. Bunamidine hydrochloride should not be given to unweaned puppies, and kittens, to male dogs within 28 days prior to their use for breeding, or to animals having cardiac or hepatic disease. Vomiting, diarrhea, and heart failure (ventricular fibrillation) are the most frequent adverse side effects. The animals should not be allowed to exercise or to become excited immediately after the administration of bunamidine hydrochloride. Bunamidine should not be administered concurrently with butamisole. An acute reaction which is sometimes fatal may ensue.

BUTAMISOLE HYDROCHLORIDE

Butamisole (STIQUIN) is an analogue of tetramisole (levamisole). Butamisole hydrochloride parenteral 1.1 per cent removes *Trichuris vulpis* and *Ancylostoma caninum* when administered subcutaneously to dogs at 2.4 mg. per kg. Butamisole is primarily effective against adult hookworms.

WARNING. Butamisole is relatively well tolerated at the recommended 2.4 mg. per kg. However, in one study of 14 dogs receiving 7.5 mg. per kg., two showed emesis and tremors, and one of these died. At 10, 12.5, and 15 mg. per kg., deaths occurred regularly. Incoordination, emesis, tremors, convulsions, and lateral recumbency were observed before the dogs died. Butamisole is a new drug. One should exercise prudence in treating very young or old and debilitated dogs with it. Adverse reactions which were sometimes fatal were reported when butamisole was administered to heartworm-infected dogs.

CAMBENDAZOLE

Cambendazole is a substituted thiabendazole. It is an odorless, white, crystalline powder, practically insoluble in water but soluble in alcohol and dimethylformamide.

Cambendazole (CAMVET) suspension, feed pellets, or paste is administered to horses at 20 mg. per kg. for the removal of adult *Strongylus vulgaris, S. edentatus,* and *S. equinus,* many species of the subfamily Cyathostominae, *Parascaris, Oxyuris,* and *Strongyloides westeri.* A number of cyathostome species have developed resistance to cambendazole at the recommended dosage level. Good activity was also observed against immature cyathostomes, *Parascaris,* and *Oxyuris.* Treatment should be repeated in six to eight weeks, depending on the weather and pasture conditions. Foals should be treated for *Parascaris* and *Strongyloides* at about 8 to 12 weeks of age; re-treatment may be necessary.

Cambendazole is well tolerated by horses. Doses up to 15 times the recommended level were administered to horses without any undesirable side effects. Pregnant mares should not be treated during the first trimester of pregnancy, however, because there may be risk of fetal damage. Cambendazole has shown embryotoxic and teratogenic activity in pregnant rats. Cambendazole is not effective against *Gasterophilus* but is compatible with trichlorfon and with carbon disulfide.

CARBON DISULFIDE

Carbon disulfide is a highly volatile, foul-smelling, colorless or straw-colored liquid that is slightly soluble in water but very soluble in organic solvents. It is very flammable and explosive.

Carbon disulfide is administered to horses by stomach tube at 5.3 ml. per 100 kg. of body weight up to a maximum dose of 30 ml. per horse following an 18 hour fast, for removal of *Gasterophilus* spp., *Habronema* spp., and *Parascaris equorum.* Carbon disulfide is also effective against swine stomach worms at 18 to 22 ml. per 100 kg. The efficacy of carbon disulfide is enhanced when it is administered on an empty stomach.

WARNING. Carbon disulfide is a strong irritant to the mucous membrane and inhalation may cause respiratory distress, depression, coma, and death. It should not be given to debilitated horses or to pregnant mares in the last two months of gestation.

COUMAPHOS

Coumaphos is a white, crystalline powder practically insoluble in water but very soluble in chloroform and aromatic hydrocarbons. Coumaphos is sold under many trade names (ASUNTOL, BAYMIX, CO-RAL, MELDANE) and in a variety of pharmaceutical forms (wettable powder, pour-on, emulsifiable concentrate, dust, feed premix, crumbles) and is registered for the control of a variety of common ectoparasites and endoparasitic nematodes of livestock. The acute oral LD_{50} for rats is 90 to 110 mg. per kg., but for mice it is only 55 mg. per kg. In cattle, the therapeutic dose is well tolerated, but single oral doses of 12.5 to 50 mg. per kg. have produced symptoms of typical organophosphorus poisoning.

BAYMIX (medicated crumbles containing 11.2 per cent coumaphos) is used as a top dressing on the feed ration of lactating and dry cows, heifers, bulls, and calves over three months old. Milk from treated cows need not be discarded. BAYMIX is fed in this manner for six consecutive days at the rate of 2 mg. per kg. for the treatment of adult gastrointestinal nematodes of the genera *Haemonchus, Ostertagia, Trichostrongylus,* and *Cooperia.* Although the Code Of Federal Regulations (April 1, 1978) indicates that this therapeutic regimen is efficacious against *Nematodirus,* a search of the literature failed to support this claim. If desired, the treatment can be repeated at 30 day intervals. Coumaphos, like other organophosphates, kills worms by inhibiting acetylcholinesterase.

WARNING. Coumaphos crumbles should not be fed to cattle less than three months old, sick animals, or animals under stress (e.g., animals in transit, those recently dehorned or castrated, or those weaned within the previous three weeks). Coumaphos is a cholinesterase inhibitor; it should not be used within a few days of exposure to other cholinesterase-inhibiting drugs or to phenothiazine tranquilizers. Coumaphos should not be used with the anthelmintic phenothiazine because it potentiates its toxicity.

DIAMPHENETHIDE

Diamphenethide, in a thixotropic formulation (CORIBAN), is used overseas for the control of acute and chronic fascioliasis. The acute oral LD_{50} for rats is more that 3000 mg. per kg. A single dose of 400 mg. per kg. produced no adverse effects in sheep. In sheep, a dose of 80 to 120 mg. per kg. is administered orally for the control of immature *Fasciola hepatica* and *F. gigantica*. For the control of adult flukes, a dose of 120 mg. per kg. should be used. Diamphenethide kills the immature flukes from the moment they reach the hepatic parenchyma. Strategic administration of this antitrematodal drug should prevent the appearance of fascioliasis in sheep. Diamphenethide is not approved by the FDA for use in the United States.

WARNING. Sheep should not be treated within seven days of slaughter. Overdosage may cause impairment of vision and loss of wool.

DICHLOROPHENE

Dichlorophene (DI-PHENTHANE 70) is a chlorinated analogue of phenylmethane. It is a white powder with a phenolic odor, practically insoluble in water, sparingly soluble in toluene, but very soluble in alcohols. It has low toxicity for mammals. The oral LD_{50} for rats is 2690 mg. per kg., and the acute oral LD_{50} in dogs is 1000 mg. per kg. Dichlorophene has bacteriostatic, fungicidal, and cestocidal properties.

Dichlorophene may be used either alone or in combination with other anthelmintic drugs for the removal of *Taenia* and *Dipylidium* tapeworms from dogs and cats. The drug may be administered orally in tablet or capsule form at 220 mg. per kg. after an overnight fast. The tapeworms are killed, digested, and eliminated in an unrecognizable form. Sheep and horse tapeworms are also susceptible to dichlorophene. Dichlorophene's activity against *Echinococcus* is erratic.

WARNING. An occasional animal may vomit or develop diarrhea.

DICHLOROPHENE AND TOLUENE

A number of small animal proprietary anthelmintic drugs (ANAPLEX, DIFOLIN, PARASITE, VERMIPLEX, WURM-KAPS) contain dichlorophene as the anticestodal ingredient and toluene (methylbenzene) as the antinematodal ingredient. Both drugs have very low mammalian toxicity.

The dichlorophene and toluene mixture is administered orally in soft capsules to dogs and cats, preferably after overnight fasting, at 220 mg. dichlorophene and 264 mg. toluene per kg. of body weight for the removal of *Toxocara canis, Toxascaris leonina, Ancylostoma caninum, Uncinaria stenocephala, Taenia pisiformis,* and *Dipylidium caninum*. The dichlorophene-toluene mixture is relatively ineffective against *Echinococcus granulosus*.

WARNING. An occasional animal may vomit or develop diarrhea. Weakness and incoordination are signs of overdosage. The owner should be informed that the tapeworms are voided in an unrecognizable form, usually within two hours after medication.

DICHLORVOS

Dichlorvos is a colorless to amber liquid, slightly soluble in water and readily soluble in most organic solvents. Hydrolyzed in water, its half-life at pH 7 is about eight hours. Dichlorvos is also rapidly degraded in mammals. The acute oral LD_{50} for rats is 80 mg. per kg. In dogs, the oral LD_{50} of unformulated dichlorvos is 28 to 45 mg. per kg., whereas the formulated (resinated) dichlorvos is of low toxicity with oral LD_{50} 387 to 1262 mg. per kg. No untoward reactions were observed in pregnant mice, rats, rabbits, sows, mares, bitches, and queens medicated with dichlorvos. Specially formulated dichlorvos is used as an anthelmintic for dogs and cats (TASK, TASK TABS), for horses (EQUIGARD, EQUIGEL, TRIDEX), and for swine (ATGARD, WORM-A-CIDE). Dichlorvos kills nematodes by inhibiting their cholinesterases.

Dogs and Cats. TASK is a slow-release formulation of dichlorvos in a non-digestible resin. TASK is administered to dogs weighing more than 1 kg. at 27 to 33 mg. per kg. This should be divided and administered in two doses 8 to 24 hours apart for old and debilitated animals. TASK TABS are administered to cats and to puppies older than ten days or weighing more than 0.5 kg. at 11 mg. per kg. TASK and TASK TABS are indicated for the removal of adult *Toxocara canis, T. cati, Toxascaris leonina, Ancylostoma caninum, A. tubaeforme, Uncinaria stenocephala,* and *Trichuris vulpis*. Dichlorvos has no activity against the migrating larvae of these worms. For more effective control of *T. vulpis,* the dog should be re-treated in 10 to 14 days. In fact, it may be necessary to treat at intervals over a period of three months, the prepatent period of *T. vulpis.*

Horses. EQUIGARD is pelleted vinyl resin impregnated with dichlorvos. Thus formulated, dichlorvos is much less toxic to horses than is the technical chemical. For horses, the resinated chemical has an oral LD_{50} of 800 to 1600 mg. per kg., whereas the technical chemical has an LD_{50} of 50 to 316 mg. per kg. When administered to horses in feed at 31 to 41 mg. per kg., EQUIGARD and TRIDEX remove *Gasterophilus intestinalis, G. nasalis, Strongylus vulgaris, S. equinus,* several genera of Cyathostominae, *Parascaris equorum, Oxyuris equi,* and *Probstmayria.* EQUIGARD and TRIDEX are only moderately effective against *Strongylus edentatus.* In debilitated horses, the dose is administered in divided doses 12 hours apart.

EQUIGEL is a thixotropic gel containing 31 per cent dichlorvos. It is administered by syringe to the dorsal surface of the tongue at 10 mg. per kg. for the removal of *Gasterophilus* bots only. The gel adheres to the tongue palate, and other oral surfaces, releasing dichlorvos which diffuses into the tissues of the mouth to destroy first and second stage *Gasterophilus* larvae, and is carried to the stomach, where it destroys the second and third stages. The manufacturer advises fasting adult horses overnight and for four to six hours after medication. Treatment may be repeated at 21 to 29 day intervals during the botfly season. EQUIGEL is also effective against *Parascaris equorum* dwelling in the intestinal lumen. TRIDEX PASTE also contains dichlorvos and has the same indication as EQUIGEL.

Swine. ATGARD consists of polyvinyl chloride resin pellets containing 9.6 per cent dichlorvos. It is used in meal type feed (not unground grain or pelleted meal) at 11.2 to 21.6 mg. per kg. for the removal of adults and fourth stage larvae of *Ascaris suum, Trichuris suis,* and *Oesophagostomum* spp., and adult *Ascarops strongylina* and *Hyostrongylus rubidus* from boars, weaners, fatteners, gilts, and sows. For best results, sows and gilts should be medicated shortly before farrowing and again at weaning. It is best to administer the medicated feed to small lots of compatibly sized pigs (e.g., single litters) at one time and watch them while feeding to ensure that all eat their share. Preliminary fasting is unnecessary, but alternative sources of feed should be excluded during the medication period. Dichlorvos treatment at 1 gram per sow per day for the last 30 days of gestation improved litter production efficiency by increasing the proportion of pigs born alive, birth weights, survival to market weight, and rate of gain even in parasite-free swine. This was a pharmacological effect completely unrelated to parasites. When administered immediately before parturition at 8.8 times the recommended dose, ATGARD produced no adverse reactions in sows.

WARNING. Dichlorvos should not be used with other cholinesterase-inhibiting chemicals, taeniacides, antifilarials, muscle relaxants, phenothiazine tranquilizers, or central nervous system depressants. Dichlorvos is contraindicated for dogs and cats showing signs of severe constipation, mechanical blockage of the intestinal tract, liver disease, or circulatory failure. Dogs with *Dirofilaria immitis* infection should not be treated with dichlorvos. Greyhound and whippet dogs are abnormally sensitive to dichlorvos. A small number of normal dogs may vomit after treatment but no other adverse reactions have been reported. Cats are more susceptible to dichlorvos. They may vomit, hypersalivate, appear apprehensive, and pass loose stools after medication.

Dichlorvos is not recommended for suckling and young weanling foals or for horses that are severely debilitated or suffering from colic, diarrhea, constipation, infectious disease, toxemia, alveolar emphysema, or other respiratory disease.

Atropine and PROTOPAM are the recommended antidotes for organophosphate poisoning.

DIETHYLCARBAMAZINE

Diethylcarbamazine citrate is an odorless, white, crystalline powder freely soluble in water and sparingly soluble in benzene, acetone, and chloroform. The oral LD_{50} for rats is 1380 mg. per kg.

Diethylcarbamazine citrate is marketed under many proprietary names (CARICIDE, CARBAM, CARBATAG, DEC TABS, DECACIDE, DECANINE, DIFIL, DIROCIDE, DIRO-FORM, FILARIBITS, NEMACIDE) and in many pharmaceutical forms (tablets, syrup, chewable tablets, powder). Diethylcarbamazine is used prophylactically in dogs to prevent infection with *Dirofilaria immitis* and for the treatment of *Toxocara canis, T. cati,* and *Toxascaris leonina* infections in dogs and cats. Diethylcarbamazine is also used for the control of *Dictyocaulus* in cattle and sheep.

For the prevention of heartworm infections, diethylcarbamazine is administered orally once a day at 6.6 mg. per kg. during the mosquito season. This regimen may be continued year-round for prevention of ascarid infection. Puppies may be started on the prevention program for heartworm at about two months of age. It is advisable to continue administration of diethylcarbamazine for the beginning until two months after the end of mosquito season. In warm climates, diethylcarbamazine should be given to dogs year round if no other means of *Dirofilaria immitis* control is available.

For removal of ascarids, diethylcarbamazine is given orally to dogs at 55 to 110 mg. per kg. as early as four weeks of age. Treatment should be repeated in 10 to 20 days.

WARNING. Dogs older than six months should be tested for microfilaremia. All those with circulating microfilariae should be freed of adult heartworms and microfilariae before starting the diethylcarbamazine prophylactic regimen. Dogs with heartworm microfilaremia may develop severe anaphylactoid reactions if treated with diethylcarbamazine. The full therapeutic dose may cause irritation of the gastric mucosa; a light meal just before medication reduces gastric irritation and emesis.

DISOPHENOL

Disophenol is a light, feathery, crystalline solid that is freely soluble in alcohol and sparingly soluble in water. The oral LD_{50} for rats is 170 mg. per kg. and the subcutaneous LD_{50} is 122 mg. per kg.

Disophenol parenteral (DNP), when administered subcutaneously to dogs and cats at 10 mg. per kg., removes adult *Ancylostoma caninum*, *A. braziliense*, *A. tubaeforme*, and *Uncinaria stenocephala* from the lumen of the small intestine. Although disophenol has a threefold margin of safety, a single dose of 36 mg. per kg. is lethal to dogs. Therefore, weigh each dog so that the dose can be calculated accurately. Because disophenol is effective only against adult hookworms, treatment should be repeated in three weeks to destroy those that have developed in the interim. Disophenol should not be used concurrently with other anthelmintics.

WARNING. An occasional dog may develop lenticular opacity. Dogs may show tachycardia, polypnea, and hyperthermia as a result of increased metabolic rate. These signs of toxicity may be controlled with antipyretics, ice baths, and intravenous administration of glucose.

DITHIAZANINE IODIDE

Dithiazanine iodide is a blue powder that is sparingly soluble in water but can be made soluble with polyvinylpyrrolidone. Dithiazanine should always be used with care. The acute oral LD_{50} for dogs is about 200 mg. per kg. but 9.2 mg. per kg. administered daily for 147 days produced liver lesions, bone marrow changes, diarrhea, malnutrition, and weight loss.

Dithiazanine iodide (DIZAN) powder or tablets is a broad spectrum nematocide and may be used for the removal of *Toxocara canis*, *Toxascaris leonina*, *Ancylostoma caninum*, *Uncinaria stenocephala*, *Strongyloides stercoralis*, *Trichuris vulpis*, and microfilariae of *Dirofilaria immitis*. The suggested oral dose for general use is 22 mg. per kg for 3 to 12 days. For heartworm microfilariae, 6.6 to 11 mg. per kg. is administered for 7 to 10 days. Dithiazanine iodide should be administered to dogs during or immediately after feeding.

WARNING. Dithiazanine iodide is contraindicated in animals that are sensitive to this particular drug and in animals with reduced renal function. The feces from treated dogs have a blue-green tint that tends to stain fabrics.

DROCARBIL

Drocarbil (NEMURAL) tablets are available in two sizes containing 18 and 54 mg. of arecoline acetarsol, respectively. Drocarbil is administered orally to dogs and cats at 4.95 mg. per kg. for the removal of *Taenia* and *Dipylidium* tapeworms. Drocarbil is best given to dogs with a piece of meat in the morning after a light meal. For adult cats, drocarbil is administered three hours after the principal meal. It is suggested that an antiemetic (e.g., promethazine 0.5 mg. per kg.) be administered 30 minutes before drocarbil. If the treated animal does not defecate within two hours, a saline or soap enema is recommended.

WARNING. Drocarbil is contraindicated in the presence of fever, catarrhal conditions of the intestines, or severe cardiac or circulatory disturbances. Puppies less than three months old and cats less than one year old should not be treated with drocarbil. In case of overdosage, adverse reactions such as salivation, restlessness, ataxia, and labored breathing appear. Atropine is antidotal.

FEBANTEL

At 6 mg. per kg. RINTAL (febantel paste and suspension) removes *Strongylus vulgaris*, *S. edentatus*, *S. equinus*, adult and immature *Parascaris equorum*, adult and fourth stage *Oxyuris equi*, and many species of cyathostomes from horses, foals, and ponies. Resistance on the part of several species of cyathostomes to the recommended dosage level of febantel has been reported. The paste may be given orally or may be mixed with a small portion of the grain ration and fed. Febantel demonstrated slight activity against *Trichostrongylus axei* at a dosage rate of 20 mg. per kg. Administration of 50 mg. per kg. was required to eliminate *Strongyloides westeri* from foals. Febantel has a wide margin of safety in young and old horses, pregnant mares, and stallions. Febantel may be administered with trichlorfon for the removal of stomach bots.

FENBENDAZOLE

Fenbendazole is an almost colorless, odorless, tasteless, crystalline powder. It is insoluble in water, slightly soluble in the usual organic solvents, but freely soluble in dimethyl sulfoxide (DMSO). The oral LD_{50} for rats and mice is higher than 10 grams per kg. Fenbendazole does not have embryotoxic or teratogenetic effects in rats, sheep, and cattle. In the rabbit, fenbendazole was fetatoxic but not teratogenic, and no carcinogenesis was observed in lifetime studies in rats and mice. In a six-month toxicity study in dogs, no effect was observed at 4 mg. per kg. or below.

Fenbendazole is a broad spectrum anthelmintic with activity against gastrointestinal nematodes and cestodes and lung nematodes of cattle, sheep, goats, and horses, and activity against a variety of helminth parasites of dogs, cats, and many zoo animals has been reported. In the United States, fenbendazole is approved for control of helminth parasites of horses, cattle, and swine.

Cattle. Fenbendazole (SAFE-GUARD) is administered orally at 5 mg. per kg. for the removal and control of adult *Dictyocaulus viviparus*, *Haemonchus contortus*, *Ostertagia ostertagi*, *Trichostrongylus axei*, *T. colubriformis*, *Bunostomum phlebotomum*, *Nematodirus helvetianus*, *Cooperia oncophora*, *C. punctata*, and *Oesophagostomum radiatum*. Overseas, the recommended dose is 7.5 mg. per kg. with additional claims of efficacy against *Trichuris*, *Strongyloides*, *Capillaria*, *Moniezia*, and eggs and immature stages of nematodes. The maximum tolerated dose is about 2000 mg. per kg. In cattle, fenbendazole is not embryotoxic or teratogenic and does not impair the fertility of bulls.

WARNING. Cattle must not be slaughtered within eight days of medication with fenbendazole, and dairy cattle of breeding age should not be treated because a suitable withdrawal time has not yet been established. In Great Britain, milk from treated cows may be consumed 72 hours after the last administration of fenbendazole.

Horses. Fenbendazole suspension (PANACUR) is administered orally to horses at 5 mg. per kg. for the control of *Strongylus vulgaris*, *S. edentatus*, *S. equinus*, *Oxyuris equi*, and many species of cyathostomes. Several species of cyathostomes have developed resistance to fenbendazole, however. For the removal of *Parascaris equorum*, 10 mg. per kg. is recommended. Pregnant mares, stallions, and foals may be treated safely with fenbendazole at the recommended dosages. Fenbendazole with trichlorfon is recommended for the removal of stomach bots in addition to susceptible nematodes.

Overseas, 50 mg. fenbendazole per kg. is recommended for treatment of *Strongyloides westeri* infections in suckling foals and 30 mg. per kg. for removal of immature cyathostomes, and 60 mg. per kg. was reported to be about 83 per cent effective against the migrating larvae of *S. vulgaris*.

Swine. Three mg. per kg. per day for three days removes *Ascaris suum*, *Hyostrongylus rubidus*, *Oesophagostomum* spp., *Metastrongylus apri*, *Trichuris suis*, and mature and immature *Stephanurus dentatus*. Higher doses are required for the removal of *Strongyloides ransomi*. There is no withdrawal time restriction.

Sheep and Goats. Overseas, oral administration of 5 mg. fenbendazole per kg. is recommended for removal of adult and immature stages of gastrointestinal nematodes and cestodes and lung nematodes. Some *Haemonchus* populations have apparently developed resistance to fenbendazole.

GLYCOBIARSOL

Glycobiarsol is a yellowish to pink, odorless, almost tasteless powder that is slightly soluble in water. It was used in man for the treatment of amebiasis and trichomoniasis. For the removal of *Trichuris vulpis*, glycobiarsol tablets (MILIBIS V) are administered to dogs daily for five days at 220 mg. per kg. up to a maximum of 5 grams per dog. In unyielding cases, a second course of therapy two to four weeks after the first is suggested. It may be necessary to repeat treatment at intervals over a period of three months, the prepatent period of *Trichuris vulpis*. Glycobiarsol is well tolerated but a few dogs may vomit. This can be avoided by crushing the tablet and mixing it with the feed.

HALOXON

Haloxon is a white, crystalline powder that is sparingly soluble in water but soluble in benzene and chloroform. It has low toxicity for mammals but is very toxic to geese. The oral LD_{50} for rats is 900 mg. per kg. This low toxicity is probably due to the high rate of spontaneous reactivation of haloxon-inhibited mammalian acetyl cholinesterase. Haloxon may cause severe delayed neurotoxicity, however. Haloxon is used in bolus form (HALOX bolus) and as a wettable powder (HALOX drench) for cattle. Haloxon is administered at 35 to 50 mg. per kg. for the removal of *Haemonchus, Ostertagia, Trichostrongylus,* and *Cooperia.* There is an ample margin of safety (three to seven times the recommended dosage level).

WARNING. Haloxon should not be administered to pregnant cows within one month of parturition. It is also contraindicated in dairy animals of breeding age. To avoid residues in edible tissues, do not treat animals within one week of slaughter. Haloxon is a mild cholinesterase inhibitor and should not be used with other anthelmintics and cholinesterase inhibitors. There are no untoward side effects when haloxon is used as directed but overdosage may cause neurotoxicity with posterior ataxia or paraplegia, particularly in older animals.

HYGROMYCIN B

Hygromycin B is an amorphous powder, freely soluble in water, ethanol, and methanol, but insoluble in nonpolar solvents. Hygromycin B (HYGROMIX) is an antibiotic with good anthelmintic activity against *Ascaris, Oesophagostomum,* and *Trichuris* when fed to pigs for at least three weeks at 12 grams per ton of feed.

WARNING. Swine fed hygromycin B continuously may develop auditory nerve impairment. Feed containing hygromycin B should be withdrawn from pigs 15 days before slaughter to allow elimination of drug residues from edible tissues. Farm dogs that eat feeds containing hygromycin B may develop hearing impairment and cataracts.

IVERMECTIN

Ivermectin is a synthetically modified derivative of the new family of antiparasitic agents known as avermectins. The avermectins are macrocyclic lactones that were isolated from the fermentation broth of *Streptomyces avermitilis.* The discovery of anthelmintic activity was made by administering the actinomycetic broth to mice infected with the nematode *Nematospiroides dubius.* Ivermectin is effective against many nematodes and arthropods. Curiously, ivermectin is very effective against immature *Dirofilaria immitis* but not at all against adult heartworms. The suggested dosage levels are 0.2 mg. per kg. for cattle, sheep, and horses and 0.3 mg. per kg. for swine. Administration of ivermectin to pregnant rats, mice, and rabbits produced teratism in fetuses only at or near maternotoxic doses. There was no teratogenesis in cattle, sheep, and dogs when ivermectin was administered to pregnant animals at four times the recommended dose. No toxicity was observed in a battery of tests. Although toxicity for aquatic animals is high, it is claimed that binding of ivermectin in soil reduces its concentration to levels that have no impact on the quality of the environment. The acute oral LD_{50} in mice varied from 11.6 to 87.2 mg. per kg. and the LD_{50} for rats was 42.8 to 52.8 mg. per kg. In a 14 week study, with rats, the "no-effect" level was 0.4 mg. per kg.

Ivermectin acts on nematodes by inhibiting transmission of signals between interneurons and excitatory motor neurons by potentiating the inhibitory neurotransmitter GABA. In arthropods, ivermectin inhibits transmission of signals at the neuromuscular junctions by the same mechanism. In both cases, death results from paralysis.

Horses. Ivermectin provides a broad spectrum of activity against nematode and arthropod parasites of horses and is administered orally (EQVALAN paste) at 0.2 mg. per kg. for control of adult *Strongylus vulgaris, S. edentatus, S. equinus, Triodontophorus* spp., *Cyathostomum* spp., *Cylicocyclus* spp., *Cylicostephanus* spp., *Cylicodontophorus* spp., *Gyalocephalus capitatus, Trichostrongylus axei, Oxyuris equi,* and *Parascaris equorum;* fourth stage larvae of *Strongylus vulgaris, S. edentatus,* and *Oxyuris equi;* microfilariae of *Onchocerca cervicalis,* and all larval stages of *Gasterophilus* spp. Ivermectin is active against benzimidazole-resistant populations of cyathostomes.

Administration of 10 to 15 times the recommended dose of ivermectin produced temporary visual impairment, but three times the recommended dose did not interfere with reproduction in either mares or stallions. Some horses develop transitory swelling at the site of injection or edema of the ventral midline; these are interpreted as anaphylactoid reactions to *Onchocerca* microfilariae killed by ivermectin. A number of horses injected with ivermectin developed fatal clostridial myositis; the oral paste formulation is to be preferred.

Cattle. Ivermectin (IVOMEC) is licensed for treatment of infections with gastrointestinal nematodes, lungworms, cattle grubs, mange, and sucking lice in beef cattle and nonlactating dairy cattle. Ivermectin is administered subcutaneously at 0.2 mg. per kg. Efficacies exceeding 95 per cent were obtained against adult and immature *Haemonchus contortus, Ostertagia lyrata, O. ostertagi* (including inhibited fourth stage larvae), *Cooperia oncophora, C. punctata, C. pectinata, Oesophagostomum radiatum, Dictyocaulus viviparus, Trichostrongylus axei, T. colubriformis, Nematodirus spathiger, N. helvetianus,* and *N. helvetianus* (adults only), and all larval stages of *Hypoderma bovis* and *H. lineatum. Linognathus vituli, Haematopinus eurysternus,* and *Sarcoptes scabiei* infestations were eliminated in seven days, and *Psoroptes ovis* infestation eliminated in 14 days. Control of *Boophilus microplus* was achieved by daily administration of 0.015 mg. per kg. to cattle. Ivermectin at 0.2 mg. per kg. was found to be highly effective against *Dermatobia hominis* infections.

WARNING. In France, a few cattle infected with *Hypoderma* died with acute esophagitis and others developed posterior paresis as a consequence of spinal cord hemorrhages. Cattle should not be slaughtered for at least 35 days after treatment with ivermectin.

Sheep. Ivermectin is not currently licensed in the United States for use in sheep. Ivermectin has about the same spectrum of activity in sheep as in cattle and is also effective against *Oestrus ovis* larvae. Efficacy of IVOMEC drench against external parasites was erratic, however.

Swine. Ivermectin is not currently licensed in the United States for use in swine. Ivermectin administered subcutaneously at 0.3 mg. per kg. was highly effective against adult and immature *Ascaris suum, Hyostrongylus rubidus, Oesophagostomum* spp., *Metastrongylus* spp., and adult *Strongyloides ransomi; Sarcoptes scabiei* and *Haematopinus suis* infestations were cleared within 14 days of treatment. Activity against *Trichuris suis* was only moderate. Adult and larval *Stephanurus dentatus* were very susceptible to a single subcutaneous dose of 0.5 mg. per kg. No signs of toxicity occurred in pigs given 50 times the recommended dose, but at 30 mg. per kg. lethargy, ataxia, mydriasis, intermittent tremors, labored breathing, and recumbency were observed.

Dogs. Ivermectin is not currently licensed in the United States for use in dogs. The equine injectable preparation is toxic to dogs and should not be used in this species. Subcutaneous injection of ivermectin at 0.05 mg. per kg. was effective against *Ancylostoma caninum* and *A. brazieliense.* For complete removal of *Trichuris vulpis,* 0.1 mg. per kg. was required. Ascarids proved more refractory; 0.2 mg. per kg. removed only 90 per cent of *Toxocara canis* and efficiency against *Toxascaris leonina* was disappointing. A single subcutaneous injection of 0.05 to 0.2 mg. per kg. completely cleared all microfilariae from the blood but ivermectin is not active against mature *Dirofilaria immitis* worms. A single oral dose of 0.05 mg. per kg. prevented maturation of *D. immitis* larvae if administered within two months of exposure but when delayed beyond that point, administration of even 0.2 mg. per kg. failed to prevent establishment of *D. immitis* infection. *Sarcoptes scabiei* and *Otodectes cynotis* were eliminated 7 and 14 days, respectively, after a single injection of 0.2 mg. per kg.

A single oral dose of 2 mg. per kg. and 0.5 mg. per kg. per day for 14 weeks were well tolerated by dogs. Mydriasis, depression, tremors, ataxia, coma, and death have been observed following doses in excess of 20 mg. per kg. No teratism was observed in fetuses when pregnant bitches received repeated oral doses of ivermectin of 0.5 mg. per kg.

LEVAMISOLE

Levamisole, the levoisomer of tetramisole, is a crystalline powder soluble in water (21 per cent). Levamisole hydrochloride (RIPERCOL L, LEVASOLE, TRAMISOLE) is administered orally as a bolus, wettable powder, or feed premix to cattle, sheep, and swine for the control of gastrointestinal and lung nematodes. The preferred preparation for horses is an aqueous solution of levamisole hydrochloride and piperazine dihydrochloride (RIPERCOL L-PIPERAZINE) for administration by stomach tube. An aqueous solution of levamisole phosphate (13.6 per cent or 18.2 per cent) is recommended for subcutaneous injection in cattle; this preparation is particularly handy for fractious range cattle and the like. The recommended dose in all animals is 8 mg. per kg. In cattle, the injectable form may be administered at 6 mg. per kg. with about the same effect.

The acute oral LD_{50} for rats is 480 mg. per kg. and for mice, 210 mg. per kg. Some sheep dosed orally with tetramisole at 80 mg. per kg. died. Subcutaneous injection is more toxic than oral administration. Signs of cholinergic toxicity such as lip licking, salivation, lacrimation, head shaking, ataxia, and muscle tremors may occur at lower dosage levels. At the recommended dosage level, an occasional animal may show transitory muzzle foam and licking of the lips. At twice the therapeutic dosage level, calves may show increased alertness, salivation, head shaking, and muscle tremors.

The anthelmintic mode of action of levamisole was formerly thought to involve the inhibition of fumarate reductase, an important enzyme in the metabolism of carbohydrates. However, more recent experiments suggest that levamisole paralyzes the worms by inducing continuous muscle contractions.

Cattle. Levamisole hydrochloride administered orally as a drench, bolus, or gel is highly effective against *Haemonchus, Ostertagia, Trichostrongylus, Cooperia, Nematodirus, Bunostomum,* and *Oesophagostomum* in the alimentary tract and *Dictyocaulus* in the lungs. Levamisole phosphate 13.15 per cent injectable solution is injected subcutaneously in the mid-neck region at 2 ml. per 45 kg. for the control of these same nematodes. Arrested early fourth stage larvae of *Ostertagia* are refractory to levamisole.

WARNING. A slight nonpersistent reaction may occur at the site of injection of levamisole phosphate. Cattle should not be slaughtered within seven days of injection, within 6 days of oral medication with levamisole hydrochloride gel, or within two days of oral medication with other preparations. Levamisole is not used in dairy animals of breeding age in order to avoid drug residues in milk.

Sheep. Orally administered levamisole removes *Haemonchus, Ostertagia, Trichostrongylus, Cooperia, Nematodirus, Bunostomum, Oesophagostomum,* and *Chabertia* from the alimentary tract and *Dictyocaulus* from the lungs. Levamisole is also efficacious against the immature stages of *Haemonchus, Nematodirus, Bunostomum, Oesophagostomum, Chabertia,* and *Dictyocaulus.*

WARNING. Levamisole has an ample therapeutic margin but an occasional sheep will show side effects (e.g., lip licking, salivation, increased alertness, muscle tremors) even at the recommended dose. Debilitated sheep appear to be more susceptible to toxicity. Sheep should not be slaughtered within 72 hours of treatment.

Swine. Levamisole administered to swine in water or feed removes *Ascaris, Oesophagostomum, Strongyloides, Metastrongylus,* and *Hyostrongylus.* Levamisole is also effective against the immature forms (including migrating larvae) of *Ascaris* and *Metastrongylus.* The label for levamisole resinate indicates effcacy against *Stephanurus dentatus.*

WARNING. Levamisole should be administered to pigs of weanling to market age after an overnight fast. Pigs should not be treated within three days of slaughter. Salivation or muzzle foam is occasionally observed after treatment. Pigs infected with adult lungworms may vomit or cough. These reactions may be caused by the expulsion of paralyzed lungworms from the bronchi.

Horses. An aqueous solution of levamisole hydrochloride and piperazine dihydrochloride is administered by drench or stomach tube for control of *Strongylus vulgaris, S. edentatus, Parascaris equorum, Oxyuris equi,* and species of the subfamily Cyathostominae. This preparation can be administered to horses of any age and is compatible with trichlorfon and carbon disulfide.

WARNING. Horses dosed with approximately three times the recommended therapeutic level may develop hyperexcitation, tremors, and incoordination. Levamisole has a narrow margin of safety for horses and rather low efficacy against their parasites.

MEBENDAZOLE

Mebendazole is an off-white, amorphous powder practically insoluble in water but soluble in formic acid. Mebendazole powder or paste is used for the control of intestinal helminth parasites in horses and dogs. Overseas, mebendazole is also used as an anthelmintic in sheep, swine, and cats. Mebendazole has a wide margin of safety for domestic animals but was found to be teratogenic and embryotoxic in rats and mice.

The mode of action of mebendazole is rather complex. There is an inhibition of glucose uptake, depletion of endogenous glycogen, and alteration of cytoplasmic microtubles in nematodes exposed to this drug.

Horses. Mebendazole powder, paste, or suspension (TELMIN) is administered orally at 8.8 mg. per kg. for the removal of *Strongylus vulgaris, S. edentatus, S. equinus, Parascaris equorum,* species of the subfamily Cyathostominae, and mature and immature *Oxyuris equi.* Mebendazole is compatible with trichlorfon and carbon disulfide. TELMIN B, a combination product containing mebendazole and trichlorfon, is available for the control of stomach bots and susceptible nematodes. It has been reported that a single dose of 15 mg. per kg. of micronized mebendazole is highly effective against *Anoplocephala perfoliata* but experience has varied; 35.2 mg. per kg. was without effect in one experiment. Mebendazole is very safe in horses; doses as high as 400 mg. per kg. were well tolerated.

Dogs. Mebendazole powder (TELMINTIC) is administered in the food once a day for three to five consecutive days at 22 mg. per kg. for the removal of *Toxocara canis, Ancylostoma caninum, Uncinaria stenocephala, Trichuris vulpis,* and tapeworms of the genera *Taenia* and *Echinococcus.* Mebendazole is not effective against *Dipylidium caninum.* A single oral dose of up to 650 mg. per kg. was well tolerated. The most prevalent adverse reactions noted in the clinical trials were vomiting and mild diarrhea. A number of case reports indicate that dogs may develop sometimes fatal hepatic dysfunction, especially following re-treatment with mebendazole. However, Van Cauteren and coworkers (1983) administered mebendazole to dogs at 110 mg. per kg. for 17 days without producing hepatic impairment. Mebendazole is also well tolerated by cats.

MORANTEL TARTRATE

Morantel is the 3-methyl analog of pyrantel. Morantel tartrate (RUMANTEL, NEMANTEL) was recently approved by FDA for the control of gastrointestinal nematodes in cattle. Morantel tartrate is a white, odorless, crystalline solid that is soluble in water. The acute oral LD_{50} is 437 mg. per kg. in

male mice and 926 mg. per kg. in male rats. Morantel tartrate boluses are administered to cattle at 9.7 mg. per kg. for the removal of adult *Haemonchus, Ostertagia, Trichostrongylus, Cooperia, Nematodirus,* and *Oesophagostomum.* Activity against larval stages of these nematodes appears to be variable. Overseas, morantel tartrate in a sustained release bolus (PARATECT BOLUS) provides control of gastrointestinal nematodes throughout the grazing season.

WARNING. Morantel is not approved for use in dairy animals of breeding age. Cattle should not be slaughtered within 14 days after treatment.

N-BUTYL CHLORIDE

Normal butyl chloride is a colorless, highly flammable liquid. It is a relatively safe compound; the oral LD_{50} for rats is 2670 mg. per kg. Normal butyl chloride is administered orally to dogs and cats after an 18 to 24 hour fast at approximately 0.22 to 0.44 ml. per kg. of body weight up to a maximum of 5 ml for animals over 18 kg. for the removal of *Toxocara canis, T. cati,* and *Toxascaris leonina,* and as an aid in the control of *Ancylostoma caninum, A. tubaeforme,* and *Uncinaria stenocephala.* Higher dosage levels, e.g., 2.2 ml. per kg., showed good activity against *Trichuris vulpis.* The administration of *n*-butyl chloride should be followed in about one hour with a cathartic in order to maximize its anthelmintic effect. Dogs and cats can be fed their regular feed within four to eight hours after treatment. Treatment may be repeated in 7 to 14 days. An occasional animal may vomit but no other untoward side effects have been reported.

NICLOSAMIDE

Niclosamide (YOMESAN) is a yellow, crystalline, tasteless powder that is insoluble in water and sparingly soluble in ethanol and chloroform. Niclosamide is available in tablets of various sizes and is administered orally to dogs and cats at 157 mg. per kg. for the removal of *Dipylidium caninum, Taenia pisiformis, T. hydatigena,* and *Hydatigera taeniaeformis.* Its activity against *Dipylidium* is not always satisfactory. An overnight fast is recommended. Niclosamide is safe to use in young puppies and kittens and in pregnant females. Expulsion of dead tapeworms usually occurs within 6 to 48 hours after administration of niclosamide.

WARNING. Niclosamide is contraindicated in animals with intestinal atony or acute diarrhea.

NITROSCANATE

Nitroscanate (LOPATOL) is a crystalline solid that is insoluble in water but soluble in organic solvents. The acute oral LD_{50} of the normal particle size preparation for rats is higher than 10 grams per kg.; of the micronized preparation (particles 2 to 3 μm, 95 per cent less than 5 μm) it is 3.5 grams per kg. of body weight. Nitroscanate is not approved by FDA for use in the United States.

Dogs and Cats. Nitroscanate is indicated for the control of the cestodes *Taenia hydatigena, T. pisiformis, T. ovis, Echinococcus granulosus,* and *Dipylidium caninum,* and nematodes *Toxocara canis, T. cati, Toxascaris leonina, Ancylostoma caninum, A. tubaeforme,* and *Uncinaria stenocephala.* Nitroscanate is administered orally to dogs and cats at 50 mg. per kg. for most purposes. To remove immature ascarids from 3 to 14 day old pups, administer a second 50 mg. per kg. dose 24 hours later. To remove *Echinococcus granulosus,* administer two 200 mg. per kg. doses 24 hours apart. Nitroscanate has poor activity against *Trichuris vulpis.*

WARNING. The most outstanding adverse effect at therapeutic dosage levels is delayed vomiting in 10 per cent or more of dogs 4 to 16 hours after administration of nitroscanate. It is claimed that vomiting does not adversely affect the efficacy of the drug. Dogs dosed with 1 gram per kg. vomited and developed diarrhea, anorexia, tranquilization, and slight transitory elevation of SGOT, SGPT, and SAP. Vomiting was observed more frequently in greyhounds. In cats, 400 mg. per kg. produced anorexia, occasional vomiting, and reversible paralysis.

NITROXYNIL

Nitroxynil is a yellow, crystalline solid, sparingly soluble in water but moderately soluble in most organic solvents. The glucamine salt of nitroxynil (TRODAX) is readily soluble in water. The aqueous solution is stable but will precipitate in the presence of calcium. It is administered subcutaneously at 10 mg. per kg. for the control of adult *Fasciola hepatica, F. gigantica,* and *Haemonchus contortus* in cattle and sheep. The maximum tolerated dose for cattle is 50 mg. per kg. and for sheep, 40 mg. per kg.

WARNING. Lactating cows should not be treated. Cattle and sheep should not be treated within 30 days of slaughter. In case of overdosage, administer glucose and saline solution intravenously. Nitroxynil increases the metabolic rate, which in turn results in hyperthermia. It is therefore beneficial to keep the animal in a cool place and to sprinkle it with cold water if necessary. A transient reaction may develop at the injection site. Nitroxynil is not approved by FDA for use in the United States.

OXFENDAZOLE

Oxfendazole is a white or off-white, crystalline powder that is insoluble in water. The oral LD_{50} is over 1600 mg. per kg. for beagle dogs and over 6400 mg. per kg. for rats and mice. Oxfendazole is active against a variety of helminth parasites but is approved only for horses in the United States. Oxfendazole powder (BENZELMIN, SYNANTHIC) is administered at 10 mg. per kg. either by stomach tube or by sprinkling the powder on the grain ration. Oxfendazole is effective against *Strongylus vulgaris, S. edentatus. S. equinus, Parascaris equorum, Oxyuris equi,* and many species of the subfamily Cyathostominae. Populations of several species of cyathostomes are reported to have developed resistance to oxfendazole.

OXIBENDAZOLE

Oxibendazole is a stable, white, odorless powder that is insoluble in water and only slightly soluble in most organic solvents. The acute oral LD_{50} is greater than 10 grams per kg. in guinea pigs, hamsters, and rabbits and greater than 32 grams per kg. in mice. A single dose of 600 mg. per kg. was well tolerated by cattle, sheep, and ponies and no adverse reactions were observed in rats and dogs treated with up to 30 mg. per kg. daily for three months. No evidence of teratogenicity or embryotoxicity was observed in rats, mice, sheep, cattle, and horses. In sheep, peak plasma concentration of oxibendazole was reached at 6 hours, and 34 per cent of the dose was eliminated in the urine by 24 hours.

Horses. Oxibendazole paste or suspension (ANTHELCIDE EQ) is administered to horses at 10 mg. per kg. for the removal and control of *Strongylus vulgaris, S. edentatus,* and *S. equinus,* species of *Triodontophorus, Cyathostomum, Cylicocyclus, Cylicostephanus,* and *Cy-*

licodontophorus, Gyalocephalus capitatus, Paras-caris equorum, and adults and larvae of *Oxyuris equi.* The dose must be increased to 15 mg. per kg. for treatment of *Strongyloides westeri* infection. Oxibendazole is not of itself effective against stomach bots but is compatible with carbon disulfide and organophosphates. Oxibendazole is highly efficient against populations of benzimidazole-resistant cyathostomes.

PHENOTHIAZINE

Phenothiazine is an odorless, tasteless, yellow, amorphous powder that is toxic to various bacteria, insects, and helminths. Phenothiazine is readily oxidized by sunlight and by the process of manufacture of finely divided, wettable preparations. Oxidized phenothiazine has a greenish-brown color. Phenothiazine is readily absorbed from the alimentary tract and excreted along with its oxidation products, thionol and leucothionol, in the urine, bile and milk. For about three days, the urine is colored red when voided or turns red on exposure to air. Consequently, if it is necessary to confine sheep after treatment, ample bedding should be provided to minimize wool staining. Spillage during administration should be avoided for the same reason. Phenothiazine is insoluble in water. Micronized phenothiazine (particle size 2 to 3 μm) is used as an anthelmintic for the control of gastrointestinal nematodes in cattle, sheep, poultry, and horses. The acute LD_{50} for rats is 5000 mg. per kg. The mode of action remains to be elucidated. After the introduction of phenothiazine, field reports indicated that *Haemonchus contortus* was becoming resistant, especially when phenothiazine was administered continuously at low dosage levels. However, it was then shown that the efficacy of phenothiazine is a function of its particle size and purity and that phenothiazine-exposed *Haemonchus* were just as susceptible to therapeutic doses of purified and micronized phenothiazine as were unexposed *Haemonchus.*

Cattle. When administered orally as a drench or bolus, phenothiazine shows consistently high efficacy against adult *Haemonchus* and *Oesophagostomum. Ostertagia, Trichostrongylus,* and *Bunostomum* are somewhat less susceptible. The recommended dose is 220 to 440 mg. per kg. up to a maximum of 60 to 80 grams in adult cattle and 40 grams in young cattle. One may supplement the therapeutic treatment with continuous prophylactic administration of 2 grams of phenothiazine per day in salt lick, feed block, or supplement feed. This will materially reduce the egg laying capacity of the female worms, render the eggs less hatchable, and kill the few larvae that do hatch in the manure. The continuous low level use of phenothiazine also kills face fly and horn fly larvae in bovine manure.

WARNING. Dairy cattle should be treated when dry, but if lactating, their milk should not be used for human consumption for a period of four days following treatment. Some cattle may develop photosensitivity and corneal opacities leading to permanent blindness. Unthrifty cattle are especially susceptible to phenothiazine. Phenothiazine should not be used concurrently with organophosphates. Other general drawbacks of phenothiazine are large dose volume, narrow spectrum of activity, and low margin of safety.

Sheep and Goats. Satisfactory control of nematodes is achieved by drenching sheep with phenothiazine suspension (25 grams for sheep over 30 kg.; 12.5 grams for lambs under 30 kg.) and following this with 0.5 to 1 gram per individual per day in the feed supplement or salt lick. Phenothiazine has retained a high degree of efficacy against *Haemonchus* and *Oesophagostomum* and satisfactory activity against *Ostertagia, Trichostrongylus, Bunostomum,* and *Chabertia.*

WARNING. Although sheep generally tolerate this drug much better than do other animals, they may develop photosensitivity following the administration of phenothiazine. Malnourished sheep and sheep exposed to hot and dry weather conditions are prone to show increased susceptibility to the toxic effects of phenothiazine.

Horses and Mules. Phenothiazine administered in a single dose of 55 mg. per kg. or continuously at the rate of 2 grams per day is recommended for the control of large and small strongyles. Phenothiazine is used most frequently in combination with piperazine and carbon disulfide (PARVEX PLUS) or piperazine and trichlorfon (DYREX T.F.).

WARNING. Phenothiazine is much more toxic to horses than to ruminants. Dullness, weakness, anorexia, colic, constipation, fever, and tachycardia are some of the side effects that phenothiazine occasionally produces. There may be anemia, icterus, or hemoglobinuria following medication.

Horses showing gastrointestinal disorders and diarrhea, and mares in the last month of gestation should not be treated with products that contain phenothiazine.

PHTHALOFYNE

Phthalofyne is a crystalline solid slightly soluble in water. The sodium salt of phthalofyne is very soluble in water, however. Phthalofyne (WHIPCIDE) is formulated as tablets and as intravenous solution for the removal of *Trichuris vulpis* from dogs. Administration of phthalofyne tablets is recommended either as a single oral dose of 200 mg. per kg. after a 24 hour fast or as two 200 mg. per kg. doses, one in the morning and one in the afternoon following a light meal. In general, the presence of intestinal contents reduces phthalofyne's trichuricidal activity. Phthalofyne 25 per cent solution is occasionally used intravenously at 250 mg. per kg. Intravenous injection of phthalofyne is carried out slowly and the dog should be watched closely for several hours afterward.

WARNING. Oral administration of phthalofyne frequently leads to vomiting. Intravenous administration may cause persistent vomiting, ataxia, severe depression, coma, and shock. Anaphylaxis, tetany, and collapse have been observed in some dogs and should be treated symptomatically. It was reported that the feces of treated dogs emit a piercing, skunklike odor. Phthalofyne should not be administered to dogs suffering from chronic nephritis, hepatitis, pancreatitis, or cardiac insufficiency.

PIPERAZINE

Various salts of piperazine (hexahydrate, monohydrochloride, dihydrochloride, citrate, phosphate, adipate, and dipiperazine sulfate) are used as anthelmintics in swine, poultry, horses, cattle, dogs, cats, and zoo animals. Piperazine is also one of the active ingredients in a number of combination anthelmintic products. Piperazine is marketed as tablets, solution, and powder under several proprietary names (CANDIZINE, F-W WORMER, HEXANTHELIM, PARLAMATE, PIPCIDE, PIPERSOL, PIPERTAB, PIP-POP 320, PIPZINE, PIP 10, and SYRAZINE). Piperazine is practically nontoxic. The oral LD_{50} for rats is 4920 mg. per kg. and for chickens 8000 mg. per kg. Piperazine can be administered to animals of all ages. Piperazine paralyzes worms by blocking the action of acetylcholine at the neuromuscular junctions and the worms are then eliminated by intestinal peristalsis.

Dogs and Cats. Piperazine administered orally at 110 to 200 mg. per kg. is effective against adult *Toxocara canis, T. cati, Toxascaris leonina,* and *Uncinaria stenocephala* but only slightly effective against *Ancylostoma caninum.*

Horses. Piperazine is effective against *Parascaris equorum* at 110 mg. per kg. Reasonable efficacy was also observed against *Strongylus vulgaris, Oxyuris equi,* and many species of small strongyles at 220 to 275 mg. per kg. Foals should first be treated when they are eight weeks old. The treatment may be repeated every four weeks, if necessary.

Swine. Piperazine in medicated feed or water is offered to pigs at 110 mg. per kg. for the removal of *Ascaris suum* and *Oesophagostomum* spp.

PICADEX

Picadex is a piperazine-carbon disulfide complex. It is marketed as a ready-to-use liquid (PARVEX) containing 250 mg. per ml. Picadex is recommended for the treatment of *Parascaris, Gasterophilus, Oxyuris equi,* and large and small strongyles in horses and ponies at a dosage rate of 165 mg. per kg. by stomach tube after an overnight fast. Feed and water should also be withheld for a few hours after treatment. Efficacy of picadex against *Gasterophilus* is enhanced when administration is followed by 500 ml. of vinegar or 0.5 per cent hydrochloric acid.

WARNING. Picadex should not be administered to horses, ponies, or foals suffering from colic, diarrhea, or infectious disease. In debilitated animals, it is suggested that one half of the recommended dose be administered and repeated in two to three weeks, but it is probably best to avoid administering picadex to debilitated or anemic horses. Injectable corticosteroids should be administered promptly if adverse reactions occur.

PICADEX WITH PHENOTHIAZINE

Piperazine-carbon disulfide complex with phenothiazine (PARVEX PLUS) is used to treat infections with *Parascaris, Gasterophilus, Oxyuris, Strongylus* spp., and species of Cyathostominae. PARVEX PLUS is administered by stomach tube and should be followed by 500 ml of 0.5 per cent hydrochloric acid to help hydrolyze the complex. Overnight fasting seems to enhance the efficacy of PARVEX preparations against *Gasterophilus* spp.

WARNING. This drug should not be administered to sick animals, especially those with gastrointestinal disorders.

PRAZIQUANTEL

Praziquantel is a colorless and practically odorless, crystalline powder with a bitter taste. It is only slightly soluble in water, sparingly soluble in alcohol, but soluble in chloroform and in dimethyl sulfoxide. Praziquantel displays marked anthelmintic activity against a wide range of adult and larval cestodes and trematodes of the genus *Schistosoma*. Praziquantel is a very safe anthelmintic. Rats tolerated daily administration of up to 1000 mg. per kg. for four weeks and dogs tolerated up to 180 mg. per kg. per day for 13 weeks. Vomition is typically observed at high dosage rates. Praziquantel did not induce embryotoxicity, teratogenesis, mutagenesis, or carcinogenesis, nor did it affect the reproductive performance of test animals. The mode of action of praziquantel is not fully understood but it appears to disturb the cation balance of parasites and this may in turn adversely affect the membrane potential of muscle cells. *In vitro,* high concentrations produced rapid paralysis, while low concentrations stimulated activity that might lead to displacement of worms *in vivo. In vitro* studies also demonstrated that praziquantel produced vacuolization of the worm tegument.

Dogs and Cats. Praziquantel (DRONCIT) is administered orally at 2.5 to 5 mg. per kg. for the removal of *Hydatigera taeniaeformis, Taenia pisiformis, T. hydatigena, Mesocestoides corti, Echinococcus granulosus,* and *E. multilocularis.* Higher dosage is required for *Spirometra.* Praziquantel is also highly active when injected subcutaneously or intramuscularly. Praziquantel is not intended for use in puppies or kittens less than four weeks old.

PYRANTEL

Pyrantel tartrate is a white, crystalline powder soluble in water. Pyrantel pamoate is a yellow, crystalline powder insoluble in water. Pyrantel tartrate is used as a powder and pellets in horses and swine. Pyrantel pamoate is marketed as a ready-to-use suspension and as tablets for dogs and horses. Pyrantel salts are stable in solid form but photodegrade when dissolved or suspended in water, resulting in reduction of potency. Pyrantel is a depolarizing neuromuscular blocking substance and probably kills the parasites by inducing continuous contractions of the musculature, leading to rigid paralysis. Pyrantel also inhibits cholinesterases. In *Ascaris* single muscle cell preparations, pyrantel and piperazine are mutually antagonistic.

Pyrantel tartrate is well absorbed after oral administration in the rat, dog, and pig. Plasma levels peak within 2 to 3 hours and the drug is rapidly metabolized and eliminated in the urine. Pyrantel pamoate is poorly absorbed from the intestine.

Dogs. Pyrantel pamoate, as a palatable suspension or as tablets (NEMEX), is indicated for the removal of *Toxocara canis, Toxascaris leonina, Ancylostoma caninum,* and *Uncinaria stenocephala* from dogs and puppies. The recommended dose of 5 mg. per kg. of NEMEX suspension is administered in the dog's feed bowl either by itself or mixed with a small amount of feed. For animals weighing 2.25 kg. or less, the dose is increased to 10 kg. per kg. Tablets may be administered directly or placed in a small portion of ground meat. NEMEX has been shown to be safe in nursling and weanling pups, pregnant bitches, males used for breeding, and dogs infected with *Dirofilaria immitis.* The oral LD_{50} is greater than 690 mg. per kg. in dogs. No significant morphological changes were induced in dogs given 94 mg. per kg. daily for 90 days. Pyrantel pamoate is compatible with organophosphates and other antiparasitic and antimicrobial agents.

Horses. A paste or caramel-flavored suspension of pyrantel pamoate, (IMATHAL, STRONGID-T, STRONGID-P) administered at 6.6 mg. of pyrantel base per kg. eliminates *Strongylus vulgaris, S. edentatus, S. equinus, Oxyuris equi, Parascaris equorum,* and several species of the subfamily Cyathostominae including populations resistant to benzimidazoles. Pyrantel pamoate can be administered as a single dose to horses by stomach tube or mixed with the grain ration. Pyrantel tartrate powder (STRONGID) or pellets may also be used as an equine anthelmintic at 12.5 mg. of pyrantel base per kg. Pyrantel is safe to use in horses and ponies of all ages, including sucklings, weanlings and pregnant mares. It can be used concurrently with insecticides, carbon disulfide, tranquilizers, muscle relaxants, and CNS depressants. At 13.2 mg. per kg, it was 98 per cent effective against *Anoplocephala perfoliata.*

Swine. Pyrantel tartrate (BANMINTH), when fed continuously at 96 grams per U.S. ton of feed as the sole ration, prevents the migration and establishment of *Ascaris suum* and *Oesophagostomum* spp. When fed to pigs for three consecutive days, this medicated feed removes the adults and fourth stage larvae of *Ascaris*. Pyrantel tartrate is also mixed with feed at the rate of 800 grams per U.S. ton and fed to pigs for the treatment of *Ascaris* and *Oeosphagostomum* for one day at the rate of 1 kg. feed per 40 kg. body weight up to 2.3 kg. of feed for pigs 91 kg. and over. Pyrantel is the only approved anthelmintic that, when administered continuously, prevents the appearance of milk spots on the liver of pigs; it does so by killing the larvae of *A. suum* in the lumen of the gut as they hatch from eggs.

WARNING. Pyrantel should not be given to pigs within 24 hours of slaughter. Because the drug is photodegradable, it should be used immediately after the package is opened. Pyrantel tartrate should not be mixed with rations containing bentonite. Because pyrantel and piperazine appear to be pharmacological antagonists, they probably should not be used concurrently.

Cattle, Sheep, and Goats. Pyrantel tartrate is not approved by FDA for use in cattle, sheep, and goats but is effective against the economically important nematode parasites of these ruminants at 25 mg. per kg.

RAFOXANIDE

Rafoxanide is a whitish, crystalline powder, sparingly soluble in water. It is formulated as a 3 per cent drench suspension (FLUKANIDE) and in combination with thiabendazole (RANIZOLE). The LD$_{50}$ for rats is about 2300 mg. per kg. Rafoxanide is not approved by FDA for use in the United States.

Cattle. Rafoxanide is administered orally at 7.5 mg. per kg. for the removal of adult *Fasciola hepatica* and *F. gigantica*. Rafoxanide also affords reasonable control of immature liver flukes. FLUKANIDE injection is administered subcutaneously at 6.6. mg. per kg.

WARNING. Adverse side effects may be produced at dosages of 58 mg. per kg. and above. At 75 mg. per kg., equatorial cataracts and blindness may occur. Animals should not be treated with the drench within 28 days or with the injection within 21 days of slaughter. Lactating dairy cows must not be treated with rafoxanide.

Sheep. Rafoxanide is administered to sheep at 7.5 to 10 mg. per kg. for the control of acute and chronic fascioliasis caused by immature and adult *Fasciola hepatica* and *F. gigantica*. Rafoxanide is also highly efficacious against *Haemonchus contortus*, including benzimidazole-resistant populations, and against the sheep nasal bot *Oestrus ovis*.

WARNING. Sheep should not be treated within 28 days of slaughter. Dosage levels over 45 mg. per kg. produce adverse side reactions such as anorexia, diarrhea, equatorial cataracts, and blindness.

RESORANTEL

Resorantel is a colorless powder, insoluble in water, hydrocarbons, and vegetable oils, slightly soluble in ethyl and methyl alcohols, and very soluble in dimethylformamide.

Resorantel is administered orally to sheep as a drench or bolus (TERENOL) at 65 mg. per kg. for removal of *Moniezia* and *Paramphistomum*. Excellent efficacy against these parasites was also reported for cattle and goats. Sheep receiving three times the therapeutic dose did not develop adverse reactions. Resorantel is not approved by FDA for use in the United States.

STYRYLPYRIDINIUM CHLORIDE AND DIETHYLCARBAMAZINE

Styrylpyridinium in combination with diethylcarbamazine (STYRID-CARICIDE) is administered to dogs as liquid, edible tablets, or complete food as an aid in the control of *Toxocara canis*, *Ancylostoma caninum*, and *Dirofilaria immitis* infections. The recommended dosage level for styrylpyridinium is 5.5 mg. per kg. and for diethylcarbamazine 6.6 mg. per kg. For heartworm control, STYRID-CARICIDE must be given daily during the mosquito exposure season. STYRID is active against adult *Ancylostoma caninum* and CARICIDE is active against adult *Toxocara canis*.

WARNING. STYRID-CARICIDE should not be given to dogs with microfilaremia.

TETRACHLOROETHYLENE

Tetrachloroethylene is a colorless, nonflammable liquid with ethereal odor. It is marketed in capsules (NEMA) of various sizes for different species of domestic animals. The capsules are administered to dogs and adult cats at 0.2 ml. per kg. to a maximum of 5 ml. per animal for the removal of hookworms and ascarids. The animals must be weighed to assure accurate dosage. The capsule should be carefully placed well back in the animal's mouth. Tetrachloroethylene is very irritating to the mucous membranes, so avoid breaking the capsule.

WARNING. Fatty foods, including milk, must be withheld from the animal's diet for at least two days before and four hours after the administration of NEMA capsules. A saline laxative must be given right after dosing. If worms are not eliminated within three to four hours after administration of tetrachloroethylene, an enema of warm, soapy water is recommended. Animals suffering from gastroenteritis or kidney or liver diseases and undernourished animals should not be treated with this drug. Absorption of tetrachloroethylene may cause dizziness, incoordination, liver damage, and even death. Tetrachloroethylene should not be administered to pregnant females. Oil laxatives are contraindicated. Finally, nurslings and pups and kittens weighing less than one kilogram should not be treated. If the clinician cannot adhere to these conditions, it would be better to select one of the many safer anthelmintics.

THENIUM CLOSYLATE

Thenium is a bitter, colorless, crystalline powder, sparingly soluble in water. Thenium closylate tablets (CANOPAR) are indicated for the removal of adult *Ancylostoma caninum* and *Uncinaria stenocephala* from dogs. One tablet containing 500 mg. thenium base is administered orally to dogs weighing 4.5 kg. and over. For dogs weighing 2.3 to 4.5 kg., the tablet is broken in two and half given at each end of the day.

WARNING. Thenium closylate should not be administered to suckling puppies or recently weaned puppies weighing less than 2.3 kg. An occasional dog may vomit following administration of thenium, but its efficacy is not reduced if emesis occurs more than two hours after dosing. Anaphylactoid or toxic reactions may rarely occur following administration of thenium.

THENIUM CLOSYLATE AND PIPERAZINE PHOSPHATE

A combination of thenium closylate and piperazine phosphate is indicated for the removal of adults and fourth stage larvae of *Ancylostoma caninum*, *A. braziliense*, *Uncinaria stenocephala*, and *Toxocara canis* from weaned puppies and adult dogs. It is believed that thenium and piperazine act synergistically.

The tablet is administered orally but the dog should not be allowed to chew it because the bitter taste will result in salivation. Overdosed animals always vomit, a safety feature of this drug.

THIABENDAZOLE

Thiabendazole is a white, crystalline powder sparingly soluble in water and slightly soluble in alcohols, esters, and chlorinated hydrocarbons. It is a very safe compound. The acute oral LD_{50} for rats is 3100 mg. per kg. Thiabendazole is used as an anthelmintic in sheep, goats, cattle, horses, swine, and other animals in which it is active against the adult and some immature forms of nematodes and inhibits embryonation of nematode eggs. It is also active against fungi and mites. Owing to its wide margin of safety, thiabendazole has been used in animals of all ages and in pregnant and debilitated animals. Thiabendazole is available in a variety of pharmaceutical forms (wettable powder, suspension, feed premix, paste, feed block, top dressing pellets, bolus, feed crumbles) and different proprietary names (EQUIZOLE, OMNIZOLE, THIBENZOLE). Thiabendazole kills parasites probably by interfering with their energy metabolism. It inhibits fumarate reductase, an important enzyme for the degradation of sugars in nematodes.

Cattle. Thiabendazole is administered orally as a drench, bolus, or paste, or in feed at 66 mg. per kg. for the control of *Haemonchus*, *Ostertagia*, *Trichostrongylus*, *Nematodirus*, and *Oesophagostomum*. In severe cases of these parasitisms or in cases involving *Cooperia*, 110 mg. per kg. is recommended. Thiabendazole is not active against the hypobiotic early fourth stage larvae of *Ostertagia*.

WARNING. Milk drawn within 96 hours after thiabendazole medication must not be used for human food. Cattle must not be treated within 30 days of slaughter.

Sheep and Goats. Thiabendazole is indicated for the control of *Haemonchus*, *Ostertagia*, *Trichostrongylus*, *Nematodirus*, *Cooperia*, *Bunostomum*, *Chabertia*, *Oesophagostomum*, and *Strongyloides* at 44 to 66 mg. per kg. A number of reports indicate that thiabendazole is not as effective against *Haemonchus* and *Trichostrongylus* as it was when first introduced for general use. Until very recently, *Haemonchus* has kept the secret of its increasing resistance to benzimidazole anthelmintics well. However, biochemical research has recently uncovered the key to this wormy secret. Thiabendazole, at least *in vitro*, inhibits the fumarate reductase in thiabendazole-sensitive *Haemonchus*, but does not inhibit the fumarate reductase of thiabendazole-resistant *Haemonchus*.

Horses. Thiabendazole, at 44 mg. per kg. in drench, paste, or feed additive formulations, is recommended for the removal of *Strongylus vulgaris, S. edentatus, S. equinus*, species of the subfamily Cyathostominae, *Oxyuris equi*, and *Strongyloides westeri*. For removal of *Parascaris equorum*, 88 mg. per kg. must be used. For activity against migrating fourth stage larvae of *S. vulgaris*, thiabendazole is administered at 440 mg. per kg. on two consecutive days. Populations of cyathostomes have developed resistance to thiabendazole and other benzimidazole anthelmintics.

Thiabendazole 44 mg. per kg. and piperazine 55 mg. per kg. is administered by stomach tube as a ready-to-use suspension (EQUIZOLE A) for the control of susceptible nematodes, including *Parascaris*.

EQUIZOLE B (thiabendazole 44 mg. per kg. and trichlorfon 40 mg. per kg.) is recommended for the removal of thiabendazole-susceptible nematodes, *Parascaris*, and *Gasterophilus*. EQUIZOLE B may be given by stomach tube, by drench, or in feed.

WARNING. The trichlorfon in EQUIZOLE B is a cholinesterase inhibitor. It should not be used in sick or debilitated horses, in foals under four months of age, or in mares in the latter months of pregnancy. Intravenous anesthetics and muscle relaxants should not be used for two weeks after the administration of EQUIZOLE B. EQUIZOLE B should not be administered to animals within a day of exposure to other cholinesterase-inhibiting chemicals. Overdosage of trichlorfon may produce ataxia and colic. Atropine and 2-PAM are antidotal.

Swine. Thiabendazole paste is used for the control of *Strongyloides ransomi* infections in newborn pigs at 63 to 88 mg. per kg. Added to feed, thiabendazole is used to prevent infections with *Ascaris suum*. It is fed at 0.05 to 0.1 per cent of the grain ration for two weeks and then continued at 0.005 to 0.02 per cent for 8 to 14 weeks. This practice should prevent the appearance of pneumonia due to migrating *Ascaris* larvae but has no effect on the larval migrations through the liver and therefore does not prevent formation of "milk spot" lesions. Pigs should not be treated within 30 days of slaughter.

TOLUENE (METHYLBENZENE)

Toluene is a flammable, refractive liquid with a benzenelike odor. It is sparingly soluble in water but miscible with alcohol, chloroform, glacial acetic acid, and carbon disulfide. It is quite safe for mammals; the oral LD_{50} for rats is 7.5 ml. per kg.

Dogs and Cats. Toluene at 220 mg. per kg. in gelatine capsules (METHACIDE CAPSULES) is used in dogs and cats for the removal of *Toxocara canis, T. cati, Toxascaris leonina, Ancylostoma caninum*, and *A. braziliense*. Toluene is about 75 per cent effective against *Trichuris vulpis*. Fasting is suggested for 12 hours before and 4 hours after medication.

WARNING. Toluene is a relatively safe drug but overdosage produces transitory incoordination, muscle tremors, vomiting, and central nervous system depression. Warm water gavage, administration of mineral oil, and oxygen therapy are suggested in severely depressed animals. Digestible oils, alcohol, and adrenalin should be avoided.

TRICHLORFON

Trichlorfon is a white, crystalline powder, soluble in water but insoluble in petroleum oils. It is stable in acidic media but is converted to dichlorvos in alkaline media. Trichlorfon is the active ingredient in a variety of products intended for the control of helminth and insect parasites of domestic animals.

Horses. ANTHON SOLUBLE POWDER, COMBOT ORAL LIQUID, COMBOT PASTE, DYREX, AND P/M TRICHLORFON are indicated for the removal of *Gasterophilus intestinalis, G. nasalis, Parascaris equorum*, and *Oxyuris equi* from horses at approximately 40 mg. per kg. The liquid form is administered with a stomach tube; the powder and granular forms are mixed thoroughly in water or in enough feed to be consumed at one feeding.

As a slow release tablet (DYREX CAP-TAB), trichlorfon is claimed to be effective against the previously listed parasites, *Strongylus vulgaris*, and various species of small strongyles. A similar broad spectrum of activity has been demonstrated with DYREX T.F. (trichlorfon 16.8 per cent, phenothiazine

11.5 per cent, and piperazine dihydrochloride 68.2 per cent). DYREX T.F. is dissolved in water and administered to horses by stomach tube. See also EQUIZOLE B, above.

WARNING. Trichlorfon is a cholinesterase inhibitor and should always be used with prudence in horses. Trichlorfon should not be administered to horses that have been exposed to other cholinesterase-inhibiting chemicals. Trichlorfon should not be administered to foals under four months of age, to mares in the last month of pregnancy, or to horses that are severely debilitated, suffering from diarrhea or severe constipation, infectious diseases, toxemia, or colic. A horse may develop diarrhea, colic, or ataxia soon after administration of the recommended dose. Atropine and PAM or 2-PAM are antidotal. We recommend that trichlorfon be used in horses only for the removal of *Gasterophilus* larvae and that one of the many safe broad-spectrum anthelmintics be used against helminths.

Dogs. Trichlorfon plus atropine tablets (FREED) is recommended for removal of *Toxocara, Ancylostoma, Trichuris, Ctenocephalides* spp., and *Demodex canis* from dogs. FREED is administered orally after a regular feeding. The recommended dose is 75 mg. per kg.; half is administered in the morning and half in the afternoon. For maximum anthelmintic effect, one should administer three such treatments at three- to four-day intervals. Occasionally, dogs may develop nausea, excessive salivation, vomiting, weakness, and incoordination. Atropine 0.05 to 0.1 mg. per kg. and 2-PAM or PROTOPAM CHLORIDE should be administered as antidotes. Keep treated dogs in a quiet place.

WARNING. Trichlorfon should not be given to cats, greyhound or whippet dogs, sick or debilitated dogs, dogs heavily infected with heartworm, or dogs that have been recently exposed to cholinesterase-inhibiting chemicals. Safer chemicals than trichlorfon are available for the control of canine parasites.

REFERENCES

Anon. (1983): Code of Federal Regulations. 21 Food and Drugs, Parts 500 to 599. Washington, D.C. The Office of the Federal Register.

Anon. (1983): Compendium of Data Sheets for Veterinary Products. London. Pharmind Publications Limited.

Anon. (1983): Controlling Insects and Mites of Livestock and Other Animals. Bulletin 256, revised 1982. Cooperative Extension Service, University of Maryland. College Park, MD.

Anon. (1983): Controlling Insects and Mites on Dairy and Beef Cattle. Special Circular 230. The Pennsylvania State University. College of Agriculture Extension service. University Park, PA.

Anon. (1978): Controlling Insects and Mites on Swine. The Pennsylvania State University. College of Agriculture Extension Service. University Park, PA.

Anon. (1983): Farm Chemicals Handbook. Willoughby, Ohio, Meister Publishing Co.

Anon. (1983): Feed Additive Compendium. Minneapolis. The Miller Publishing Co.

Anon. (1983): Freedom of Information Summary NADA No. 127-443. Merck Sharp and Dohme Laboratories.

Anon. (1983): 1984 Insect Pest Management Guide. Circular 898, Cooperative Extension Service, University of Illinois at Urbana-Champaign.

Anon. (1976): Pesticide Index. Edited by Wiswesse, W. J. College Park, MD. Entomological Society of America.

Anon. (1979): Pesticide Profiles. Part One: Insecticides and Miticides. Bulletin 267. College Park, MD. Cooperative Extension Service, University of Maryland.

Anon. (1978): Styquin Butamisole for control of whipworms and hookworms. Technical Bull. 37r. Cyanamid Agricultural de Puerto Rico, Inc.

Anon. (1977): Telmintic (Mebendazole) Powder, NADA 102-987. Freedom of Information Summary, FDA BVM, Washington, D.C.

Boray, J. C., Strong, M. B., Allison, J. R., Orelli, M. von., Sarasin, G., and Gfeller, W. (1979): Nitroscanate, a new broad spectrum anthelmintic against nematodes and cestodes of dogs and cats. Australian Vet. J., 55, 45-53.

Bowers, W. S. (1976): Hormone mimics. *In* The Future for Insecticides: Need and Prospects. Edited by Metcalf, R. L., and McKelvey, J. J., Jr. New York. John Wiley and Sons, pp. 421-441.

Brooks, G. T. (1974): Chlorinated Insecticides. Vol. II. Biological and Environmental Aspects. Cleveland. CRC Press.

Brown, A. W. A. (1978): Ecology of Pesticides. New York. John Wiley and Sons.

Campbell, W. C., Fisher, M. H., Stapley, E. O., Albers-Schönberg, G., and Jacob, T. A. (1983): Ivermectin: A potent new antiparasitic agent. Science, 221, 823-828.

Casida, J. E. (1973): Biochemistry of the pyrethrins. *In* Pyrethrum: The Natural Insecticide. Edited by Casida, J. E. New York. Academic Press, pp. 101-120.

Corbett, J. R. (1974): The Biochemical Mode of Action of Pesticides. New York. Academic Press.

Duncan, J. (1982): Internal parasites of horses: Treatment and control. In Practice (November), 183-188.

Eaton, L. G., Siegmund, O. H., Rankin, A. D., and Bramel, R. G. (1969): The veterinary use of thiabendazole. Texas Rep. Biol. Med., 27 (suppl. 2), 693-708.

Eto, M. (1974): Organophosphorus Pesticides: Organic and Biological Chemistry. Cleveland. CRC Press.

Gaenssler, J. G., and Reinecke, R. K. (1970): The anthelmintic efficacy of resorantel. J. S. Afr. Vet. Med. Assoc., 41, 214-221.

Gibson, T. E. (1975): Veterinary Anthelmintic Medication, 3rd ed. Technical Communication No. 33. Farnham Royal, England. Commonwealth Institute of Helminthology, St. Albans. Commonwealth Agricultural Bureaux.

Goodman, L. S., and Gilman, A. (1980): The Pharmacological Basis of Therapeutics, 6th ed. New York. The Macmillan Co.

Gosselin, R. E., Hodge, H. C., Smith, R. P., and Gleason, M. N. (1976): Clinical Toxicology of Commercial Products, 4th ed. Baltimore. The Williams and Wilkins Co.

Hall, M. C., and Schillinger, J. E. (1923): Some critical tests of arecoline hydrobromide as an anthelmintic. J. Am. Vet. Med. Assoc., 63, 454-463.

Harris, R. L., Frazer, E. D., and Younger, R. L. (1973): Hornflies, stable flies, and house flies. Development in feces of bovines treated orally with juvenile hormone analogs. J. Econ. Entomol., 66, 1099-1102.

Harwood, P. D., Jerstad, A. C., Underwood, P. C., and Schaffer, J. M. (1940): The efficacy of N-butyl chloride for the removal of intestinal nematodes, especially whipworms from dogs. N. Amer. Vet., 21, 35-41.

Hass, D. K. (1970): Dichlorvos—an organophosphate anthelmintic. In Topics in Medicinal Chemistry, Vol. III, edited by Rabinowitz, J. L. and Myerson, R. M. New York. John Wiley and Sons, pp. 171-202.

Hass, D. K., and Collins, J. A. (1975): Feline anthelmintics: A comparative evaluation of six products. Vet. Med. Small Anim. Clin., 70, 423-425.

Hatton, C. J. (1965): A new taeniacide, bunamidine hydrochloride: Its efficacy against Taenia pisiformis and Dipylidium caninum in the dog and Hydatigera taeniaeformis in the cat. Vet. Rec., 77, 408-411.

Horak, I. G. (1976): The control of ticks, fleas, and lice on dogs by means of a sendran-impregnated collar. J. S. Afr. Vet. Assoc., 47, 17-18.

Horak, I. G., Louw, J. P., and Raymond, S. W. (1971): Trials with rafoxanide. 3. Efficacy of rafoxanide against the larvae of the sheep nasal bot fly Oestrus ovis. J. S. Afr. Vet. Med. Assoc., 42, 337-339.

Jackson, R. F. (1963): Two-day treatment with thiacetarsamide for canine heartworm disease. J. Am. Vet. Med. Assoc., 142, 23-26.

Kelly, J. D. (1977): Canine Parasitology. Veterinary Review No. 17. Sydney. The University of Sydney, The Post-Graduate Foundation in Veterinary Science.

Kenaga, E. E., and Emd, C. S. (1974): Commercial and Experimental Organic Insecticides. Special Publ. 74-1. College Park, Maryland. Entomological Society of America. 77 pp.

Khan, M. A. (1973): Toxicity of systemic insecticides: Toxicological considerations in using organophosphorus insecticides. Vet. Rec., 92, 411-419.

Kirkwood, A. (1983): Insecticides and dips for farm animals. In Practice (November), 198-201.

Kuhr, R. J., and Dorough, H. W. (1976): Carbamate Insecticides: Chemistry, Biochemistry, and Toxicology. Cleveland. CRC Press.

Magat, A., Cottereau, Ph., and Faure, N. (1968): Accidents after treatment of bovine hypodermatosis with organophosphorus compounds. Revue Med. Vet., 119, 595-605.

Malkin, M. F., and Camacho, R. M. (1972): The effect of thiabendazole on fumarate reductase from thiabendazole-sensitive and resistant Haemonchus contortus. J. Parasitol., 58, 845-846.

Martin, C. L., Christmas, R., and Leipold, H. W. (1972): Formation of temporary cataracts in dogs given a disophenol preparation. J. Am. Vet. Med. Assoc., 161, 294-301.

Miller, J. E., Baker, N. F., and Colburn, E. L., Jr. (1977): Insecticidal activity of propoxur- and carbaryl-impregnated flea collars against Ctenocephalides felis. Am. J. Vet. Res., 38, 923-925.

Miller, R. W., Gordon, C. H., Bowman, M. C., Beroza,

M., and Morgan, N. O. (1970): Gardona as a feed additive for control of fly larvae in cow manure. J. Econ. Entomol., 63, 1420-1423.

Miller, T. A. (1966): Anthelmintic activity of tetrachloroethylene against various stages of Ancylostoma caninum in young dogs. Am. J. Vet. Res., 27, 1037-1040.

Morrow, G. L. (1978): Clinical evaluation of febantel and trichlorfon paste formulations in the horse. Vet. Med. Small Anim. Clin., 73, 1388-1393.

Nelson, D. L., Allen, A. D., Mozier, J. O., and White, R. G. (1967): Diagnosis and treatment of adverse reactions in cattle treated with grubs with a systemic insecticide. Vet. Med. Small Anim. Clin., 62, 683-684.

O'Brien, R. D. (1967): Insecticides: Action and Metabolism. New York. Academic Press.

O'Brien, R. D., and Yamamoto, I. (1970): Biochemical Toxicology of Insecticides. New York. Academic Press.

Ogbourne, C. P., and Duncan, J. L. (1977): Strongylus vulgaris in the Horse: Its Biology and Veterinary Importance. Farnham Royal, England. Commonwealth Institute of Helminthology. Commonwealth Agricultural Bureaux.

Otto, G. F., and Maren, T. H. (1947): Possible use of an arsenical compound in the treatment of heartworm in dogs. Vet. Med., 42, 128.

Palmer, J. S., and Danz, J. W. (1964): Tolerance of Brahman cattle to organic phosphorus insecticides. J. Am. Vet. Med. Assoc., 144, 143-145.

Poynter, D. (1956): A comparative assessment of the anthelmintic activity in horses of four piperazine compounds. Vet. Rec., 68, 291-297.

Reedy, L. (1977): Ectoparasites. In Current Veterinary Therapy VI. Philadelphia. W. B. Saunders Company. p. 547.

Roelofs, W. L. (1976): Pheromones. In The Future for Insecticides, Needs and Prospects. Edited by Metcalf, R. L., and McKelvey, J. J., Jr. New York. John Wiley and Sons, pp. 445-461.

Rossoff, I. S. (1974): Handbook of Veterinary Drugs. New York, Springer Publishing Co.

Scott, D. W., Schultz, R. D., and Baker, E. (1976): Further studies on the therapeutic and immunologic aspects of generalized demodectic mange in the dog. J. Am. Anim. Hosp. Assoc., 12, 203-213.

Scott, P. (1977): A review of some modern equine anthelmintics. N. Z. Vet. J., 25, 373-378.

Shaw, R. D. (1970): Tick control on domestic animals. II. The effect of modern methods of treatment. Trop. Sci., 12 29-36.

Spinelli, J. S., and Enos, L. R. (1978): Drugs in Veterinary Practice. St. Louis. The C. V. Mosby Co.

Theodorides, V. J., Gyurik, R. J., Kingsbury, W. D., and Parish, R. C. (1976): Anthelmintic activity of albendazole against liver flukes, tapeworms, lung and gastrointestinal roundworms. Experientia, 32, 702.

Thomas, H., and Andrews, P. (1977): Praziquantel—a new cestocide. Pestic. Sci., 8, 556-560.

Ulmann, I., Ed. (1972): Lindane, Monograph of an Insecticide. Freiburg im Briesgall, Verlag K. Schillinger.

Van Cauteren, H., Marsboom, R., Vandenberghe, J., and Will, J. A. (1983): Safety studies evaluating the effect of mebendazole on liver function in dogs. J. Am. Vet. Med. Assoc., 183, 93-98.

Van den Bossche, H. (1976): The molecular basis of anthelmintic action. In Biochemistry of Parasites and Host-Parasite Relationships. Edited by Van den Bossche, H. Amsterdam. North Holland Publishers. pp. 553-572.

Van den Bossche, H., and Janssen, P. A. (1969): The

biochemical mechanism of action of the antinematodal drug tetramisole. Bichem. Pharmacol., *18*, 35-42.

Ware, G. W. (1978): Pesticides—Theory and Application. San Francisco. W. H. Freeman and Co.

Warren, B. C., and Yeoman, G. H. (1977): Phosmet as a warble control agent. Vet. Rec., *101*, 504-505.

Wood, I. B., Pankavich, J. A., Wallace, W. S., Thomson, R. E., Burkhart, R. L., and Waletzky, E. (1961): Disophenol, an injectable anthelmintic for canine hookworms. J. Am. Vet. Med. Assoc., *139*. 1101-1105.

Woodard, G. T. (1957): The treatment of organic phosphate insecticide poisoning with atropine sulfate and 2-P.A.M. (2-Pyridine Aldoxine Methiodide). Vet. Med., *52*, 571-578.

Yamamoto, I. (1973): Mode of action of synergists in enhancing the insecticidal activity of pyrethrum and pyrethroids. *In* Pyrethrum, The Natural Insecticide. Edited by Casida, J. E. New York, Academic Press.

Yarborough, J. H., and Yarborough, J. H., Jr. (1968): A clinical evaluation of cythioate, a new oral systemic parasiticide for dogs. Vet. Med. Small Anim. Clin., *63*, 584-586.

THREE

DIAGNOSTIC PARASITOLOGY

Jay R. Georgi and Marion E. Georgi

As busy veterinarians, we would like to be able to achieve reasonably accurate identification of parasites with a reasonable expenditure of effort. The conventional system and the one on which the organization of Chapters 12 and 13 is based, is to take advantage of the site and host specificities of parasites and list them according to their customary locations in or on their customary hosts. In using this system, it is well to recognize that it must fail in abnormal cases. Whenever doubt arises or the exact identity of a parasite is essential (e.g., as for publication), recourse must be had to detailed morphological study, preferably by a recognized expert.

The diagnostic categories used in the following chapters do not adhere consistently to any particular level of taxonomic nomenclature. This is because the goals of typological taxonomy differ from those of applied parasitology. The taxonomist strives to arrange living organisms into ranks and files in a way that, to his tastes at least, best displays the phylogenetic relationships among them. But the needs of clinicians and clinical parasitologists are best served by diagnostic categories that do not happen to coincide consistently with any particular level of the taxonomist's classification scheme. Thus, we identify an egg from one of several dozens of species of canine tapeworms as a taeniid egg rather than as a *Taenia pisiformis* egg because it is practically impossible to carry the identification of such eggs below the family level. Fortunately, all members of this particular family except *Echinococcus* respond in about the same way to anthelmintic therapy and the infective larvae of all develop in vertebrate intermediate hosts. Therefore, the diagnostic category "taeniid" is adequate to the needs of effective treatment and control. In another instance, the recognition of a worm as a member of its particular phylum may suffice. For example, an acanthocephalan from a pig is almost certain to be *Macracanthorhynchus hirudinaceus*. In still other instances, however, species identification is necessary. For example, the distinction between *Toxocara canis* and *Toxascaris leonina* is important from the standpoints of both animal parasite control and public health.

Unfortunately, there are many important practical distinctions that transcend even the lowest levels of conventional systematics. There exist infraspecific races of many nematodes that may differ remarkably in pathogenicity, antigenicity, and response to pharmacological agents yet, on morphological grounds, fall into the same species. Here we must make our way with whatever criterion proves helpful.

12

ANTEMORTEM DIAGNOSIS

QUALITATIVE FECAL EXAMINATION

Specimen Preparation

DIRECT SMEAR

The direct smear made by breaking up a very small particle of feces in a drop of water is a simple, quick method. When examining outpatients, many small animal practitioners routinely smear the feces adhering to the rectal thermometer directly on a microscope slide. A coverslip improves the optics, subdues eddy currents, and helps prevent soiling of the objective lens of the microscope. Because the resulting suspension must be thin enough to read through, only a small particle of feces can be examined, but limited efficiency is the only shortcoming of this technique. Negative findings are inconclusive, but positive results are just as valid as those obtained with the more efficient concentration techniques. In fact, the smear presents advantages over concentration techniques in dealing with delicate forms such as nematode larvae and protozoan trophozoites, which are distorted or destroyed by concentration media, and with particularly heavy eggs that fail to float in them. As a rule, the concentration techniques should supplement rather than supplant the smear but, in practice, one or the other technique is adopted as a matter of routine.

FLOTATION CONCENTRATION OF EGGS AND CYSTS

All flotation techniques take advantage of a difference in the bouyancy of parasites relative to food residues. If some feces are suspended in water, the eggs and solid fecal particles will settle out, allowing the supernatant fats and dissolved pigments to be decanted. If the sediment is then resus-pended in a solution intermediate in density between the eggs and fecal debris, the former will float, while the latter will sink. In general, techniques based on the flotation principle work well for nematode and cestode eggs and protozoan cysts but fail to float some trematode eggs and distort protozoan trophozoites and certain nematode larvae beyond recognition. Zinc sulfate (specific gravity 1.18) is superior to sucrose of equal density for floating protozoan cysts and nematode larvae because it is slower to shrink and distort them.

Feces puddling is by no means an exact science; the actual procedure followed is less important than a show of respect for the basic principles involved. A workable procedure is outlined as follows:

(1) Mix a teaspoonful or so of feces with enough water to make a semisolid suspension. Use a tongue depressor and a paper cup.

(2) Place a wire tea strainer over a second paper cup and empty the fecal suspension into it. Use the tongue depressor to press out most of the liquid; return solid waste to the first cup and discard. Wash strainer in hot, running water.

(3) Pinch the rim of the second paper cup to form a pouring spout and transfer contents to 15 ml. centrifuge tubes.

(4) Centrifuge for three minutes and decant the supernatant containing fats and dissolved pigments.

(5) Add concentrated sucrose solution (specific gravity 1.33) to 1 cm. from the top of the tube and resuspend the sediment with an applicator stick. Stopper and mix by four or more inversions. The viscosity of the sugar solution impedes mixing but the solution must, nevertheless, be thoroughly mixed with the sediment.

(6) Centrifuge for five minutes. Without removing the tube from the centrifuge, pick up the surface film containing eggs and cysts by touching it gently with a glass "nail" or wire loop. Transfer the surface film to a microscope slide and add a coverslip.

Variant. Alternatively, after step 5 has been completed, the centifuge tube may be filled to the brim with saturated sucrose solution and a coverslip applied to the top. After centrifuging, remove the coverslip by lifting it straight up and place it and its adherent film of sugar solution on a glass slide. This variant will not work with fixed angle-head centrifuges.

(7) Scan the slide under 100x magnification. To avoid omission or overlap of fields, start by scanning along one edge of the coverslip from one corner to the other. Then shift one field width and continue scanning. The shift can be executed precisely by concentrating attention on any object that happens to lie at or near the edge of the field and moving that object to the other edge with the mechanical stage adjustment. As skill in identification is acquired, the scanning may be done under 50X magnification with considerable saving of time.

Gravitational force may be used in lieu of centrifugal but it is weaker and therefore takes longer. Several commercially available, disposable fecal analysis kits that work by gravity afford satisfactory results. If sodium nitrate solution (specific gravity 1.20) is used as flotation medium, the preparation is ready for microscopic examination in 10 minutes. Saturated sucrose solution, because of its greater viscosity, requires 15 to 20 minutes to yield equivalent results. A disadvantage of sodium nitrate is that the slide must be examined promptly; otherwise, osmotic distortion may have rendered the parasites difficult to identify or crystallization of the medium may have totally obscured the microscopic field.

CONCENTRATION OF NEMATODE LARVAE BY THE BAERMANN TECHNIQUE

In the Baermann technique, advantage is taken of the inability of most nematode larvae to swim against gravity. The vertical migrations of nematode larvae on vegetation occur in moisture films where surface tension translates their sinusoidal body movements into effective locomotion. By contrast, nematode larvae tend to gradually sink in an appreciable body of water within which there is no surface tension. A typical Baermann apparatus is illustrated in Figure 12-1. Break up a fairly large fecal specimen (5 to 15 grams), place it in a tea strainer or wrap it in cheesecloth, and place it in lukewarm water in the funnel. The warmth stimulates larval motility and many larvae will come to the surface of the fecal mass, fall off, and descend

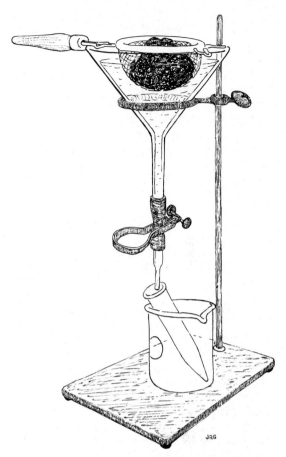

Figure 12–1. Baermann apparatus for separating and concentrating nematode larvae from feces, minced tissues, and soil samples. The specimen is placed in the basket of a tea strainer or wrapped in cheesecloth and immersed in lukewarm water in the funnel. Nematode larvae unable to swim against gravity descend to the pinch clamp and may then be recovered in a small volume of water. A few minutes to several hours may be required, depending on the kind of larvae and the degree of infection.

to the pinch clamp. In heavy infections, larvae can be drawn off in a drop of water after an hour or so, but when few larvae are present, it may be necessary to leave the "Baermann" set up overnight. If more than a single drop of water is drawn for examination, it will be necessary to centrifuge, decant, and pipette a drop of sediment. There are many refinements and modifications of this technique, but the same simple principle underlies them all.

The infective first stage larvae of *Filaroides osleri* and *F. hirthi* are lethargic and do not migrate out of the fecal mass. The Baermann technique is therefore an utter failure with respect to *Filaroides* larvae, and it is necessary to resort to the flotation concentration technique using zinc sulfate (specific gravity 1.18) as flotation medium.

CULTURE OF NEMATODE LARVAE

Generic identification of strongylid eggs usually requires rearing infective stage larvae. Well-formed horse and sheep feces contain just the right amount of water and can usually be successfully cultured merely by placing a few pellets in a covered jar that has been rinsed with 0.1 per cent sodium carbonate solution to inhibit mold growth and storing the jar in a drawer or dark shelf at room temperature for a week to ten days. The walls of the jar should always be covered with droplets of condensed moisture. If the culture appears to be drying out, add a few drops of water or sodium carbonate solution. When the jar is returned to the light after incubation, larvae will soon be found squirming about in the condensation droplets on the walls of the jar.

Cattle feces of similar consistency can also be cultured without further preparation, but usually cattle feces are more fluid and require addition of vermiculite or sand to produce a damp but not wet culture.

All fecal cultural techniques are essentially qualitative because various species of nematodes have differing optimum conditions for hatching, development, and survival. As a result, the relative abundances of species of third stage larvae harvested from cultures is not a simple function of the relative abundances of species of strongylid eggs that were present at the start. *Haemonchus contortus* or *Strongyloides papillosus* larvae tend to predominate in culture whenever eggs of either of these species are present in the feces, and the possible clinical importance of *Trichostrongylus* or *Cooperia* should not be discounted because they are represented by only a small number of larvae.

Culture of dog feces for the demonstration of *Strongyloides stercoralis* filariform larvae consists of merely storing the specimen in a jar at room temperature. Filariform larvae of the homogonic generation appear by 24 to 48 hours but, if the isolate under study is principally or entirely heterogonic, substantial numbers of filariform larvae will not appear in less than 96 hours.

When larvae can be seen swimming in droplets of condensed moisture on the walls of the culture jar, rinse the walls of the jar with a small volume of water, collect the rinsings, and concentrate the larvae by centrifugation. Few larvae will be lost with the supernatant if the decanting is done by simply inverting the centrifuge tube in a single motion. Sediment containing the larvae can then be taken up in the small volume of water retained by cohesion and transferred with a bulb pipette to a microscope slide.

Nutrient agar plates provide excellent cultural conditions for certain nematode eggs or larvae that have been separated from feces and concentrated by the techniques already described. For example, rhabditiform larvae that have been concentrated from dog feces by the Baermann technique are deposited on the surface of the agar in a small volume of water and are incubated at room temperature. If these are *Strongyloides* larvae, the culture will be found teeming with infective filariform larvae and/or rhabditiform adult worms in less than two days.

Identification of larvae often requires that they be killed in an extended posture. This is easily accomplished by judicious warming of the droplet of water before applying the coverslip. Hold a lighted match below the slide and view the cessation of motion and extension of larvae from above. "Relaxation" is the customary euphemism applied to the thermal death of nematodes. Since *Strongyloides* tend to revive, it may be necessary to heat them up again. Avoid overheating the larvae, because this distorts them. As an alternative to heating, a drop of Lugol's solution may be added at the edge of the coverslip. This both relaxes and stains the larvae.

Whenever measurements are critical, the coverslip must be supported or it will press upon the larvae and distort them. Ring the coverslip with petroleum jelly to avoid this effect and to retard evaporation. The coverslip may be ringed quickly and conveniently as follows: Spread some petroleum jelly in a thin film on the heel of the left hand. Then, holding a coverslip edgeways between the thumb and forefinger of the right hand, draw each edge of the coverslip in turn through the film to obtain a uniform dam of petroleum jelly all about the perimeter.

CULTURE OF COCCIDIAN OOCYSTS FOR SPORULATION

Mix a small amount of feces or concentrated suspension of oocysts with 1 per cent potassium dichromate solution and make a shallow pool of this mixture in a Petri dish.

Sporulating oocysts need a lot of air, so the pool must be shallow to favor diffusion of oxygen, but do not let the culture dry out; add more dichromate solution, if necessary. Sporulation is usually complete after two to four days incubation at room temperature but some species require weeks.

MICROMETRY

Measuring the lengths of parasites with a microscope equipped with a calibrated eyepiece micrometer sometimes provides the most efficient means of reaching a diagnosis. An *object micrometer* is a glass microscope slide etched with a linear scale 1 or 2 mm. long and subdivided in units of 10 μm (0.01 mm.). An *eyepeice micrometer* is a glass disc etched with a scale of arbitrary units. The disc is inserted into the microscope eyepiece and the scale may be used to compare linear dimensions of objects in the microscopic field. For example, the ratio of length to width of a particular kind of egg may be determined. In order to measure absolute lengths, however, the eyepiece micrometer must first be calibrated for each objective magnification against the scale of the object micrometer.

(1) Focus the 10x objective on the scale of the object micrometer.
(2) Rotate the eyepiece until the eyepiece scale and objective scale are parallel.
(3) Align their zero marks by adjusting the mechanical stage (Fig. 12-2).

(4) Locate any point past the halfway mark where the two scales are in perfect register. The ratio of the object length to the number of eyepiece scale divisions up to this point provides a factor for converting all subsequent eyepiece micrometer measurements made with the 10x objective to absolute units. In Figure 12-2, 40 eyepiece scale divisions correspond exactly to 170 μm of the object micrometer scale, yielding a ratio of 4.25 μm per scale division.
(5) Repeat the calibration procedure for all objective magnifications.

N. B.: Microscopes with variable tube lengths and other sources of variation in secondary magnification must be brought into the same state of adjustment each time measurements are taken or else they must be recalibrated anew. Any variation of the interpupillary distance of the binocular microscope alters the tube length and is easily overlooked as a source of error.

IDENTIFICATION OF EGGS, CYSTS, AND LARVAE

Parasite vs. Pseudoparasite. One must first learn to distinguish between parasites and superficially similar but unrelated objects such as air bubbles, pollen grains, hair, plant fibers, fat droplets, and corn smut spores. Identification of *pseudoparasites* may occasionally shed light on the host's recent dietary adventures. Suppose, for example, that we find *Moniezia expansa* eggs in a specimen of

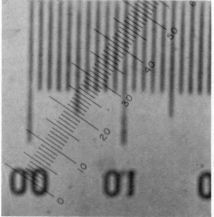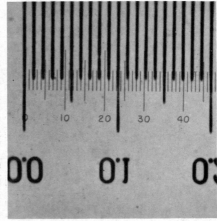

Figure 12–2. Eyepiece micrometer calibration. In the left picture, the object micrometer scale is out of focus and the eyepiece micrometer scale is about one eighth turn out of alignment. In the right picture, the scales have been made parallel by rotating the eyepiece, the object scale has been brought into focus, and the zero line (0.0) of the object scale has been aligned with the zero (0) line of the eyepiece scale by adjustment of the mechanical stage. Notice that 0.17 mm. (170 μm) equals 40 eyepiece divisions (measuring consistently from the right edges of the rather thick object scale lines) so that, at this magnification, each ocular division equals 4.25 μm. An oocyst measuring 9 by 5.5 divisions would thus be 38.2. μm long by 23.4. μm wide.

dog feces. We know then that the dog has recently eaten sheep feces because *M. expansa* is a parasite of sheep and never of dogs. Actually, because, *M. expansa* is a true parasite when it is in a sheep, its egg should be called a *spurious parasite* rather than a pseudoparasite when it is found in dog feces, but perhaps that distinction is a bit too pedantic. For practical purposes, if a dog or cat is passing an unidentifiable object in its feces,

give the animal an enema, confine it for 24 to 36 hours, and do another fecal examination. If the unidentifiable object is still there, chances are it is a parasite, whereas if it is gone, it was probably a pseudoparasite. I deliberately resisted including photomicrographs of pseudoparasites in previous editions of this book because I believed that learning to identify the *bona fide* parasites while simply ignoring the irrelevant rubbish

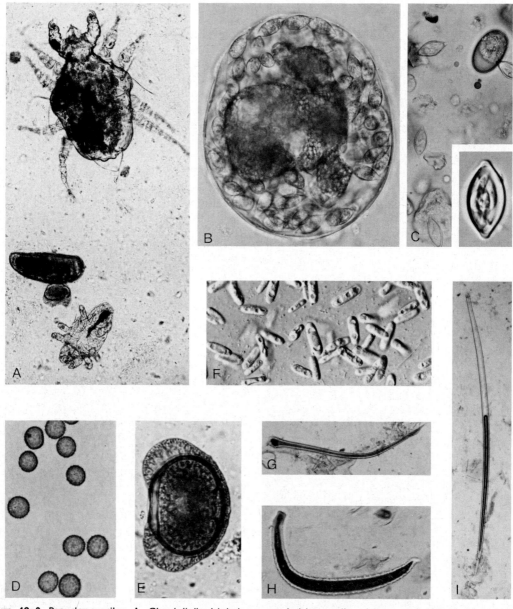

Figure 12–3. Pseudoparasites. A. *Cheyletiella blakei*, an arachnid parasite of the cat (x108). B. *Monocystis*, a protozoan parasite of the earthworm. C. *Monocystis* and ruminant *Eimeria* cysts in dog feces (x425). Inset: Sporulated *Monocystis* (x1000). D. Corn smut spores (x630). E. Pine pollen (x425). F. *Saccharomycopsis gutulatus*, normal alimentary yeast of rabbits (x425). G. Plant hair (x168), H. Plant hair (x63), I. Plant hair (x63).

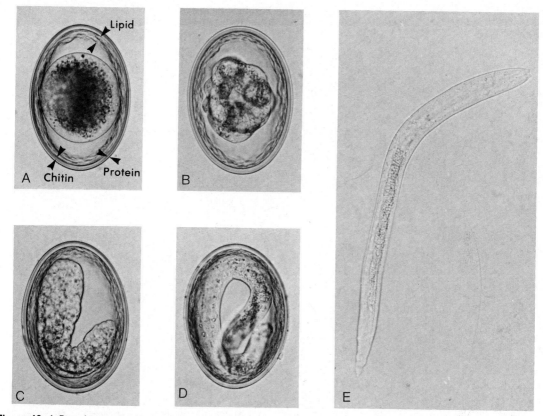

Figure 12–4. Development of a *Toxascaris leonina* egg from a tiger. A. One cell stage typically found in fresh fecal specimens with shell layers indicated by opposed arrow heads. B. Morula stage. C. Early vermiform embryo. D. Infective larva in egg shell. E. Infective larva artificially hatched *in vitro*. Hatching of ascarid eggs does not normally occur until they have been ingested by a host (x425).

scattered about them was more efficient than trying to identify all objects in the microscopic field. I still believe this but, out of respect for the opinions of others, have included examples of the more common pseudoparasites in Figure 12-3.

In acquiring diagnostic skill, one must not be content with merely comparing general impressions of the microscopic image with a set of pictures in a book. Persons basing their diagnoses on superficial appearances often confuse *Toxascaris* eggs with *Isospora canis* cysts less than half as large. In Figure 12-6, a *T. leonina* egg x425 and an *Isospora canis* oocyst x1000 have been placed side by side to show how easily this mistake could be made. The matter may be resolved with an ocular micrometer or, more simply, by observing whether a distinct lipid layer (Fig. 12-4A) is present (*Toxascaris*) or absent (*Isospora*).

Fecal specimens for parasitological examination should be fresh and not contaminated

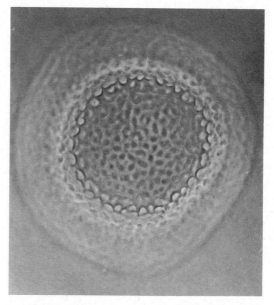

Figure 12–5. Surface of a *Toxocara canis* egg cleared in Berlese solution to show the distinctive dimpled pattern of the protein layer (phase contrast x660).

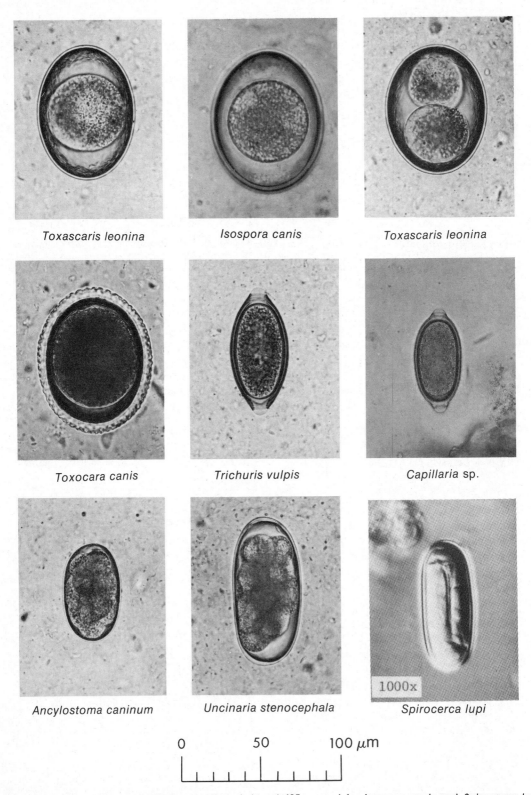

Figure 12–6. Eggs of some nematode parasites of dogs (x425, except for *Isospora canis* and *Spirocerca lupi*). *Toxascaris leonina* produces a colorless, subspherical to ellipsoidal egg shell with a smooth shell surface and a prominent lipid layer containing one or sometimes two cells in fresh specimens. *Isospora canis*, a coccidian oocyst and not a nematode egg, is portrayed here x1000 to illustrate how easily it might be confused with *T. leonina* unless the difference in size or the absence of a lipid layer is noticed. *Toxocara canis* produces a yellowish brown, subspherical egg with a uniformly pitted shell surrounding a single cell in fresh specimens.

Legend continued on opposite page.

with soil or bedding. If feces are allowed to stand, single cells develop into morulae, larvae hatch, and oocysts begin to sporulate. Identification of developmental stages other than those usually encountered is possible but requires greater skill. Contamination with soil or bedding is likely to lead to confusion because the specimen may be invaded by free-living nematodes and arthropods, Starting, on the other hand, with a fresh, uncontaminated specimen, one may frequently reach a more specific identification by observing the subsequent development in fecal culture.

PARASITES OF DOGS

The common internal parasitisms of dogs can usually be diagnosed on the basis of the microscopic appearance of eggs, cysts, or larvae found in the feces. Micrometry or fecal culture may be necessary when more specific identification is required than can be accomplished on the basis of microscopic appearance alone.

Nematode Eggs

The shell proper of the nematode egg is a smooth, homogeneous, transparent capsule of chitin (Fig. 12-4A). Its external surface is covered with a layer of protein that may be smooth (Fig. 12-4), rough (*Parascaris*, Fig. 12-32), or uniformly and distinctively patterned (Fig. 12-5). An internal lipid layer (vitelline membrane) and a narrow fluid-filled space separate the capsule from its contained embryo. Eggs of some nematode parasites of dogs are shown in Figures 12-6 and 12-7.

The stage of embryonic developent of eggs found in fresh fecal specimens varies among nematode species and thus provides us with a diagnostic criterion. In fresh fecal specimens *Toxacara*, *Toxascaris*, *Trichuris*, and *Capillaria* eggs contain a single cell; the *Ancylos-*

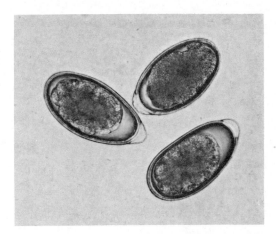

Figure 12–7. *Gnathostoma spinigerum* from a dog (x425). This dog belonged to a pet shop owner who occasionally fed it defunct tropical fish. Probably, infection with this exotic parasite was acquired by eating one of these fish.

toma or *Uncinaria* embryo has already segmented to produce a morula; many spirurid eggs contain first stage larvae; and *Strongyloides* and *Filaroides* have already hatched and appear in the feces as first stage larvae. The development of a typical nematode egg is portrayed in Figure 12-4.

Unfortunately, the range of sizes of eggs, cysts, and larvae precludes adoption of one standard magnification for all. In the following pages, most of the nematode eggs are represented x425, most protozoan cysts x1000, and nematode larvae either x250 or x425. The scale at the bottom of Figs. 12-6, 12-20, 12-23, and 12-32 corresponds to magnification x425.

Nematode Larvae

If the canine fecal sample is fresh and not contaminated with soil or extraneous organic material, larvae found swimming about the microscopic field may be either *Strongyloides*

Figure 12–6 (Continued). *Trichuris vulpis* and *Capillaria* spp. eggs are lemon-shaped and have bipolar plugs. *Trichuris vulpis* eggs average more than 75 μm whereas those of *Capillaria* spp. average less than 75 μm in length. Recovery of *C. aerophila* eggs from respiratory mucus by tracheal swab requires general anesthesia. The presence of *C. plica* eggs in fresh fecal specimens represents contamination with urine. Urine specimens may also contain eggs of *Dioctophyme renale* (no photomicrograph available) but these have much larger and rougher shells than do the eggs of *C. plica*. *Ancylostoma* and *Uncinaria* eggs have a smooth, clear, colorless, ellipsoidal shell and contain an embryo in the morula stage of development. *Ancylostoma caninum* eggs average under 65 μm, whereas *Uncinaria stenocephala* eggs average more than 70 μm in length. Mixed infection with these two common species is easily recognized by the simultaneous presence of eggs of disparate size. De Faria (1910), who first described *A. braziliense*, gave the dimensions of that egg as 65 by 32 μm. *Caution:* the eggs of strongyle parasites of domestic herbivores frequently find their way into dog feces through coprophagy and may be confused with hookworm eggs. Eggs of the order Spirurida are usually smooth-walled and contain a larva. The most important of these, *Spirocerca lupi*, produces very small (30 by 12 μm), cylindrical eggs with rounded ends.

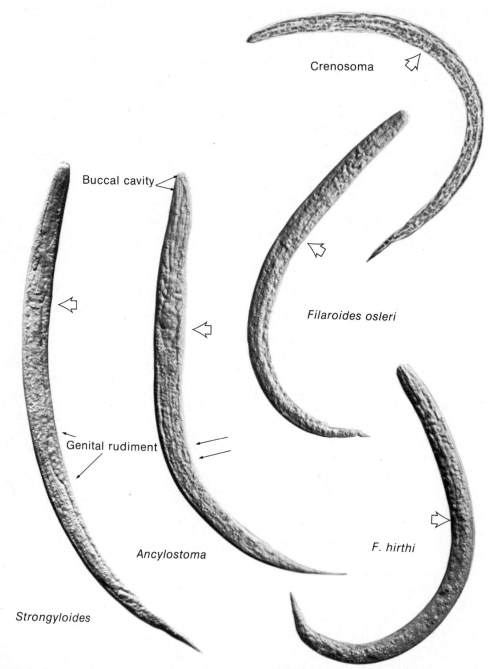

Figure 12–8. First stage larvae of some nematode parasites of dogs. *Crenosoma* and *Filaroides* spp. are metastrongyloid lungworms and usually undergo no development in fecal cultures. *Strongyloides* and *Ancylostoma* first stage larvae can be distinguished by differences in the relative sizes of their genital rudiments and relative lengths of their buccal cavities. In fecal cultures, both *Strongyloides* and *Ancylostoma* develop to the infective stage (see Fig. 12–9).

stercoralis or one of the following metastrongyloids: *Filaroides osleri*, *F. hirthi*, *Crenosoma* sp., or *Angiostrongylus vasorum*. The esophagus of metastrongyloid larvae is longer than the rhabditiform esophagus of the first stage *Strongyloides* larva and the tail may have a slight kink as in *Filaroides* or a dorsal spine as in *Angiostrongylus*, whereas the tail of the *Strongyloides* and *Crenosoma* first stage larva taper smoothly to a point (Fig. 12-8).

If the sample is stale, hookworm larvae may have developed and hatched. These somewhat resemble *Strongyloides* rhabditiform larvae but have a longer buccal capsule and smaller genital rudiment (Fig. 12-8). Should doubt remain, culture the feces for the development of infective stages. The infective sheathed third stage larvae of hookworms do not begin to appear until after five to seven days incubation at room temperature, whereas homogonic *Strongyloides* filariform larvae appear as early as 24 to 36 hours, and heterogonic filariform larvae appear in about four days. *Strongyloides* filariform larvae are slender, have a very long esophagus, and the tip of their tail appears notched or truncated (Fig. 12-9). If the specimen is contaminated with soil or extraneous organic material, free-living nematodes and their larvae may confuse the issue. Under such circumstances, the best course is to obtain a fresh sample directly from the dog's rectum.

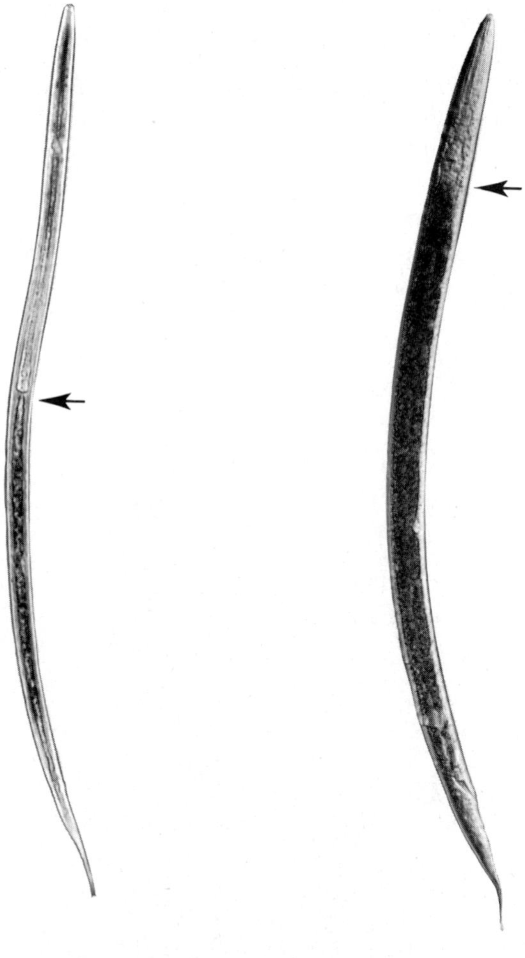

Strongyloides   *Ancylostoma*

Figure 12–9. Third stage infective larvae of *Strongyloides* and *Ancylostoma*. *Strongyloides* infective larvae have a very long esophagus and the tip of the tail appears to be "notched" (actually, it is composed of four small projections of the double lateral alae). *Ancylostoma* infective larvae are usually enclosed in the uncast cuticle ("sheath") of the second stage, here seen extending slightly beyond the tail of the third stage.

Tapeworm Segments

Detached segments of eucestode tapeworms are often found crawling about on the perineum or fresh feces of infected dogs (and cats). Hand lens inspection permits identification for practical purposes. Owners sometimes submit for identification shriveled objects that are actually dehydrated tapeworm segments (Fig. 12-10A). If these are soaked in water, they will usually regain their familiar appearance (Fig. 12-10B). Should doubt remain, the "reconstituted" segment may be squashed between two microscope slides bound together with adhesive tape. The segment may then be identified by the microscopic appearance of its eggs and such organs (e.g., genital pore, uterine diverticulae or capsules, paruterine organ) as may persist in gravid segments of various species. Taeniid segments are roughly rectangular with a single, lateral genital pore, and contain taeniid eggs (Figs. 5-9, 12-11 and 12-14A). *Dipylidium* segments are shaped somewhat like cucumber seeds, have a genital pore on each lateral margin, and contain eggs clustered in packets (uterine capsules) (Figs. 12-12 and 12-14D). *Mesocestoides* segments have a dorsal genital pore and eggs massed in a central, thick-walled paruterine organ (Fig. 12-13).

Eucestode Eggs

Taeniid eggs are spherical or subglobular with a radially striated embryophore (a shell-like covering) and contain an embryo (oncosphere or hexacanth embryo) with three pairs of hooks (Figs. 5-9 and 12-14A). If the hooks are not clearly visible, they may sometimes be demonstrated by pressing a needlepoint on the coverslip to break the embryophore (Figs. 12-14B and 12-14C). The eggs of *Echinococcus* are a serious menace to human health and cannot be distinguished from those of *Taenia* and *Multiceps*. In *Echinococcus* endemic areas, therefore, the discovery of taeniid eggs in canine fecal samples demands prompt anthelmintic therapy and caution in the handling and disposal of feces. The eggs of Dipylidiidae are spherical or subspherical with an unstriated embryophore, contain an oncosphere, and are enveloped in a uterine capsule. In *Dipylidium*

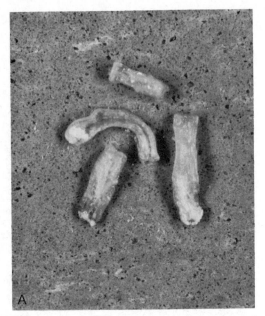

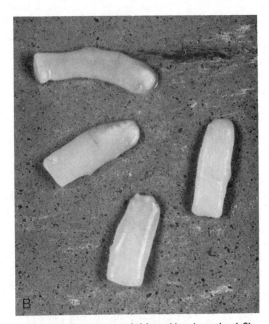

Figure 12–10. A. Dehydrated taeniid segments. B. Same segments after an overnight soaking in water (x2).

there may be up to 29 eggs per capsule (Fig. 12-14D); in *Joyeuxiella* and *Diplopylidium* there is only one egg per uterine capsule. The eggs of *Mesocestoides* are oval and thin-shelled and contain an oncosphere.

Diphyllobothriid Eggs

Diphyllobothriid eggs are discharged continuously through the uterine pores of many segments along the body of the worm and hence are passed independently of any detached segment. *Diphyllobothrium* eggs are oval with an operculum at one pole and a small button at the other (Fig. 12-15A).

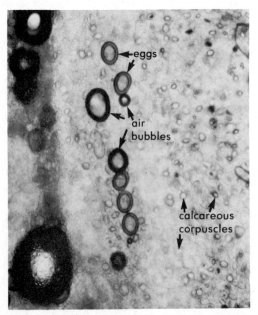

Figure 12–11. Taeniid segment in squash preparation (x150).

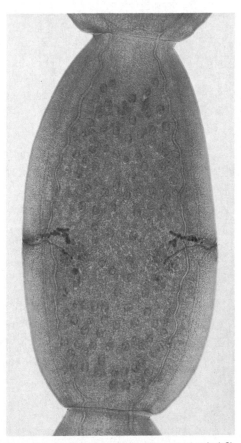

Figure 12–12. *Dipylidium caninum* segments (x2).

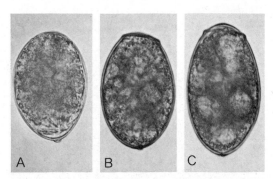

Figure 12–15. Operculate eggs (x425). A. *Diphyllobothrium* egg. B. and C. Unidentified eggs; their prominent opercula suggest that, except for their small size, these might be *Paragonimus* eggs (see Fig. 12–17). This figure illustrates the difficulty of distinguishing *Diphyllobothrium* eggs from those of certain trematodes.

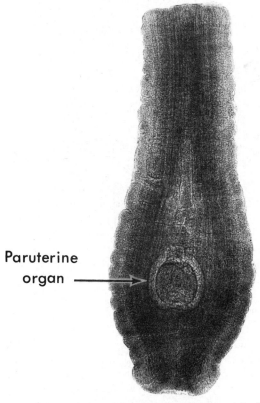

Paruterine organ ———→

Figure 12–13. *Mesocestoides* sp. gravid segment; fresh, unrelaxed, and viewed with transmitted light (x35).

Acanthocephalan Eggs

Acanthocephalan eggs have a thick outer and thinner inner shell enclosing an embryo called an acanthor. The external surface of the egg of *Macracanthorhynchus* is elegantly patterned (Fig. 12-16).

Trematode Eggs

Eggs of most digenetic trematodes have an operculum at one pole and contain an embryo whose stage of development varies with the species in question (Fig. 12-17). Schistosome eggs, on the other hand, lack an operculum and contain a fully developed miracidium that hatches shortly after the egg comes in contact with water. Many, but not all, schistosome eggs have a sharp spine. If a dog has fed recently upon trematode-infected tissues such as sheep liver infected with *Dicrocoelium* or *Fasciola*, or rabbit entrails in-

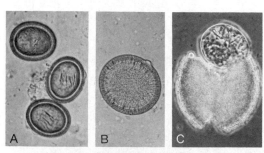

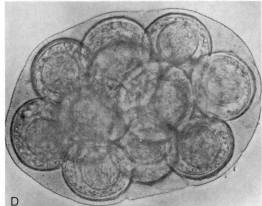

Figure 12–14. Eucestode eggs. A. Three taeniid eggs. B. Taeniid egg, hooks not visible. C. Oncosphere emerging from the broken embryophore of the taeniid egg at left. D. *Dipylidium* egg capsule (x380).

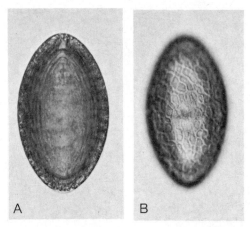

Figure 12–16. *Macracanthorhynchus ingens* (Acanthocephala) egg (x425). A. Acanthor in focus. B. Surface of shell in focus.

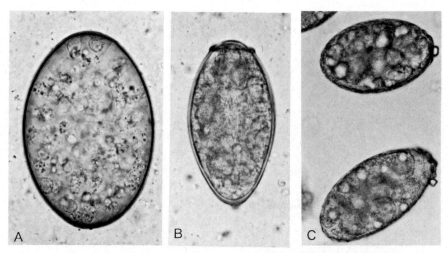

Figure 12–17. Trematode eggs (x425). A. *Alaria* sp. B. *Paragonimus kellicotti*. C. *Nanophyetus salmincola*.

fected with *Hasstilesia*, the presence of myriads of trematode eggs in its fecal specimen may lead to misdiagnosis.

Coccidian Oocysts and Sporocysts

Isospora. *Isospora* spp. oocysts have colorless, ovoid or ellipsoidal, smooth-surfaced walls without micropyle or polar cap, and contain a single sporont when passed in the feces of the host (Fig. 12-6). Sporulation occurs in two to four days at room temperature. The fully sporulated *Isospora* oocyst then contains two sporocysts, each of which contains four sporozoites (Fig. 12-18A). Because dogs tend to be coprophagic, oocysts of various other coccidia, especially *Eimeria* spp. of herbivores, are very common pseudoparasites

in dog feces. If the *Eimeria* spp. in question have micropyles, polar caps, or other distinguishing features, they present no diagnostic problem (Fig. 12-18B), but a few species are difficult to differentiate from *Isospora* spp. Differentiation of *Eimeria* and *Isospora* may be accomplished by fecal culture for oocyst sporulation. Sporulated *Eimeria* oocysts contain four sporocysts, each of which contains two sporozoites (Fig. 12-18C).

Identification of species of *Isospora* requires micrometry. Oocyst dimensions in μm for four species infecting dogs are as follows: *Isospora canis*, 32-42 x 27-33; *I. ohioensis*, 19-27 x 18-23; *I. burrowsi*, 17-22 x 16-19; *I. heydorni*, 10-13 x 10-13.

Sarcocystis. *Sarcocystis* spp. sporulate within the host and the fragile oocyst wall

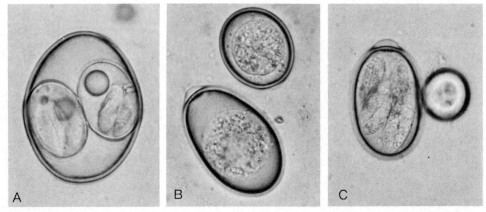

Figure 12–18. Coccidian oocysts (x1000). A. *Isospora canis*, sporulated. B. *Eimeria* spp., one cell stage. C. *Eimeria* sp., sporulated. *Isospora* spp. sporulated oocysts contain two sporocysts, each of which contains four sporozoites. *Eimeria* spp. sporulated oocysts contain four sporocysts, each of which contains two sporozoites. See Figure 12–6. for *Isospora canis* one cell stage.

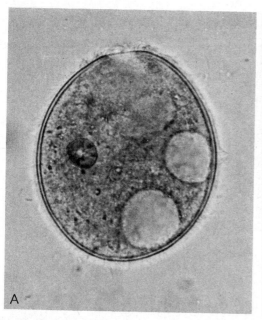
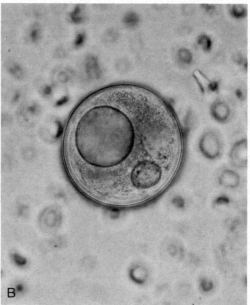

Figure 12–19. *Balantidium coli.* A. Trophozoite (electronic flash photomicrograph of motile ciliate x700). B. Cyst (x425). Trophozoites abound in the large intestine of normal swine, and cysts are passed in their feces. *Balantidium coli* has been incriminated in human colonic disease ranging from mild colitis to an ailment resembling amebic dysentery.

often breaks so that the sporocyst containing four sporozoites is the form usually found in the feces (Fig. 12-22). Sporocysts measure 11-18 x 7-13 μm but it is not possible to distinguish species of *Sarcocystis* by micrometry of sporocysts (see Table 3-1).

Amoebas

Entamoeba histolytica, a serious human pathogen, may appear in canine fecal specimens as either trophozoite or cyst. The trophozoites are more likely to be encountered in diarrheal feces and the cysts in formed fecal specimens. Trophozoites of the large race of *Entamoeba histolytica* are 10 to 30 μm across and their nuclei have marginated chromatin and a small central endosome. *Entamoeba histolytica* trophozoites display ameboid movement and often ingest erythrocytes. The mature cysts are 10 to 20 μm in diameter and contain four nuclei.

Entamoeba coli trophozoites are 20 to 30 μm in diameter; their nuclei have a relatively large eccentric endosome. Erythrocytes are not found in *E. coli* trophozoites. As many as eight nuclei may be counted in *E. coli* cysts.

Entamoeba gingivalis, a parasite of the oral cavity, infects both man and dog. Only trophozoites, ranging in size from 5 to 35 μm, are found in oral scrapings.

Flagellates

Giardia sp. trophozoites are less than 21 μm long, bilaterally symmetrical, and pear-shaped. Two nuclei with large central endosomes look like a pair of eyes (Fig. 12-35). *Giardia* cysts are less than 12 μm long, are ellipsoidal, and contain four nuclei.

Trichomonas and related genera do not form cysts and occur in feces (usually diarrheal) only as mononucleate trophozoites.

Ciliates

Balantidium coli. *Balantidium coli* trophozoites are ovoid with a cytostome at one end; measure 25 to 150 μm in diameter; contain one macronucleus and one micronucleus, two contractile vacuoles, and inclusions; and are covered with rows of cilia (Fig. 12-19A). Cysts are spherical or ovoid, measure 40 to 60 μm in diameter, and have a wall consisting of two membranes (Fig. 12-19B).

PARASITES OF CATS

Cats share a few parasites (e.g., *Toxascaris leonina, Capillaria aerophila, Dipylidium caninum, Paragonimus kellicotti*) with dogs, and cross-infections with others may occur on rare occasions. However, the commonest cat parasites (Figs. 12-20, 12-21, and 12-22) are

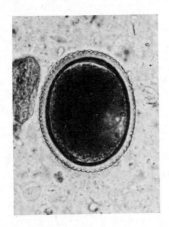
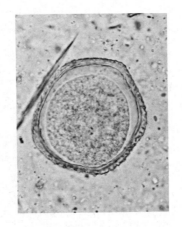
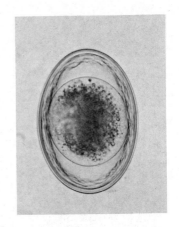

Toxocara cati   *T. cati* (infertile)   *Toxascaris leonina*

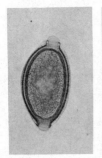
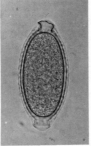
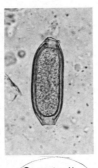
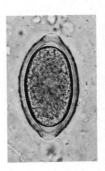

C. aerophila   *C. feliscati*   *C. putorii*   *Trichuris* spp.

Capillaria spp.

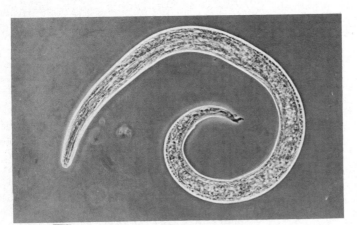
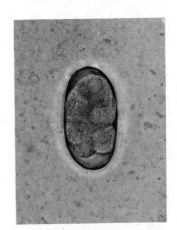

Aelurostrongylus abstrusus   *Ancylostoma tubaeforme*

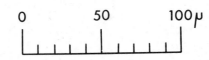

0   50   100μ

Figure 12–20 *See legend on opposite page*

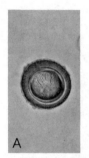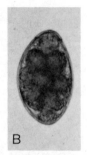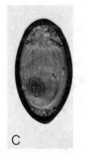

Figure 12–21. Eggs of cat platyhelminths. A. *Hydatigera taeniaeformis.* This taeniid cestode egg has a radially striated embryophore and contains a fully developed oncosphere. B. *Spirometra mansonoides.* This diphyllobothriid cestode egg has an operculate capsule and contains an undeveloped embryo. C. *Platynosomum fastosum.* This dicrocoeliid trematode egg also has an operculate capsule but contains a fully developed miracidium.

different species of the genera found in dogs (e.g., *Toxocara cati, Ancylostoma tubaeforme, Isospora felis).* Pseudoparasitism in cats is usually the result of predation rather than coprophagy. For example, the eggs of *Capillaria hepatica* accumulate in infected rodent livers and may be found in the feces of a cat that has eaten such a rodent (Fig. 14-89). Feline *Trichuris* infection often excites lively debate because its rare appearances in North American cats violate a time-honored belief that it does not exist at all. In any case, it is certainly of little practical importance aside from its tendency to complicate the differential diagnosis of pulmonary and vesical capillariasis.

Isospora, Hammondia, Besnoitia, and *Toxoplasma*

Until about fifteen years ago, it was thought that cats and dogs shared three species of coccidia, *Isospora felis, I. rivolta,* and *I. bigemina.* Two "races" of *I. bigemina* were

supposed to exist: a smaller one shed as unsporulated oocysts and a slightly larger one shed as sporulated oocysts. Gradually, it has developed that the species of *Isospora* infecting cats are entirely distinct from those infecting dogs, that the larger, sporulated oocyst of *I. bigemina* represents a growing list of species of the elusive *Sarcocystis,* and that the smaller, unsporulated oocyst of *I. bigemina* represents *Toxoplasma gondii* and at least two other genera of coccidians. With this has come the revelation that the life cycles of cat and dog coccidia involve either facultative or obligatory intermediate hosts (see Chapter 3). Careful micrometry affords differentiation of some species of oocysts but, unfortunately, the most important species, *Toxoplasma,* remains confounded with *Hammondia.* Until this dilemma is resolved, oocysts smaller than 14 μm should be regarded as *Toxoplasma,* just to be on the safe side (Fig. 12-22).

Species	Oocyst Dimensions (μm)
Isospora felis	38-51 x 27-39
I. rivolta	21-28 x 18-23
Besnoitia besnoiti	14-16 x 12-14
B. darlingi	11-13 x 11-13
B. wallacei	16-19 x 10-13
Toxoplasma gondii	11-13 x 9-11
Hammondia hammondi	11-13 x 10-12

Sarcocystis. Sarcocystis sporulates within the host and the fragile oocyst wall often breaks. Therefore, the sporocyst measuring 9-12 x 7-12 μm and containing four sporozoites is the form usually found in the feces (Fig. 12-22). It is not possible to distinguish species of *Sarcocystis* by micrometry (see Table 3-1).

Cryptosporidium. The oocysts of *Cryptosporidium* are best floated in saturated sucrose

---

Figure 12–20. Nematode parasites of cats. *Toxocara cati* eggs are smaller and more delicate than *T. canis* eggs (Fig. 12–6). *Toxascaris leonina* is a parasite of both cats and dogs. The egg in this figure came from a tiger. *Capillaria* spp. eggs may be those of *C. aerophila* in the lungs, *C. feliscati* or *C. plica* in the urinary bladder, or *C. putorii* in the stomach and small intestine. Recovery of eggs from respiratory mucus or urine therefore aids in identification. *Capillaria hepatica* (Fig. 14-89) is a common pseudoparasite of cats when this parasite is endemic in the local rodent population. *Trichuris* spp. are rare parasites of North American cats. The *Trichuris* egg at left was observed in the feces of a cat from Puerto Rico that was found on necropsy examination to contain three female *Trichuris* sp. worms. The egg at its right, from a New York State cat, was presumptively identified as *Trichuris* sp. because of its close resemblance (except for smaller size) to *Trichuris vulpis* (Fig. 12–6). *Aelurostrongylus abstrusus* larvae may be identified by their curiously shaped tail. *Ancylostoma tubaeforme, A. braziliense,* and *Uncinaria stenocephala* all produce typical strongyle eggs. *Strongyloides* spp. rhabditiform larvae (Fig. 12–8) and *Trichinella spiralis* prelarvae and defunct adults are sometimes found in the feces of cats.

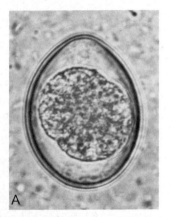
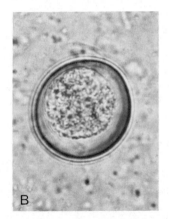
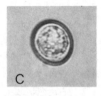
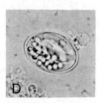

Figure 12–22. Coccidian cysts of cats (×1000). A. *Isospora felis.* B. *I. rivolta.* C. *Toxoplasma gondii.* D. *Sarcocystis* sp. *Sarcocystis* sporocysts released by rupture of the oocyst wall are only slightly larger than *T. gondii* but are ovoid rather than subspherical and contain four sporozoites. *Sarcocystis* sp. photomicrograph from Dubey, J. P.: J. Am. Vet. Med. Assoc., *162* (10), 876, 1973.

solution. Because they are a mere 5 μm in diameter, slides must be scanned at high dry magnification. *Cryptosporidium* oocysts tend to lie in the focal plane immediately below the coverslip.

PARASITES OF RUMINANTS

The Strongyle Egg

Females of the superfamilies Strongyloidea, Trichostrongyloidea, and Ancylostomatoidea lay rather thin-walled ellipsoidal eggs containing an embryo in the morula stage of development, and this same stage is found in the host's feces. In this text, such eggs are collectively referred to as "strongyle" eggs because that is what most clinicians and diagnostic parasitologists call them. The eggs of Metastrongyloidea are also thin-walled and ellipsoidal but the developmental stage deposited in the host's tissues by different species of female metastrongyloids varies from a single cell (e.g., *Muellerius*) to a first stage larva that is ready to hatch (e.g., *Filaroides*). Even those that are laid in the single cell stage develop to the first stage and may have hatched by the time they appear in the feces. Therefore, one finds either larvated eggs (e.g., *Metastrongylus*) or first stage larvae in the feces of hosts with patent metastrongyloid infections.

A Diagnostic Dilemma

With a few exceptions, the generic identity of individual strongyle eggs cannot reliably be established by microscopic inspection or by micrometry (Fig. 12-23). *Nematodirus* eggs stand out because of their large size and *Bunostomum* eggs have sticky surfaces that accumulate debris, but the rest look very much alike. Investigators working with cultures reared from identified female worms develop considerable skill in differentiating strongyle eggs from nuances of color, shape, and shell thickness but, for practical purposes, it is usually necessary to resort to fecal culture or necropsy to obtain an accurate diagnosis. An ingenious stochastic technique involving the measurement of at least 100 eggs permitted species identification of egg populations or, expressed another way, permitted estimation of the relative abundances of species in mixed infections (Cunliffe and Crofton, 1953). This technique is limited in application to the eight species of sheep nematodes studied and, in principle, is strictly valid only on a geographical basis. It is mentioned here in the hope that the basic principles might find fruitful application elsewhere and to illustrate the nature of the diagnostic dilemma posed by strongyle eggs.

Necropsy of a few animals to establish an accurate diagnosis is justifiable if the unit value of the animal is sufficiently low or the herd sufficiently large. Owners of valuable animals are understandably reluctant to sacrifice them, however, and recourse must be had to larval identification. Whenever the situation is too urgent to afford the necessary delay of culturing, the clinical signs should be clear enough to suggest a reasonably accurate diagnosis.

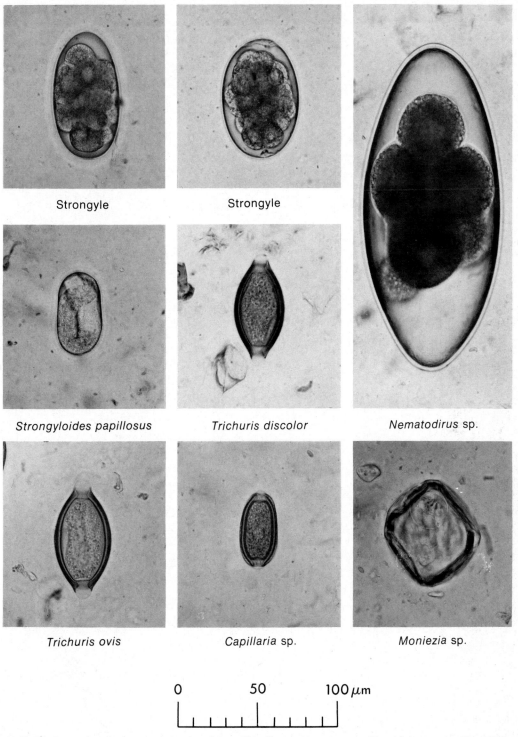

Strongyle

Strongyle

Strongyloides papillosus

Trichuris discolor

Nematodirus sp.

Trichuris ovis

Capillaria sp.

Moniezia sp.

0   50   100 μm

Figure 12–23. Eggs of some common ruminant parasites. Strongyle eggs are ellipsoidal, are smooth-walled, and contain a morula. *Nematodirus* spp. eggs are very large but some species are considerably smaller than the one shown here. *Marshallagia marshalli* eggs (not shown) are also very large but differ from *Nematodirus* eggs in having more parallel sides and less pointed poles. *Strongyloides papillosus* eggs are slightly smaller than strongyle eggs and contain a rhabditiform larva in fresh fecal specimens. On incubation, the larvae soon hatch and develop into infective filariform larvae (Fig. 12–24) or free-living adult males and females, predominantly the latter. *Trichuris* spp. eggs of ruminants are more than 60 μm long; those of *Capillaria* spp. are less than 60 μm long. *Moniezia* spp. eggs contain a pear-shaped embryophore containing an oncosphere. *Thysanosoma* spp. eggs (not shown here) are grouped in uterine capsules.

Identification of Strongyle Infective Larvae

Identification of third stage infective larvae in cultured ruminant feces is challenging but not formidable. Usually, two or more genera are present and one can best determine just how many there are by scanning the slide at low power and mentally grouping those of similar appearance. Certain species stand out from the crowd. For example, *Strongyloides* larvae are more slender than any of the others, lack a sheath, and have a long, cylindrical esophagus and truncated tail. Two sizes, of which the larger is "standard," are

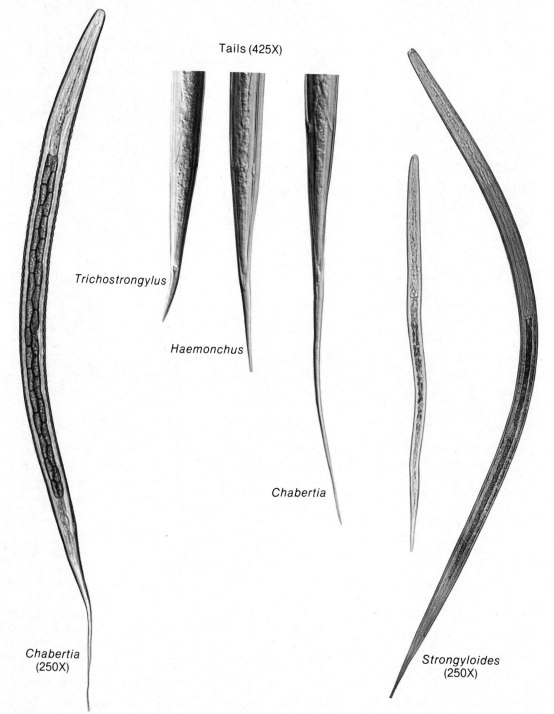

Tails (425X)

Trichostrongylus

Haemonchus

Chabertia

Chabertia (250X)

Strongyloides (250X)

Figure 12–24. Infective, third stage larvae of nematode parasites of sheep. Both large and small *Strongyloides* infective larvae are represented at the same magnification.

| Tricho-strongylus | Oster-tagia | Buno-stomum | Haem-onchus | Cooperia | Oesopha-gostomum |

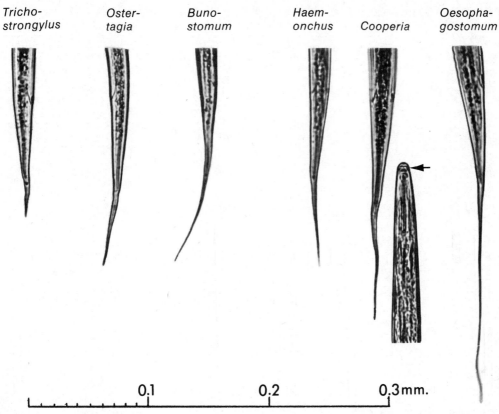

0.1   0.2   0.3 mm.

Figure 12–25. Tails of infective, third stage larvae of nematode parasites of cattle and the anterior end of a *Cooperia* larva showing the "conspicuous oval bodies" (arrow) which represent optical cross-sections of a bundle of fibers surrounding the buccal capsule (x350). Photomicrographs from J. H. Whitlock, 1960.

portrayed in Figure 12-24. I have encountered both sizes in a single culture. Similarly, *Bunostomum* spp. are distinguished from other sheathed strongyle larvae by their smaller size. Other genera of sheathed larvae may be grouped according to the length of their caudal sheath extension (the extension of the sheath beyond the tip of the larva's tail): Short, *Trichostrongylus* and *Ostertagia;* medium, *Haemonchus* and *Cooperia;* and long, *Oesophagostomum* and *Chabertia,* as illustrated in Figures 12-24 and 12-25. Within these groupings, further identification depends on micrometry and observation of such morphological details as the caudal tubercles of *Trichostrongylus,* the "oval bodies" of *Cooperia,* and the number and shape of the intestinal cells of *Oesophagostomum* and *Chabertia.* The odd larva may defy identification but accurate diagnosis of the predominating genera in a culture is not a difficult task. Proceed as follows:

Place a drop of larval suspension on a microscope slide. Relax the larvae by gentle warming or by adding a drop of Lugol's solution (5 grams iodine crystals and 10 grams potassium iodide in 100 ml. distilled water). Ring the coverslip with petroleum jelly for support and thus prevent distortion of the larvae. Avoid higher magnifications at first but instead scan the slide under low power to get an impression of how many different kinds of larva are present. Then seek representatives of each kind, examine these under higher power, and take whatever measurements may be necessary for generic or specific diagnosis. The data of Table 12-1 are taken from the works of Dikmans and Andrews (1933, sheep) and Keith (1953, cattle). The number of intestinal cells is 16 except as otherwise noted. Taxa grouped with braces are similar in appearance and require more care for their differentiation than comparisons among groups.

Other Nematodes

Eggs of the following ruminant nematodes are not illustrated in Fig. 12-23: *Toxocara vitulorum* (parasite of cattle) eggs are subglob-

Table 12–1 TABLE OF MEASUREMENTS OF INFECTIVE THIRD STAGE LARVAE OF STRONGYLES INFECTING SHEEP AND CATTLE

Genus (Sensu Latu)	Measurements (Microns)			Special Morphological Features
	Overall	Tail of Sheath*	Extension of Sheath†	
Strongyloides				
sheep	574–710		sheath	Length of esophagus at least ⅓ length
cattle	524–678		absent	of body, caudal extremity of larva truncated (Fig. 11–21)
Trichostrongylus				
sheep	622–796	76–118	21–40	Tiny tubercles on tip of tail
cattle	619–762	83–107	25–39	
Ostertagia				
sheep	797–910	92–130	30–60	
cattle	784–928	126–170	55–75	
Haemonchus				
sheep	650–751	119–146	65–78	Sheath kinked at tip of tail; anterior
cattle	749–866	158–193	87–119	end tapers
Cooperia oncophora				
sheep	804–924	124–150	62–82	Two conspicuous oval bodies at ante-
cattle	809–976	146–190	79–111	rior end of esophagus
Cooperia spp.				
sheep	711–850	97–122	39–52	Two conspicuous oval bodies at ante-
cattle	666–866	109–142	47–71	rior end of esophagus
Nematodirus				
sheep	922–1118	310–350	250–290	Unlikely to be encountered in cultures
cattle	1095–1142	296–347	207–266	less than two weeks old; forked tail with rodlike process, intestine has 8 cells
Bunostomum				
sheep	514–678	153–183	85–115	Small size, long tail sheath
cattle	500–583	129–158	59–83	
Oseophagostomum				
sheep	771–923	193–235	125–160	16–24 triangular intestinal cells
cattle	726–857	209–257	134–182	
Chabertia				
sheep	710–789	175–220	110–150	24–32 rectangular intestinal cells

*Anus to tip of sheath.
†Tip of larva to tip of sheath.

ular with a uniformly pitted surface and one cell. *Note:* Patent *Ascaris suum* infections are occasionally reported from sheep and cattle. *Ascaris suum* eggs (Fig. 12-34) are easy to distinguish from those of *Toxocara vitulorum*. *Gongylonema* eggs are thick-walled, have bipolar opercula, and contain vermiform embryos. *Skrjabinema ovis* eggs are typical pinworm eggs with one side slightly flattened.

Lungworm Larvae. *Dictyocaulus viviparus* is the only lung nematode of cattle. *Dictyocaulus filaria*, *Protostrongylus rufescens*, and *Muellerius capillaris* are common lung nematodes of sheep and goats in North America. Differential diagnosis is based on morphological features of the first stage larvae found in the host's feces (Fig. 12-26). *Dictyocaulus* spp.

larvae are tough enough to be countable by the Cornell-McMaster egg counting technique, but the counting should be done promptly to avoid osmotic shriveling of the larvae. For sensitive qualitative diagnosis of lungworm infections, the Baermann is the technique of choice.

Trematode Eggs

Trematode eggs may fail to float in the concentrations of sugar solutions ordinarily used. They are best concentrated by washing feces through sieves to remove coarse debris, then centrifuging the washings. The eggs will be found in the sediment. The operculum of trematode eggs is sometimes difficult to see.

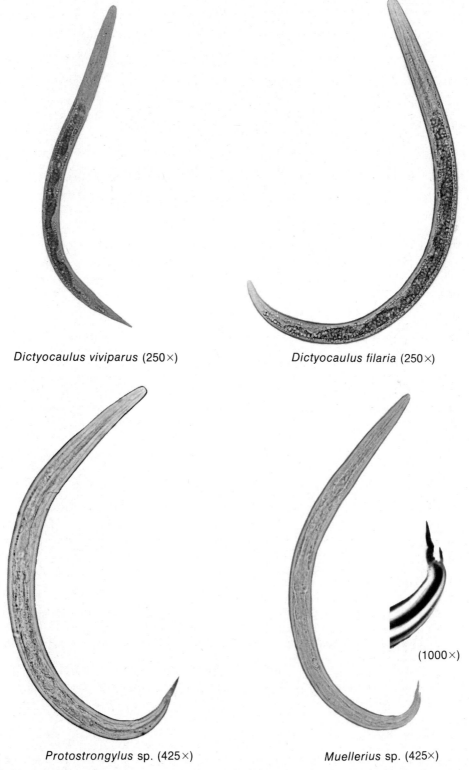

Dictyocaulus viviparus (250×)

Dictyocaulus filaria (250×)

Protostrongylus sp. (425×)

Muellerius sp. (425×)

(1000×)

Figure 12–26. First stage larvae of ruminant lungworms. *Dictyocaulus viviparus* is the only lungworm of cattle and *D. viviparus* first stage larvae are the only larvae of parasitic nematodes found in fresh cattle dung. Notice the prominent granules. *Dictyocaulus filaria* first stage larvae from sheep are large and have bluntly rounded tails and a "button" at the mouth, and likewise have prominent granules. *Protostrongylus rufescens* larvae are rather stout and have conically tapering tails without spines. *Muellerius capillaris* larvae have a curiously shaped tail with a dorsal spine (inset).

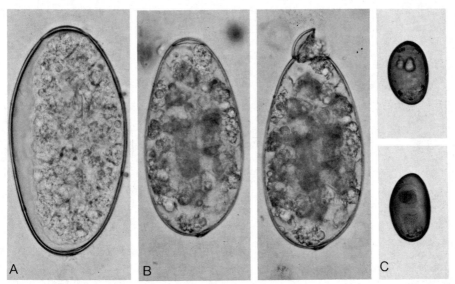

Figure 12–27. Eggs of some trematode parasites of ruminants (x425). A. *Fasciola hepatica.* B. Paramphistominae. C. *Dicrocoelium dendriticum.*

When in doubt, press the coverslip with a pencil point. Usually, the type of operculum found on trematode eggs will pop open under such pressure (Fig. 12-27B).

Fasciola hepatica eggs are large (up to 150 μm) and operculate, and contain a cluster of yolk cells (Fig. 12-27A). *Fasciola gigantica* (Africa, Hawaii, Philippines, and India) are like those of *F. hepatica* but larger (more than 150 μm). Eggs of *Fascioloides magna*, normally a parasite of deer, resemble those of *F. hepatica* but are infrequently found in the feces of infected domestic ruminants because the eggs are trapped in the hepatic cysts containing the adult worms in cattle and because the flukes fail to mature in sheep and goats. Paramphistomatid (rumen fluke) eggs are large and easily confused with those of *Fasciola* spp. (Fig. 12-27B). *Dicrocoelium dendriticum* eggs are small (50 μm), lopsided, and yellowish brown, and contain a miracidium (Fig. 12-27C). *Eurytrema pancreaticum* (Far East) eggs resemble those of *Dicrocoelium dendriticum.* Schistosome eggs lack an operculum, contain a fully developed miracidium, and are armed with a spine.

Coccidia of Ruminants

Oocysts of *Eimeria* spp. are often found in considerable numbers in the feces of healthy ruminants. Even experimental lambs raised on wire become infected with coccidia. Despite their frequent occurrence in healthy animals, coccidia are quite capable of causing serious disease in cattle, sheep, and goats. At times, severe disease signs appear before oocysts are shed in the feces. Diagnosis of clinical coccidiosis must be based not only on identification of the oocysts in the feces (Figs. 12-28 and 12-29) but also on consideration of the case history and clinical signs.

Cryptosporidium. The oocysts are best concentrated by floatation in saturated sucrose solution. Because they are a mere 5 μm in diameter, the slide must be scanned under high dry magnification. *Cryptosporidium* oocysts tend to lie in the focal plane immediately below the coverslip.

PARASITES OF HORSES

The intestinal parasites of horses form a unique group. There is only one coccidian species *Eimeria leuckarti* (Fig. 12-30), three species of tapeworms all belonging to the family Anoplocephalidae (Fig. 12-31), and a group of nematodes (Fig. 12-32) that includes one ascarid, two pinworms, one species of *Strongyloides*, three spirurids of the subfamily Habronematinae, and many strongylids. There are no hookworms or whipworms, but 54 species of strongylids more than make up for these deficiencies. The diagnostic dilemma associated with strongyle eggs is thus accentuated in the case of the horse. How-

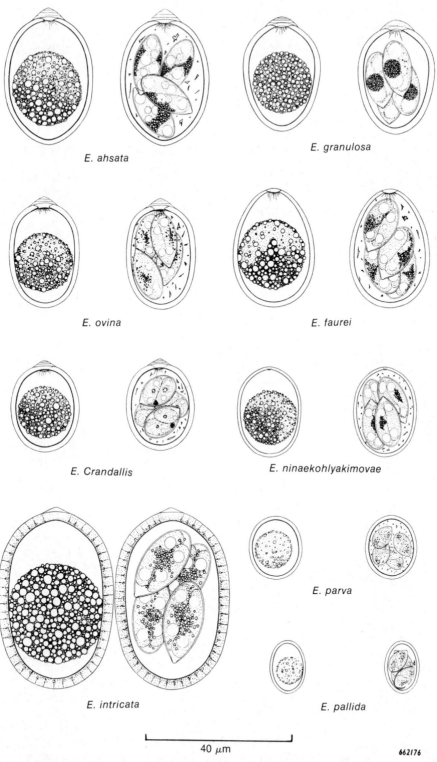

E. ahsata

E. granulosa

E. ovina

E. faurei

E. Crandallis

E. ninaekohlyakimovae

E. intricata

E. parva

E. pallida

40 μm

662176

Figure 12–28. Unsporulated and sporulated oocysts of nine species of *Eimeria* of sheep (x1000). From Joyner *et al.*: Parasitology, *56*, 533, 1966. Crown copyright. Reproduced by permission of the Controller of Her Britannic Majesty's Stationery Office.

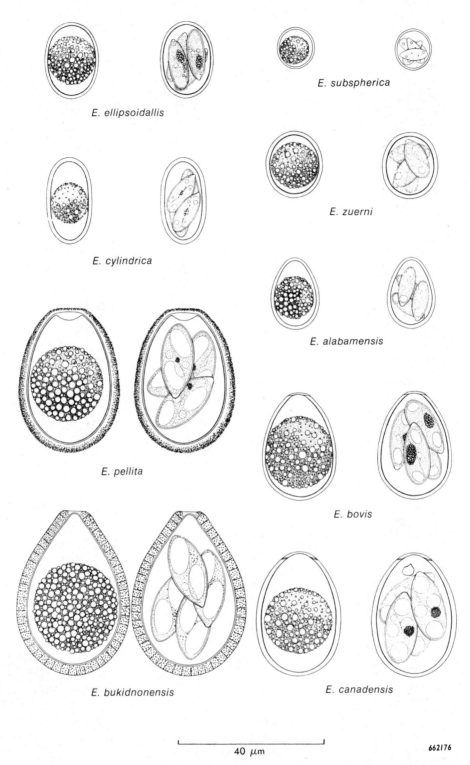

Figure 12–29. Unsporulated and sporulated oocysts of 12 species of *Eimeria* of cattle (x1000). From Joyner *et al.*: Parasitology, *56*, 536, 1966. Crown copyright. Reproduced by permission of the Controller of Her Britannic Majesty's Stationery Office.

Illustration continued on opposite page

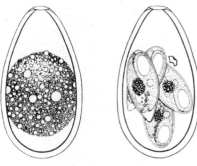

E. auburnensis

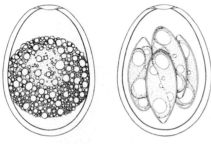

E. wyomingensis

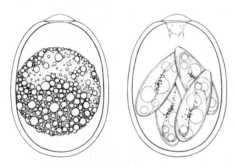

E. brasiliensis

Figure 12–29 Continued

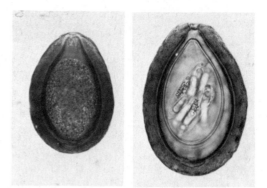

Figure 12–30. Eimeria leuckarti unsporulated (left) and sporulated (right) oocysts (x425).

ever, the major diagnostic categories can be identified by fecal culture and reference to Figure 12-33.

PARASITES OF SWINE

The following nematodes are not represented in Figure 12-34: *Stephanurus dentatus* eggs are large and morulated and are found in urine specimens from infected swine. The last urine voided contains the highest concentration of eggs. *Strongyloides ransomi* eggs resemble those of *S. papillosus* (Fig. 12-23). *Ascarops* and *Physocephalus* produce thick-walled, larvated eggs.

Intestinal protozoa include *Eimeria* spp., *Isospora suis*, *Entamoeba* spp., *Iodamoeba buetschlii*, *Endolimax nana*, *Giardia* spp., other flagellates, and the ciliate *Balantidium coli* (Fig. 12-19).

PARASITES OF LABORATORY ANIMALS

A few of the more common parasites of rodents, rabbits, and primates are represented in Figures 12-35 and 12-36.

Text continued on page 258

Figure 12–31. *Anoplocephala magna* (left) and *A. perfoliata* (right) eggs (x425). The oncospheres are enclosed by pear-shaped embryophores. The egg of *Paranoplocephala mamillana* is only three-fourths as large as these.

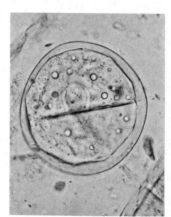

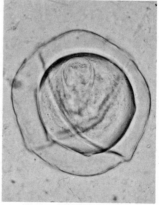

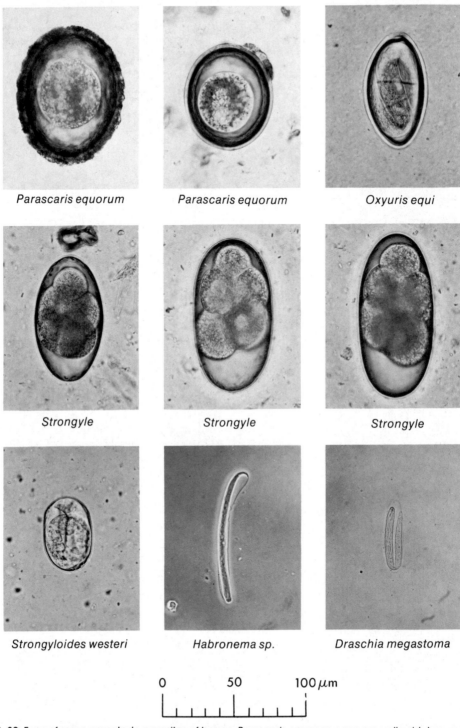

Figure 12–32. Eggs of some nematode parasites of horses. *Parascaris equorum* eggs are yellowish brown with thick, subspherical, rough-surfaced shell walls and contain one cell. Eggs are often found with their external protein layer partially or completely detached. The exposed portions of such shells are smooth and clear. *Oxyuris equi* eggs are more likely to be recovered from anal scrapings than from fecal specimens. The egg shown here was collected by momentarily pressing the adhesive side of a piece of Scotch tape against a horse's anus, then mounted by sticking the tape to a microscope slide. Strongyle eggs present the usual differential diagnostic problem. Recourse may be had to fecal culture and identification of infective third stage larvae (Fig. 12–33). *Strongyloides westeri* eggs are smaller than strongyle eggs and contain a rhabditiform larvae in fresh specimens. *Draschia* and *Habronema* eggs are cigar-shaped and contain a vermiform embryo. Such eggs are difficult to demonstrate in feces. If a technique for antemortem diagnosis of gastric habronemiasis is essential, resort to xenodiagnosis using *Musca domestica* larvae for *D. megastoma* and *H. muscae*, and *Stomoxys calcitrans* larvae for *H. microstoma*.

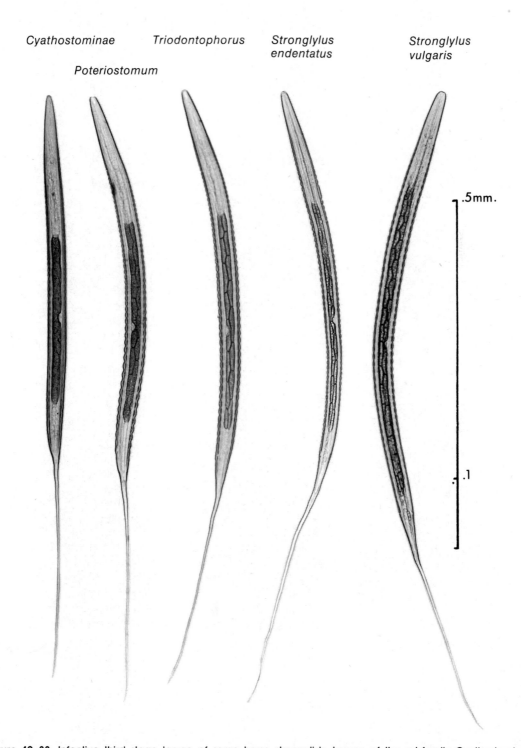

Cyathostominae

Poteriostomum

Triodontophorus

Stronglylus endentatus

Stronglylus vulgaris

.5mm.

.1

Figure 12–33. Infective third stage larvae of some horse strongylids. Larvae of the subfamily Cyathostominae, represented here by *Cyathostomum catinatum,* have 8 intestinal cells. *Gyalocephalus capitatus* (not shown) has 12, *Poteriostomum* has 16, *Triodontophorus* has 18 (but the *T. serratus* larva shown here has only 16), *Strongylus edentatus* has 18 to 20, and *S. vulgaris* has 32 intestinal cells. *Strongylus vulgaris* is easily distinguished from all the rest by its large size and long column of intestinal cells.

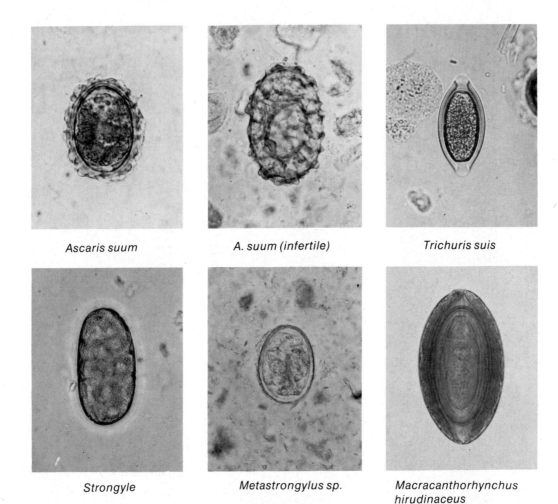

Ascaris suum   A. suum (infertile)   Trichuris suis

Strongyle   Metastrongylus sp.   Macracanthorhynchus hirudinaceus

Figure 12–34. Eggs of some parasites of swine (x425). *Ascaris suum* eggs have a rough, bile stained, external protein layer. Infertile *A. suum* eggs are common. Strongyle eggs may represent infection with *Hyostrongylus rubidus*, *Oesophagostomum* spp. , *Globocephalus urosubulatus*, or *Necator americanus*, but, most commonly, only the first two. *Trichuris suis* are typical of the genus. *Trichuris suis* and *T. trichiura* (human whipworm) are possibly nonspecific. *Metastrongylus* spp. eggs are small and subglobular and contain a larva. *Macracanthorhynchus hirudinaceus* (Acanthocephala) eggs have three concentric, ellipsoidal shells surrounding the acanthor embryo.

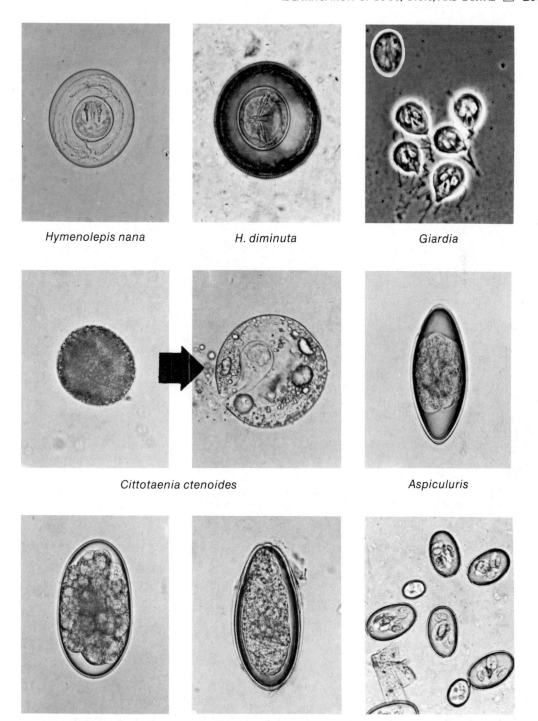

Hymenolepis nana   *H. diminuta*   *Giardia*

Cittotaenia ctenoides   *Aspiculuris*

Obeliscodes cuniculi   *Passalurus ambiguus*   *Eimeria*

Figure 12–35. Common parasites of laboratory mice, rats, and rabbits. For a more comprehensive listing of laboratory animal parasites by host and organ, see Chapter 13. MOUSE AND RAT: *Hymenolepis nana* and *H. diminuta* (Hymenolepidae) are also parasites of man. *Hymenolepis nana* infection in rodent colonies is directly infective to human beings; no intermediate host is required by this tapeworm. Various beetles and cockroaches serve as intermediate hosts for *H. diminuta* and, facultatively, for *H. nana*. *Giardia* (Mastigophora) trophozoites (group of five, center) and cysts (inset, upper left) are common parasites of mice. RABBIT: *Cittotaenia ctenoides* (Anoplocephalidae) eggs appear as amorphous spheres (left of arrow) until crushed by pressure on the coverslip (right of arrow), whereupon the oncosphere and pear-shaped embryophore become visible. *Obeliscoides cuniculi* eggs are typical strongyle eggs. *Passalurus ambiguus* (Oxyuridae) are somewhat asymmetrical and have a cap at one end. *Eimeria*, sporulated oocysts. Avoid mistaking *Saccharomycopsis gutulatus* (see Fig. 12–3) for a bona fide parasite of the rabbit. All x425 except *Giardia* (x1000).

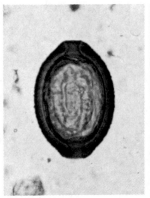
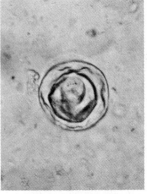
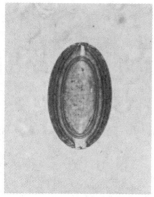

Anatrichosoma cynomolgi   Anoplocephalidae   Prosthenorchis elegans

Figure 12–36. Three parasites of primates. For a more complete listing of simian parasites by host and organ, see Chapter 13. *Anatrichosoma cynomolgi* adult worms tunnel in the nasal mucosa. Anoplocephalid eggs have a pear-shaped embryophore surrounding the oncosphere. *Prosthenorchis elegans* (Acanthocephala) eggs have a thick outer shell and thin inner shells enclosing the embryo (acanthor).

QUANTITATIVE FECAL EXAMINATION

The Cornell-McMaster dilution egg counting technique as described in the following paragraphs is based on the work of Stoll (1923 and 1930), Gordon and Whitlock (1939), Whitlock (1941), and Kauzal and Gordon (1941).

Briefly, a sample of feces is weighed and vigorously mixed with water in the proportion of 1 gram per 15 ml. Aliquots of 0.3 ml. are drawn from this suspension and mixed with equal parts of saturated sucrose solution in a counting chamber. The parasite eggs float in this medium and come to rest at the undersurface of the chamber cover. In this way, all the eggs in a 0.02 gram subsample are brought into the same focal plane of a microscopic field that is relatively free of fecal debris. The number of eggs counted in this aliquot is multiplied by 50 to yield an estimate of the number of eggs per gram of feces.

MATERIALS REQUIRED

1. Balance sensitive enough to indicate a change of as little as 0.1 gram in sample weight.

2. Mixing apparatus (Fig. 12-37) consisting of a 250 to 300 ml. graduated cylinder with a height to diameter ratio of about 2 to 1 (the cylinder of Figure 12-37 was made by sawing off a 500 ml. plastic cylinder at the 300 ml. mark) and an electric hand drill with a special beater. The beater may be easily fabricated using a brass rod for the shank and a strip of old inner tube for the beater. The beater shank should glide freely through a hole in a rubber stopper that fits the graduated cylinder.

3. Counting chamber (Fig. 12-38). Two micro-

scope slides separated by two thicknesses of slide cut into narrow strips and cemented together with aquarium cement. The upper and lower slides should be offset slightly to facilitate filling the chamber. To clean the chamber, rinse under a stream of cold water.

4. Avian tuberculin syringe, 1 ml. The needle hub may be ground off to avoid plugging by coarse debris.

5. Saturated sucrose solution. Add granulated table sugar to boiling water, stirring continuously until no more will dissolve. Cool. Add a few

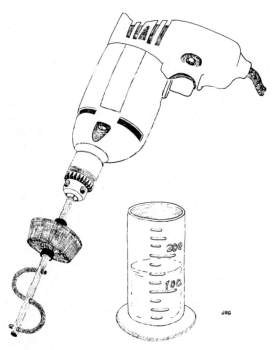

Figure 12–37. Mixing apparatus for preparing fecal suspensions.

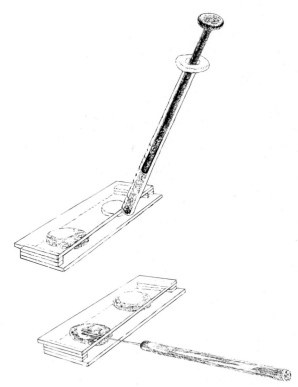

Figure 12–38. Loading the counting chamber. Two 0.3 ml. volumes of saturated sucrose solution are placed in the counting chamber. Then a 0.3 ml. aliquot of fecal suspension is added to each volume of sucrose solution and thoroughly mixed with a dissecting needle.

phenol crystals to inhibit mold growth. The specific gravity at room temperature should be at least 1.31.

6. Paper cups, tongue depressors. and dissecting needles.

PROCEDURE

1. Weigh out 10 grams of feces in a paper cup (correct for tare) and add to 150 ml. water in the graduated cylinder. If less than 10 grams of feces is available, reduce the volume of water to preserve the 1:15 proportion.

2. Mix feces and water thoroughly. With the hand drill mixer, only a few seconds are required.

3. (Optional) The suspension may be passed through a tea strainer to remove coarse debris that might interfere with microscopic examination. This is often necessary when examining horse manure but should be avoided if possible because it may yield lower counts.

4. Place 0.3 ml. saturated sucrose solution in each half of the counting chamber (Fig. 12-38).

5. Stir the fecal suspension, withdraw two 0.3 ml. aliquots, and add one to each pool of sucrose solution in the counting chamber.

6. Mix each aliquot-sucrose pool thoroughly with a dissecting needle and allow the preparation to stand for about 15 minutes.

7. Count all the eggs in each pool while scanning with the low power of the microscope. The focal plane containing the eggs may be quickly located by the presence of air bubbles. Take care to include eggs lying in the optically darkened borders of the pools.

Variations of this technique employing calibrated chambers overcome the difficulty of counting eggs in the optically darkened borders of the pools. Unfortunately, such chambers often prove difficult to obtain commercially and some of those that have been available in the past were inaccurately calibrated.

INTERPRETATION OF EGG COUNT DATA

Statistical Considerations

If it were possible to obtain a *uniform* distribution of parasite eggs in the fecal suspension, we could expect to find the same number of eggs in all aliquots. However, as we mix the suspension, the distribution of eggs does not become *uniform* but instead becomes *random* and stays *random* as long as we continue mixing. Aliquots from a thoroughly mixed suspension thus represent fair samples drawn from a random distribution and the numbers of eggs counted in replicate aliquots vary in a predictable fashion.

When relatively rare objects are distributed at random in space (or relatively infrequent events are distributed at random in time), the number of objects to be found in each sample volume (or the number of occurrences in each sample time interval) follows a Poisson distribution. In a 150 ml. fecal suspension there is room for well over a billion eggs, yet even in acute haemonchosis, there will rarely be more than a half million present. This means that for every 2000 volumes the size of a *Haemonchus* egg, no more than one volume will actually contain an egg. Certainly then, eggs counted in aliquots drawn from a well mixed fecal suspension meet the specifications for "relatively rare objects distributed at random in space," and we can expect the number counted in each sample volume to follow a Poisson distribution.

The mean and variance of a Poisson distribution are equal. This fact can be turned to practical advantage because it provides a criterion by which we can assess the adequacy of our technique. If the variance of a series of aliquot counts turns out to be much greater

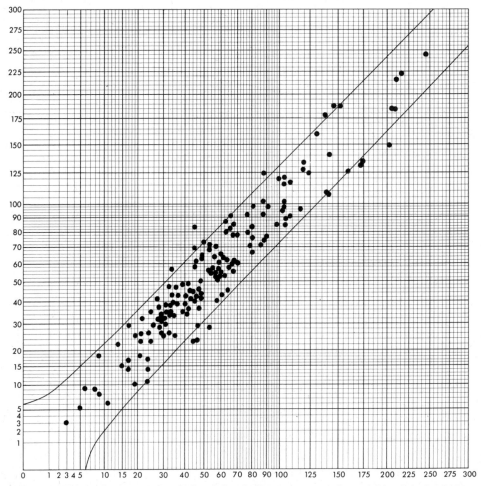

Figure 12–39. Plot of 151 duplicate egg counts. According to theory, no more than eight points should have fallen outside the diagonal boundary lines. More careful mixing, sampling, and counting could improve the picture.

than the mean, we may conclude that the mixing, sampling, or counting has been carelessly done. If, on the other hand, the sample variance turns out to be much smaller than the mean, we may conclude that someone has "fudged" the data. Chi-square analysis provides an objective numerical method for testing how well replicate egg counts fit the Poisson distribution (Hunter and Quenouille, 1952), but few practitioners would be tempted to bother with the necessary calculations. A simple alternative is provided by the graph of Figure 12-39. The diagonal lines drawn on this graph enclose a zone within which 95 per cent of all points representing duplicate egg counts should fall, on the average, provided the sampling and counting are adequate. The tolerance bounds on the graph are nearly parallel instead of divergent, as might be expected in view of the equality

of means and variances inherent in the Poisson distribution, because the axes have square root scales. Square root transformation of a Poisson variate converts the variance to a constant for all but very small values of the variate. In Figure 12-39, of 151 pairs of egg counts, 19 (13 per cent) lie on or outside the boundaries of the 95 per cent zone. This is almost three times too many and we may conclude that technical performance could be improved.

Applications

Egg counting techniques may be applied, in principle, to any patent parasitic infection of any host. For practical purposes, however, they find their greatest utility in estimating levels of strongylid infections in ruminants and horses. Under conditions of ordinary husbandry, these species of domestic animals always shed strongyle eggs in their feces except when they have recently been treated with an effective anthelmintic drug. Therefore, the question is not whether or not these animals are infected with strongyles but instead, what level of infection is present.

Determining Rates of Environmental Contamination. Most contemporary methods for controlling strongylids in grazing livestock depend heavily on periodic medication with anthelmintic drugs to suppress the production of strongylid eggs and thereby curtail contamination of the pastures. Unfortunately, when populations of parasites are repeatedly exposed to anthelmintics for several years, they develop resistance to these anthelmintics and to their chemical congeners. The more frequently anthelmintic medication is applied, the more rapidly does resistance to them develop. In order to slow or stop the development of resistance, anthelmintics should only be administered when they are actually needed to reduce a significant rate of pasture contamination. This can be accomplished by performing periodic fecal egg counts on a representative sample of the herd. When egg output is low, treatment may be delayed until it has reached a point deemed significant in relationship to the extent and productivity of pasture, the stocking rate, the species and susceptibility of hosts, and the objectives of the husbandry operation. The *critical number* of eggs per gram at which the herd ought to be treated cannot be specified without taking all of these factors into consideration. For example, I would suppose that 1000 eggs per gram might be an appropriate *critical number* for clinically normal sheep grazing at low stocking rate under weather conditions favorable to *Haemonchus contortus.* On the other hand, I would not wish to exceed 100 eggs per gram for brood mares with foals at their sides grazing a small paddock. In both of these cases, the *critical number* would be subject to revision according to the results achieved and any significant modifications of management practices.

Diagnosing Clinical Illness. High egg counts, e.g., over 5000 eggs per gram for sheep and goats, or over 500 eggs per gram for cattle, are easy to interpret; they indicate that these animals are infected with many reproductively active parasites. However, high counts do not necessarily indicate that the host is suffering from clinical parasitic disease because healthy, well-nourished hosts can often support and compensate for very impressive populations of parasites. Negative egg counts indicate that the host either is uninfected or is infected with nonreproductive worms (e.g., developing or arrested larvae, infertile adults). Negative egg counts are typical of the early stages of winter ostertagiosis in cattle and peracute hookworm disease in newborn pups. Such facts tend to discredit quantitative fecal analysis in the minds of those who require short lists of simple, plausible rules. However, when interpreted by minds familiar with the biology of both host and parasite, egg counts provide one valuable insight into the interaction taking place between them.

EXAMINATION OF BLOOD AND TISSUES

FIXATION AND IDENTIFICATION OF MICROFILARIAE IN BLOOD

Diagnosis of Heartworm Infection In Dogs

The simplest procedure for diagnosing heartworm infection in dogs is to place a drop of heparinized venous blood on a slide, add a coverslip, and examine the preparation under low and high dry magnification. Microfilariae reveal their presence by agitating the erythrocytes in their immediate vicinity. In general, if more than 5 or 10 microfilariae are observed per drop of blood, they are probably *Dirofilaria immitis.* If a smaller number are observed, they may represent either heartworm or another filariid parasite infection. In North America, the only other filariid recognized in dogs is *Dipetalonema reconditum* (Newton and Wright, 1956, 1957), but in certain other parts of the world, there are still other species to contend with. The following procedure is about 15 times as sensitive as the direct smear and permits more accurate differentiation of microfilariae of *Dirofilaria immitis* and *Dipetalonema reconditum.*

TECHNIQUE OF KNOTT (1939) MODIFIED

1. Draw a sample of venous blood into a syringe containing a suitable anticoagulant such as EDTA or heparin.

2. Draw 1 to 2 ml. of air into the syringe and mix the blood and anticoagulant by rocking the

syringe so as to run the air bubble back and forth along the length of the barrel. Prolonged delay and thermal extremes are to be avoided; remix blood immediately before proceeding with Step 3.

3. Place 1 ml. of blood in a 15 ml. centrifuge tube. Add 10 ml. of 2 per cent formalin, stopper, and mix by inversion and shaking. *Note: When submitting blood samples to a laboratory for identification of microfilariae, complete only Steps 1, 2, and 3 to prepare them for shipment.*

4. Wait two or three minutes.

5. Centrifuge for about five minutes and pour off the supernatant by inverting the centrifuge tube only once.

6. Add one drop of 0.1 per cent methylene blue to the sediment, mix, and transfer some stained sediment to a slide for microscopic examination.

There are other microfilarial concentration techniques but the Knott test is preferred because it is standard, is inexpensive, and includes the best preparative technique for specimens submitted to the laboratory. The quality and concentration of the formalin solution are critical. Two per cent formalin is 2 ml. of stock 37 per cent formaldehyde solution (i.e., formalin) and 98 ml. of distilled water. This reagent tends to deteriorate in storage and should be made up fresh periodically.

Differentiation of Microfilariae. Microfilariae of *Dirofilaria immitis* are 6.0 to 7.0 μm wide, whereas those of *Dipetalonema reconditum* are less than 5.6 μm wide. Length measurement is a more tedious and less reliable differential criterion. When fixed by the preceding technique, the tails of *D. reconditum* microfilariae tend to be curved like an ovariectomy hook. The anterior end of the *D. immitis* microfilaria tapers gently, whereas that of *D. reconditum* maintains about the same diameter throughout. The *cephalic hook* of *D. reconditum* (Fig. 12-40) is demonstrable with the 40x objective of any modern, standard, compound microscope in samples prepared by the Knott technique described above. It is not necessary to resort to thick smears or special stains to demonstrate the cephalic hook. Patience is required at first but, with practice, the *cephalic hook* proves the quickest, easiest, and most reliable differential criterion.

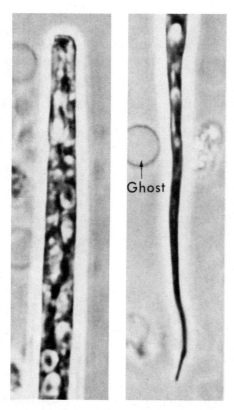

Dirofilaria immitis

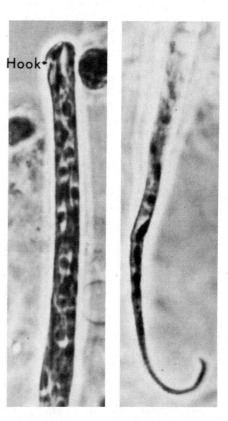

Dipetalonema reconditum

Figure 12–40. Microfilariae of *Dirofilaria immitis* and *Dipetalonema reconditum* (x2000). See text for exposition of differential characters.

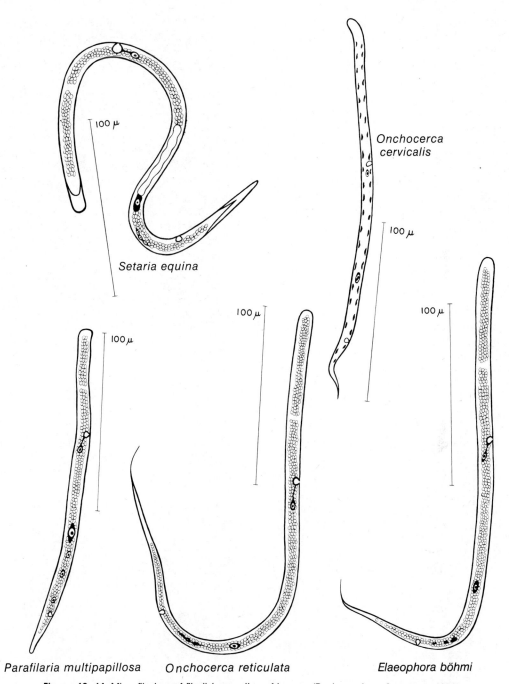

Figure 12–41. Microfilariae of filariid parasites of horses. (Redrawn from Supperer, 1953).

Identification of Equine Microfilariae

Equine microfilariae are portrayed diagrammatically in Figure 12-41.

Setaria equina. The sheathed microfilariae of *Setaria equina* may be demonstrated in blood samples by the techniques of the preceding section.

Parafilaria multipapillosa microfilariae may be found in blood discharged from "summer bleeding" nodules caused by the adult female worms. They are less than 200 μm long, are unsheathed, and have a rounded posterior extremity (Supperer, 1953).

Microfilariae of *Onchocerca cervicalis*, *O. reticulata*, and *Elaeophora böhmi* may be demonstrated by excising a small piece of skin from near the linea alba and placing it in physiological saline solution. The microfilariae of these three species will soon be observed migrating out of the dermis into the saline solution. Leave the preparation set up overnight to detect low levels of microfiladerma.

Onchocerca cervicalis microfilariae are slender, delicate, and 207 to 240 μm long.

Onchocerca reticulata microfilariae are 330 to 370 μm long and have a long, whiplike tail ending in a fine point.

Elaeophora böhmi microfilariae are 300 to 330 μm long and may be distinguished from *O. reticulata* by a difference in the distance from the genital cell to the tip of the tail, which is greater than 140 μm for *O. reticulata* and less than 120 μm for *E. böhmi*.

EXAMINATION FOR TRICHINAE

Squash Preparation

Moderate to heavy *Trichinella spiralis* infections can be diagnosed by simply squashing bits of muscle tissue between two glass slides and scanning under low power. The diaphragm and masseter muscles are especially likely to yield positive findings.

1. Detach a small scrap of meat and place it on a microscope slide.
2. Cover with a second microscope slide and press the two slides together with the thumb and forefinger, thus squashing the scrap of meat.
3. While maintaining pressure, bind the slides firmly together by wrapping each end with adhesive tape.
4. Trim off any meat protruding from between the slides to avoid contaminating the microscope stage.
5. Scan the entire field under low power. Larvae, if present, are easily visible (Fig. 12-42).

Note: This procedure is also applicable to other tissue-dwelling parasites such as the smaller lungworms of sheep and carnivorans, encysted *Toxocara* larvae, and the like.

Tissue Digestion

Peptic digestion is used to detect light infection with *Trichinella spiralis* and other nematodes in tissues. Gastric juice digests the muscle tissue but not the larvae of *Trichinella spiralis*. Pepsin-acid solution consists of 0.2 gram granular pepsin and 1.0 ml. concentrated hydrochloric acid in 100 ml. distilled water.

1. Weigh out 4 grams of tissue and mince it with a scalpel.

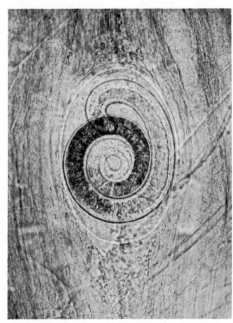

Figure 12–42. *Trichinella spiralis* cyst in a fresh squash preparation of pork muscle (×160).

2. Add 100 ml. of pepsin-acid solution and allow to stand for about one hour.
3. Decant excess supernatant carefully, suspend sediment, and transfer to a Petri plate.
4. Count larvae under a dissecting microscope. Larvae may be retrieved with a Pasteur pipette for closer study under the compound microscope.

SKIN SCRAPINGS FOR MANGE DIAGNOSIS

Skin scrapings for mange diagnosis must be obtained in a manner that takes into account both the nature of the lesion and the location of the mite in question.

For *lesions with minimal epidermal hyperplasia and lesions caused by deeply burrowing mites* (e.g., *Sarcoptes, Demodex*), dip a scalpel blade in mineral oil, pinch a fold of skin firmly between the thumb and forefinger and, holding the blade at right angles to the skin, scrape until blood begins to seep from the abrasion. Most patients do not object to deep scraping, although local anesthesia may occasionally be required. Much of the detritus will adhere to the layer of mineral oil on the scalpel blade and may be transferred to a microscope slide and searched for mites.

For *lesions with marked epidermal hyperplasia and exfoliation and lesions caused by lice and superficially dwelling mites* (e.g., *Chorioptes*), scrape the detritus into an ointment tin using the cover as a scraper. Examine scrapings under a stereoscopic microscope or with a hand lens to find the lice and mites crawling about. Dip fine-tipped thumb forceps or a dissecting needle into Berlese solution and use this sticky mounting medium to pick up mites and transfer them to a slide for closer study under the compound microscope. Berlese solution is made by mixing 200 grams chloral hydrate, 30 grams gum arabic, 20 grams glycerine, and 50 ml. distilled water, boiling this mixture for 5 to 15 minutes, and filtering through cheesecloth. Berlese solution clears the specimen and hardens to produce a permanent preparation. Unfortunately, chloral hydrate is now regulated as a narcotic and different lots of gum arabic vary considerably in quality so that good Berlese solution is becoming hard to come by. Mineral oil is a reasonably satisfactory temporary mounting medium. Five per cent sodium or potassium hydroxide solution may also be used as a temporary mounting medium that digests epidermis and hair, thus helping to clear the microscopic field of debris.

If the scraping contains much debris and no mites or lice have been found by inspection with the stereoscopic microscope or hand lens, proceed as follows:

1. Add 10 volumes of 5 per cent KOH to 1 volume of skin scrapings in a large (500 to 1000 volumes capacity) beaker, cover with a watch glass or funnel to return condensate, and heat until hair and epidermal scales dissolve. It may be necessary to boil the mixture but do not allow it to boil dry. *Beware of spattering lye!*

2. Allow to cool.

3. Transfer to a centrifuge tube, centrifuge, decant supernatant, resuspend sediment in water, and centrifuge again. These steps dispose of interfering soaps. Decant the supernatant.

4. Transfer sediment to a Petri dish and search for mites and eggs with a stereomicroscope or 10x pocket lens, or proceed with Step 5.

5. Add saturated sucrose solution to the centrifuge tube, resuspend the sediment, and centrifuge again. Pick mites off the top of the sucrose solution with a wire loop or glass nail and transfer them to a microscope slide for study under the compound microscope.

Ear mites may be removed from the external ear canal with a cotton swab. If the swab is placed on a dark background in sunlight or near an incandescent lamp, white *Otodectes* mites may be seen crawling about within a few minutes.

REFERENCES

Cunliffe, G., and Crofton, H. D. (1953): Egg sizes and differential egg counts in relation to sheep nematodes. Parasitology, 43, 275-286.

Dikmans, G., and Andrews, J. S. (1933): A comparative morphological study of the infective larvae of the common nematodes parasitic in the alimentary tract of sheep. Trans. Am. Micros. Soc., 52, 1-25.

Dubey, J. P. (1976): A review of *Sarcocystis* of domestic animals and of other coccidia of cats and dogs. J. Am. Vet. Med. Assoc., 169, 1061-1078.

Gordon, H. McL., and Whitlock, H. V. (1939): A new technique for counting nematode eggs in sheep faeces. J. Counc. Sci. and Industr. Res. (Australia), 12, 50-52.

Hunter, G. C., and Quenouille, M. H. (1952): A statistical examination of the worm egg count sampling technique for sheep. J. Helminthol. 26, 157-170.

Kauzal, G. P., and Gordon, H. McL. (1941): A useful mixing apparatus for the preparation of suspensions of faeces for helminthological examinations. J. Counc. Sci. and Industr. Res. (Australia), 14, 304-305.

Keith, R. K. (1953): Infective larvae of cattle nematodes. Australian J. Zool., 1, 223-235.

Knott, J. (1939): A method for making microfilarial surveys on day blood. Trans. Roy. Soc. Trop. Med. Hyg., 33, 191-196.

Newton, W. L., and Wright, W. H. (1956): The occurrence of a dog filariid other than *Dirofilaria immitis* in the United States. J. Parasitol., 42, 246-258.

Newton, W. L., and Wright, W. H. (1957): A reevaluation of the canine filariasis problem in the United States. Vet. Med., 52, 75-78.

Stoll, N. R. (1923): Investigations on the control of hookworm disease. XV. An effective method of counting hookworm eggs in human feces. Am. J. Hyg., 3, 59-70.

Stoll, N. R. (1930): On methods of counting nematode ova in sheep dung. Parasitology, 22, 116-136.

Supperer, R. (1953): Filariosen der Pferde in Osterreich. Weiner Tierärztliche Monatschr., 40, 214-216.

Trayser, C. V., and Todd, K. S. (1978): Life cycle of *Isospora burrowsi* n. sp. (Protozoa:Eimeriidae) from the dog *Canis familiaris*. Am. J. Vet. Res., 39, 95-98.

Whitlock, J. H. (1941): A practical dilution egg count procedure. J. Am. Vet. Med. Assoc., 98, 466-469.

13

POSTMORTEM DIAGNOSIS

NECROPSY PROCEDURES

Occasionally, severe or fatal parasitosis may escape antemortem diagnosis. For example, pups with peracute hookworm disease may bleed to death before shedding an egg. When disease breaks out in a flock of sheep, postmortem examination of a few sick animals often provides the most efficient and economical means of arriving at a diagnosis. In strongylid infections of sheep, various combinations of primary and secondary pathogens often yield a confusing array of clinical signs that may be resolved by identification and enumeration of the worms.

Necropsy findings must be correlated with the case history and clinical signs in order to arrive at a definitive diagnosis. This is especially true of parasitic diseases. For example, a diagnosis of acute haemonchosis must rest not only on the demonstration of a sufficient number of *Haemonchus contortus* worms in the abomasum but on the existence of clinical anemia as well. If there is no anemia, then there is no haemonchosis. In fact, *H. contortus* sometimes desert a moribund host so that, on necropsy examination, one finds pallor and edema of the tissues but no worms. The correct diagnosis is still *haemonchosis*.

Opening the Cadaver. Arrange a ruminant cadaver on its left side to get the rumen out of the way. Cadavers of other species are about equally accessible from either side, but you should adopt a consistent approach in order to develop a mental image of the normal appearance and location of the various organs so that any abnormal relationship will be quickly noticed. Incise the skin along the midline from the submaxillary space to the perineum. Reflect the skin from one side, including the superficial thoracic muscles and the pectoral limb with it so as to lay bare the rib cage. Cut the ribs close to the axial muscles and the costal cartilages close to the sternum. Lift away the rib cage, severing attachments to the diaphragm in the process. Incise the abdominal wall along the midline, taking pains to avoid puncturing the viscera; carry the incision across the brim of the pubis, and reflect the abdominal wall. Split the pubic symphysis or incise the ligaments of the hip joint and reflect the pelvic limb.

Thoracic Viscera. Incise the intermandibular muscles, hyoid apparatus, and other attachments and dissect the tongue, larynx, trachea, and esophagus. Removal of the heart and lungs is facilitated by traction on the trachea and esophagus; the points of attachment (aorta, cavae, azygous vein, various ligaments) are easily found and severed. Remove the thoracic viscera from the carcass. Lay open the tracheobronchial tree, heart chambers, cavae, aortic trunk, and ramifications of the pulmonary arteries, and inspect the contents and linings for macroscopic parasites. Very small metastrongyloid nematodes (e.g., *Muellerius capillaris, Aelurostrongylus abstrusus, Filaroides hirthi*) are practically invisible grossly; these may be demonstrated in squash preparations of their grayish subpleural nodules. The Baermann technique is useful for demonstrating larvae of lung nematodes (e.g., *Muellerius, Aelurostrongylus*) but usually fails in the case of *Filaroides hirthi* because the larvae of this parasite are too lethargic to migrate out of the lung tissues.

Abdominal Viscera. Examine the peritoneum for cysticerci, tetrathyridia, encysted pentastomid and acanthocephalan nymphs; *Strongylus edentatus* larvae may often be observed immediately beneath the parietal peritoneum of horses. Examine the surface of the liver for migration tracts of ascarid, taeniid, and *Fasciola* larvae, and the kidneys for encysted *Toxacara* larve. The equine pancreas is a favorite location for *Strongylus equinus* larvae. Place double ligatures about the cardia (or omasoabomasal junction), pylorus, and ileocecal junction, thus isolating the stomach, small intestine, and large intestine. These regions provide differing environments for distinct sets of parasites and valuable diagnostic information is lost by pooling the collection from the entire gut. Open one region at a time, carefully poking through the ingesta and scanning the mucosa for the smaller forms. Many parasites of dogs, cats, horses, and pigs are large enough to see with the unaided eye but there are a few very small ones that are important (e.g., *Strongyloides*, *Trichinella*). Scrape the mucosa of the small intestine and examine the scrapings for small nematodes, coccidia, and the like.

Most of the important nematode parasites of ruminants are very small and great care must be taken not to overlook them. The population of nematodes sufficient to kill a heifer may pass the notice of a careless prosector completely. The following technique accomplishes the concentration and separation of these worms from much of the ingesta and mucosal debris and, with a bit of extra effort, provides an estimate of the number of worms present.

1. Transfer all ingesta from a particular organ (the abomasum is an easy one to begin with) to a bucket, scrub or lightly scrape the mucosal surface to assure complete transfer of worms.
2. Add several quarts of tepid water, mix, and allow to stand for about five minutes so that the worms and heavy debris can settle to the bottom; then decant the supernatant. Repeat this process until the sediment consists principally of worms and coarse ingesta.
3. Transfer a *small* amount of sediment to a Petri dish and examine with transillumination, preferably under a magnifying glass or stereoscopic microscope. If the worms have been taken from the cadaver of a recently dead animal, they will become very active in the tepid water and can be easily detected and fished out with a forceps for closer examination.

The small intestine is long and the occasion fleeting. Most of the important nematode parasites of the ruminant small intestine can be collected by flushing a liter of water through its first 6 meters. Insert a funnel into the pyloric end of 6 meters of unopened small intestine and pour a beaker of water into it. Massage the water along the length

of gut and collect it at the other end; then proceed with Steps 2 and 3 above.

A popular alternative to Step 2 above is to vigorously rinse sediment over a sieve having openings small enough to retain the parasites but large enough to pass water and fine debris. The sieve may then be inverted and back-rinsed to transfer the parasites and coarse debris to a collecting vessel. If time or facilities for examining sediment for parasites is lacking, the sediment can be preserved in 10 per cent formalin and attended to later. Be sure to sieve preserved sediments once again to remove the formalin before attempting to isolate and study the parasites; this will save you a big headache.

Because we are almost certain to find parasites in sheep, young cattle, and horses, it follows that the evaluation of the necropsy findings must rest on the abundance of the parasites as well as on their identity. To obtain an estimate of worm numbers, substitute Step 3a for Step 3 and proceed as follows:

3a. Transfer the washed sediment to a graduated cylinder and fill with water to 1 liter. We now have all the worms from some particular organ suspended in 1 liter.
4. Stir the suspension thoroughly and withdraw a 50 ml. aliquot.
5. Pour a small portion of the 50 ml. aliquot into a Petri dish and count all of the worms. Continue until the 50 ml. is used up. The number of worms counted times 20 provides an estimate of the total number of worms in the particular organ.

The worm count must be interpreted in the light of other necropsy findings, especially the nutritional status of the cadaver and lesions specifically related to the parasites found. Etiological significance should be attached to *Trichostrongylus* or *Cooperia* only if it is apparent that the animal has suffered severe and protracted diarrhea. The presence of even 10,000 *Trichostrongylus* worms in a well-nourished lamb carcass with formed fecal pellets in the rectum suggests only that we should search further for the cause of death. Etiological significance should be attached to *Haemonchus* only if the carcass shows signs of anemia. Cattle suffering from ostertagiosis can become emaciated on full feed. These animals don't even lose their appetites but suffer from malabsorption that causes them to starve to death in the midst of plenty. It's just as well not to accuse the farmer of starving the animal to death when in fact *Ostertagia* is the culprit.

In the following host-organ listings of parasites, the organ systems and organs of the host are listed as centered headings and the systematic categories of the parasites are listed as side headings. Page citations refer the reader to further diagnostic information and figure citations to illustrations of the species in question or at least a member of the same genus.

PARASITES OF DOGS

Toxoplasma gondii may occur in any tissue of any host as extracellular or intracellular tachyzoites or as bradyzoites in cysts (see page 69 and Figs. 14-27 and 14-28).

Alimentary System

MOUTH

PROTOZOAN

Trichomonas canistomae (Mastigophora). Found around gum margins; nonpathogenic.

ESOPHAGUS AND STOMACH

NEMATODES

Spirocerca lupi (Spirurida). Found in fibrous nodules in the wall of the esophagus and sometimes the stomach (see page 129 and Figs. 14-80 to 14-82).

Physaloptera rara and *P. preputialis* (Spirurida) (see page 128 and Figs. 6-49 and 6-50).

Gnathostoma spinigerum (Spirurida). Relatively rare in North America (see page 127 and Fig. 6-48).

SMALL INTESTINE

NEMATODES

Toxocara canis and *Toxascaris leonina* (Ascaridoidea, page 124). *Toxocara* has a ventriculus intercalated between the esophagus and the intestine (Fig. 13-1), whereas *Toxascaris* has none (Fig. 13-2). The ventriculus is visible in transilluminated fresh specimens under the stereoscopic microscope and in fixed, cleared specimens under the compound microscope. Large, fixed specimens may be dissected to determine the presence or absence of a ventriculus. The tail of male *Toxocara* is digitiform (Fig. 13-3), whereas the tail of male *Toxascaris* tapers to a point (Fig. 13-4). Female *Toxocara* and *Toxascaris* may be

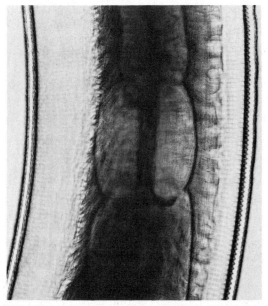

Figure 13–1. *Toxocara.* A *ventriculus* is intercalated between the esophagus and the intestine (x108).

distinguished by comparing their eggs (see Fig. 12-6).

Ancylostoma caninum, A. braziliense, and *Uncinaria stenocephala* (Ancylostomatoidea). Mature hookworms are found anchored to the mucosa by their buccal capsules unless the cadaver has cooled out or the host has died of an overdose of barbiturate, in which case

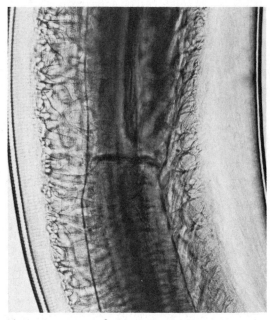

Figure 13–2. *Toxascaris.* There is no ventriculus between the esophagus and the intestine (x108).

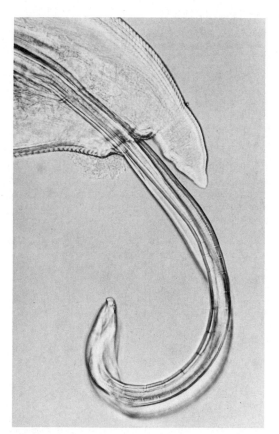

Figure 13–3. *Toxocara.* The tail of the male is fingerlike (x108).

CESTODES

Taenia pisiformis, T. hydatigena, T. ovis, Multiceps multiceps, M. serialis (Taeniidae) (see page 89 and Figs. 5-7, 5-9, 5-13, and 12-14).

Echinococcus granulosus and *E. multilocularis* (Taeniidae) (see page 89 and Fig. 5-14).

Dipylidium caninum, Diplopylidium, and *Joyeuxiella* (Dipylidiidae) (see page 94 and Figs. 5-2, 12-12, and 12-14D).

Mesocestoides spp. (Mesocestidae) (see page 95 and Figs. 5-24 and 12-13).

Diphyllobothrium latum (Diphyllobothriidae) (see page 95 and Figs. 5-5, 5-25, and 12-15A).

TREMATODES

Alaria americana (5 mm.), *A. arisaemoides* (10 mm.), *A. canis* (3.2 mm.), and *A. michiganensis* (1.9 mm.) (Diplostomatidae) (see page 81 and Fig. 4-15).

Mesostephanus appendiculatum (1.8 mm.), *M. longisaccus* (1 mm.) (Cyathocotylidae). These cyathocotylids resemble *Alaria* in having a bulbous tribocytic organ but differ in not being divided into distinct fore- and hindbody regions.

many specimens will be found unattached. Preadult *A. caninum* burrow deeply and destructively in the mucosa, and the mesenteric lymph nodes may be hemorrhagic as a result during the prepatent phase of severe infections. *A. caninum* is colored red by the blood in its gut, whereas *A. braziliense* and *U. stenocephala* are grayish white. The red color of *A. caninum* quickly fades on fixation, however. Specimens may be differentiated by microscopic examination of their buccal structures: *A. caninum* has three pairs of pointed teeth on the ventral border of the buccal capsule, *A. braziliense* has one pair of pointed teeth, and *U. stenocephala* has a pair of rounded plates instead of teeth (see page 113 and Fig. 6-10).

Strongyloides stercoralis (Rhabditoidea) (see page 100, Fig. 6-7). The tiny (2.2 mm.) parthenogenetic parasitic female worms may be found in scrapings of the mucous membrane.

Trichinella spiralis (Trichuroidea) (see page 134 and Fig. 6-59).

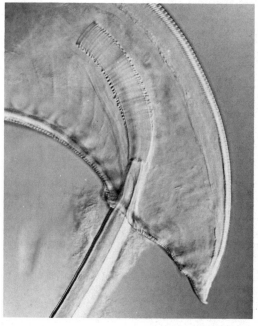

Figure 13–4. *Toxascaris.* The tail of the male tapers gradually (x168).

Echinochasmus schwartzi (2.1 mm.) (Echinostomatidae) is a slender echinostomatid with a collar of spines surrounding the oral sucker.

Apophallus venustus (1.4 mm.), *Cryptocotyl lingua* (2.2 mm.) and *Phagicola longa* (1.2 mm.) (Heterophyidae) (see page 81).

Plagiorchis sp. This small (1.2 mm.) plagiorchiid has a spindle-shaped, spinous body with well-developed suckers; the genital pore is anterior to the ventral sucker.

Nanophyetus salmincola (1.1 mm., see page 79 and Fig. 4-13) and *Sellacotyl mustellae* (0.4 mm.) are ovoid and pear-shaped respectively and have spinous bodies with well-developed suckers.

ACANTHOCEPHALANS

Oncicola canis is small (14 mm.) and spindle-shaped (see page 140 and Fig. 6-65). *Macracanthorhynchus ingens* is very large (see page 138 and Figs. 6-67 and 12-16).

PROTOZOANS

Flagellate

Giardia lamblia (see page 65 and Fig. 12-35).

Coccidian Schizonts, Gamonts, and Oocysts

Isospora canis, I. ohioensis, I. burrowsi, and *I. heydorni.* Oocysts contain a single sporont when shed in the feces (see page 67 and Figs. 12-6 and 12-18).

Sarcocystis cruzi, S. ovicanis, S. miescheriana, S. bertrami, S. fayeri, S. hemionilatrantis (see page 68, Table 3-1, and Fig. 12-22).

CECUM AND COLON

NEMATODE

Trichuris vulpis (Trichuroidea) (see page 136 and Figs. 6-63 and 12-6).

PROTOZOANS

Entamoeba histolytica and *E. coli* are cyst-forming amebas. Trophozoites of *E. histolytica* may contain phagocytosed erythrocytes.

Trichomonas spp. and *Pentatrichomonas hominis* are non-cyst-forming mucosoflagellates.

Balantidium coli (see page 65 and Fig. 12-19).

LIVER AND PANCREAS

NEMATODES

Toxocara canis and *Toxascaris leonina* sometimes invade the common bile duct erratically (see page 126).

Capillaria hepatica (see page 136 and Fig. 14-89).

NEMATODE LARVAE

Toxocara canis
Filaroides spp.

TREMATODES

Opisthorchis tenuicollis, O. viverini, Clonorchis sinensis, Metorchis albidus, and *M. conjunctus* (Opisthorchiidae) (see page 83 and Fig. 4-9).

Peritoneum and Peritoneal Cavity

CESTODE LARVA

Mesocestoides tetrathyridium (see page 95 and Figs. 14-53 and 14-54).

Respiratory System

NASAL PASSAGES

NEMATODE

Capillaria aerophila (Trichuroidea) (see page 136 and Fig. 12-20).

ARTHROPODS

Pneumonyssoides caninum (Mesostigmata) (see page 50 and Fig. 14-9).

Linguatula serrata (130 mm., Pentastomida) (see page 50). Bloodsucking, wormlike parasite of the nasal cavity and paranasal sinuses.

TRACHEA AND BRONCHI

NEMATODES

Filaroides osleri (Metastrongyloidea) (see page 119 and Figs. 6-35 and 12-8). In nodules near the bifurcation of the trachea.

Crenosoma vulpis (Metastrongyloidea) (see page 118 and Figs. 6-34 and 12-8). Small worms (16 mm.) found on bronchial and bronchiolar mucosa.

Capillaria aerophila (*Eucoleus aerophilus*) (Trichuroidea) (see page 136 and Fig 12-20).

LUNG PARENCHYMA

NEMATODES

Filaroides hirthi and *F. milksi* (*Andersonstrongylus milksi*) (Metastrongyloidea) (see page

119, Georgi, 1979, and Figs 6-31, 12-8, 14-71 and 14-72).

Dirofilaria immitis (Filarioidea) (see page 130 and Figs. 6-54 and 12-40). Large (30 cm.) worms in pulmonary infarcts.

NEMATODE LARVAE

Petechial hemorrhages, areas of focal necrosis, and nodular inflammation of lung tissue may be caused by migrating nematode larvae. Such lesions should be investigated by preparing squashes and by the Baermann technique. Identification of nematode larvae in histological preparations is considered in Chapter 14.

Angiostrongylus vasorum eggs and larvae (see page 118).

Strongyloides stercoralis (Rhabditoidea) filariform larvae (see page 101 and Fig. 12-9).

Ancylostoma caninum, A. braziliense, and *Uncinaria stenocephala* (Ancylostomatoidea) (see page 113 and Fig. 12-8).

Toxocara canis (Ascaridoidea) (see page 124 and Fig. 13-5).

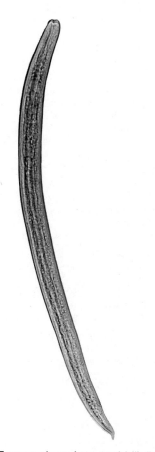

Figure 13–5. *Toxocara* larva from a rabbit's liver (x250).

TREMATODE

Paragonimus kellicotti (Troglotrematidae) (see page 80 and Figs. 4-12 and 12-17B).

Vascular System

PULMONARY ARTERY, RIGHT HEART AND VENAE CAVAE

NEMATODES

Dirofilaria immitis (300 mm., Filarioidea) (see page 130 and Figs. 6-54 and 12-40).

Angiostrongylus vasorum (25 mm., Metastrongyloidea). Much smaller than *D. immitis* and located in the pulmonary arterial branches; first stage larvae resembling those of *Aelurostrongylus* (Fig. 12-20) are shed in the host's feces.

MESENTERIC AND PORTAL VEINS

TREMATODE

Heterobilharzia americana (Schistosomatidae) (see page 78 and Fig. 4-11).

BLOOD

NEMATODE MICROFILARIAE

Dirofilaria immitis and *Dipetalonema reconditum* (Filarioidea) (see page 130 and Fig. 12-40).

PROTOZOANS

Babesia canis (piroplasm) (see page 70).

Trypanosoma cruzi (hemoflagellate). Trypomastigotes of this flagellate may be scarce in blood films. Examine heart muscle histologically for amastigotes (see Fig. 14-16).

SKELETAL MUSCLES

NEMATODE LARVAE

Trichinella spiralis (Trichuroidea) (see page 134 and Figs. 12-42 and 14-87).

Ancylostoma caninum (Ancylostomatoidea). Larvae in vacuoles in muscle fibers with little or no evidence of host reaction (see page 113 and Fig. 14-69).

CONNECTIVE TISSUES

NEMATODES

Dipetalonema reconditum (32 mm., Filarioidea) (see page 132 and Figs. 6-58 and 14-85).

Dirofilaria immitis (300 mm., Filarioidea) (see page 130 and Figs. 6-54 and 12-40).

Dracunculus insignis (360 mm., Spirurida) (see page 127 and Figs. 6-46, 6-47, and 14-84).

INSECT LARVAE

Cuterebra (30 mm., Cuterebridae) (see page 22 and Figs. 1-12, 1-21, 14-1, and 14-3).

Cochliomyia hominivorax (17 mm., Calliphoridae) (see page 17 and Figs. 1-11 and 1-20).

Phaenicia sericata, Phormia regina, Protophormia terraenovae (17 mm., Calliphoridae) (see page 17 and Figs. 1-11 and 1-20).

Wohlfahrtia vigil and *W. opaca* (Sarcophagidae) (see page 16 and Fig. 1-20).

Urogenital System

KIDNEY

NEMATODE

Dioctophyme renale (up to 1 meter! Spirurida). A giant worm in the kidney pelvis or peritoneal cavity.

NEMATODE LARVAE

Toxocara canis (see Fig. 13-5).
Ancylostoma caninum

URINARY BLADDER

NEMATODE

Capillaria plica (60 mm., Trichuroidea) (see page 137 and Fig. 12-20).

Nervous System

NEMATODES

Dirofilaria immitis (Filarioidea) (see page 130 and Figs. 6-54 and 12-40). In the anterior chamber of the eye, or epidural space, erratically.

Thelazia californiensis (19 mm., Spirurida) (see page 129 and Fig. 6-51). In the conjunctival sac and ducts of the lacrimal gland.

Skin and Hair

INSECTS

Adult dipterans (see page 27).
Linognathus setosus (Anoplura) (see page 27 and Fig. 7-1).

Trichodectes canis (Mallophaga) (see page 29 and Figs. 1-36 and 1-37).

Heterodoxus spiniger (Mallophaga) has club-shaped antennae that lie in cephalic grooves and the anterior margin of the head is pointed; restricted to warm climates.

Ctenocephalides canis, C. felis, Pulex irritans, Echidnophaga gallinacea (Siphonaptera) (see page 30 and Figs. 1-41, 1-42, and 1-44).

ARACHNIDS

Rhipicephalus sanguineus, Dermacentor variabilis, D. andersoni, Amblyomma americanum, A. maculatum, Ixodes spp., and others (Ixodidae) (see page 40 and Figs. 2-6 to 2-16).

Sarcoptes scabiei (Sarcoptidae) (see page 51 and Figs. 2-23 and 14-4).

Otodectes cyanotis (Psoroptidae) (see page 55 and Fig. 2-30).

Demodex canis (Demodicidae) (see page 58 and Figs. 2-33 and 14-7).

Cheyletiella yasguri (Cheyletidae) (see page 59 and Figs. 2-34 and 14-6).

NEMATODE LARVA

Rhabditis strongyloides (Rhabditida) (see page 99 and Figs. 6-6 and 14-57).

PARASITES OF CATS

Toxoplasma gondii may occur in any tissue of any host as extracellular or intracellular tachyzoites or as bradyzoites in cysts (see page 69 and Figs. 14-27 and 14-28). Sexual reproduction with formation of oocysts (see Fig. 12-22) occurs only in the intestinal mucosae of members of the cat family (Felidae).

Alimentary System

MOUTH

PROTOZOAN

Trichomonas felistomae (flagellate). Found around the gum margins; nonpathogenic.

STOMACH AND ESOPHAGUS

NEMATODES

Gnathostoma spinigerum (Spirurida) (see page 127 and Fig. 6-48).

Physalsoptera spp. (Spirurida) (see page 128 and Figs. 6-49 and 6-50).

Ollulanus tricuspis (1 mm.! Trichostrongyloidea) (see page 109).

Capillaria putorii (Trichuroidea) (see page 136 and Fig. 12-20).

SMALL INTESTINE

NEMATODES

Toxocara cati and *Toxascaris leonina* (Ascaridoidea) (see page 123 and Figs. 6-41, 12-20, and 13-1 to 13-4).

Ancylostoma tubaeforme, A. braziliense, Uncinaria stenocephala (Ancylostomatoidea) (see page 113 and Figs. 6-10, 12-20, and 13-6).

Strongyloides stercoralis (2.2 mm., Rhabditida) (see page 100 and Fig. 6-8).

Trichinella spiralis (Trichuroidea) (see page 134 and Fig. 6-59).

CESTODES

Hydatigera taeniaeformis (Taeniidae) (see page 90 and Figs. 5-3, 5-9, 14-43, and 14-44).

Echinococcus multilocularis (Taeniidae) (see page 89 and Fig. 5-14).

Dipylidium caninum (Dipylidiidae) (see page 94 and Figs. 5-2, 12-12, and 12-14D).

Mesocestoides latus and *M. variabilis* (Mesocestidae) (see page 95 and Figs. 5-24 and 12-13).

Spirometra mansonoides (Diphyllobothriidae) (see page 95 and Figs. 5-6 and 5-11).

TREMATODES

Alaria spp. (5 mm., Diplostomatidae) (see page 81 and Fig. 4-15).

Apophallus venustus (1.4 mm.) and *Phagicola longa* (1.2 mm.) (Heterophyidae) (see page 81).

Mesostephanus spp. (1.8 mm., Cyathocotylidae) (see page 81).

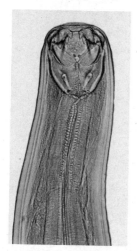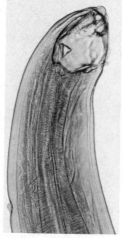

Figure 13–6. *Ancylostoma tubaeforme.* At left, the dorsoventral aspect of the stoma and at right, its lateral aspect (x78).

ACANTHOCEPHALAN

Oncicola spp. (see page 140 and Fig. 6-65).

PROTOZOANS

Isospora felis, I. rivolta, Besnoitia spp., *Hammondia hammondi, Toxoplasma gondii* (coccidia) (see page 67 and Fig. 12-22).

Sarcocystis hirsuta, S. tenella, S. porcifelis, S. leporum (coccidia) (see page 68, Table 3-1, and Fig. 12-22).

LARGE INTESTINE

NEMATODES

Strongyloides tumefaciens (5 mm., Rhabditida) (see page 100 and Fig. 6-8).

Trichuris campanula and *T. serrata* (Exotic, South America: Trichuroidea) (see page 136 and Figs. 6-63 and 12-20).

Liver, Bile Ducts, and Gall Bladder; Pancreatic Duct

NEMATODE

Capillaria hepatica (see page 136 and Fig. 14-89).

TREMATODES

Opisthorchis tenuicollis, Metorchis albidus (4.6 mm.), *M. conjunctus* (6.6 mm.), *Amphimerus pseudofelineus* (22 mm.), *Parametorchis complexus* (10 mm.), *Clonorchis sinensis* (Asia) (Opisthorchiidae) (see page 83 and Figs. 4-9 and 4-19).

Platynosomum fastosum (8 mm.), *Eurytrema procyonis* (3.3 mm.) (Dicrocoeliidae) (see page 82 and Figs. 4-18 and 12-21).

Respiratory System

NASAL CAVITY, TRACHEA, AND BRONCHI

NEMATODES

Capillaria aerophila (Trichuroidea) (see page 136 and Fig. 12-20).

Mammomonogamus spp. (Syngamidae) (see page 116 and Fig. 6-29).

LUNG PARENCHYMA

NEMATODE

Aelurostrongylus abstrusus (9 mm., Metastrongyloidea) (see page 118 and Figs. 12-20 and 14-70).

TREMATODE

Paragonimus kellicotti (Troglotrematidae) (see page 80 and Figs. 4-12 and 12-17B).

Vascular System

PULMONARY ARTERY AND RIGHT HEART

NEMATODES

Dirofilaria immitis (Filarioidea) (see page 130 and Figs. 6-54 and 12-40).
Angiostrongylus vasorum (see page 118).

BLOOD

PROTOZOON

Cytauxzoon felis (Piroplasm) (see page 71).

NEMATODE MICROFILARIA

Dirofilaria immitis (see page 262 and Fig. 12-40).

Skeletal Muscles

NEMATODE LARVA

Trichinella spiralis (Trichuroidea) (see page 134 and Figs. 12-42 and 14-87).

Connective Tissues

INSECT LARVA

Cuterebra spp. (30 mm.) (see page 22 and Figs. 1-12, 1-21, 14-1, and 14-3).

Urogenital System

URINARY BLADDER

NEMATODES

Capillaria plica (60 mm.), *C. feliscati* (32 mm.) (Trichuroidea) (see page 137 and Fig. 12-20).

Nervous System

NEMATODE

Dirofilaria immitis adults migrating erratically in meninges and ventricles (see page 130 and Fig. 6-54).

INSECT LARVA

Cuterebra spp. (30 mm.) (see page 22 and Figs. 1-12, 1-21, 14-1 and 14-3).

Skin and Hair

INSECTS

Adult dipterans (see pages 4 to 19).
Felicola subrostratus (Mallophaga) (see Fig. 7-2).
Ctenocephalides canis, C. felis, Echidnophaga gallinacea (Siphonaptera) (see page 31 and Figs. 1-41 and 1-42).

ARACHNIDS

Dermacentor spp., *Haemaphysalis leporispalustris*, *Ixodes* spp. (Ixodidae) (see pages 40 to 45 and Figs. 2-6 to 2-16).
Notoedres cati, Sarcoptes scabiei (Sarcoptidae) (see page 52 and Figs. 2-23 to 2-25)
Lynxacarus radovskyi (Listrophoroidea) (see page 56).
Cheyletiella blakei (Cheyletidae) (see page 59 and Figs. 2-34 and 12-3).
Demodex cati (Demodicidae) (see page 58 and Fig. 2-33).
Neotrombicula whartoni, Walchia americana (Trombiculidae) (see page 60 and Fig. 2-36). *Neotrombicula whartoni*, a bright red chigger, has been found in the external ear canal of cats. *Walchia americana*, normally a parasite of the gray squirrel *Sciurus carolinensis*, is capable of causing a severe and generalized dermatitis in cats.

PARASITES OF RUMINANTS

Toxoplasma gondii may occur in any tissue of any host as extracellular or intracellular tachyzoites or as bradyzoites in cysts (see page 69 and Figs. 14-27 and 14-28).

Alimentary System

MOUTH, ESOPHAGUS, AND FORESTOMACHS

PROTOZOANS

Sarcocystis sarcocysts in muscles of tongue and esophagus (see page 68 and Fig. 14-26).

CESTODE LARVAE

Taenia spp. cysticerci in muscles of tongue (see page 89, Table 5-1, and Fig. 14-46).

INSECT LARVA

Hypoderma lineatum in wall of esophagus (see page 20).

NEMATODES

Gongylonema pulchrum (150 mm.), *G. verrucosum* (100 mm.) (Spirurida) (see page 129 and Fig. 13-26). Woven in a neat, sinusoidal pattern in the esophageal (*G. pulchrum*) or ruminal (*G. verrucosum*) mucosa.

TREMATODES

Cotylophoron cotylophoron, *Paramphistomum cervi*, *P. liorchis*, *P. microbothroides* (Paramphistomatidae) (see page 80 and Fig. 4-14).

ABOMASUM

PROTOZOAN

Eimeria gilruthi megaschizonts (see page 309 and Fig. 14-24).

NEMATODES

Haemonchus contortus, *H. placei*, *H. similis*, *Mecistocirrus digitatus*, *Ostertagia ostertagi*, *O. bisonis*, *O. circumcincta*, *O. orloffi*, *O. trifurcata*, *O. (Grosspiculagia) lyrata*, *O. (G.) occidentalis*, *O. (Telodorsagia) davtiani*, *O. (Pseudostertagia) bullosa*, *Marshallagia marshalli*, and *Trichostrongylus axei* (Trichostrongyloidea) (see pages 105 to 109).

Genus	Length (mm.)	Figure(s)
Haemonchus	14 to 30	6-11, 6-18
Mecistocirrus	43	6-14
Ostertagia (s.l.)	7 to 9	6-11, 6-12
Trichostrongylus axei	7	6-11, 6-15, 14-61

SMALL INTESTINE

NEMATODES

Toxocara vitulorum (30 cm., Ascaridoidea). This exotic parasite of cattle has an esophageal ventriculus and produces subspherical eggs with a pitted shell surface. *Ascaris suum*, an occasional parasite of ruminants, lacks a ventriculus and produces ellipsoidal eggs with a mammillated shell surface.

Cooperia curticei, *C. bisonis*, *C. oncophora*, *C. pectinata*, *C. punctata*, *C. spatulata*, *C. occidentalis*, *Trichostrongylus colubriformis*, *T. longispicularis*, *T. capricola*, *T. vitrinus*, *Nematodirus helvetianus*, *N. spathiger*, *N. filicollis*, *N. abnormalis*, *N. lanceolatus*, *N. battus* (Strongylida: Trichostrongyloidea).

Genus	Length (mm.)	Figure(s)
Cooperia	6 to 16	6-11, 6-20
Trichostrongylus	6 to 7	6-11, 6-15
Nematodirus	20 to 25	6-11, 6-13, 6-19

Bunostomum phlebotomum (cattle), *B. trigonocephalum* (sheep) (25 mm., Ancylostomatoidea) (see page 113 and Fig. 6-26).

Strongyloides papillosus (6 mm., Rhabditida) (see page 100 and Fig. 6-8).

Capillaria bovis, *C. brevipes* (Trichuroidea) (see page 136 and Fig. 12-23).

Oesophagostomum spp. third and fourth stage larvae (Strongyloidea) (see page 112 and Fig. 6-25).

CESTODES

Moniezia expansa, *M. benedeni* (Anoplocephalidae) (see page 93 and Figs. 5-10, 5-21 and 12-23).

Thysanosoma actinoides, *Wyominia tetoni* (Anoplocephalidae) (see page 93).

Thysaniezia, *Stilesia*, *Avitellina* (Anoplocephalidae). Exotic anoplocephalids of ruminants.

PROTOZOANS

Eimeria spp. (coccidia) (see page 67 and Figs. 12-28, 12-29, and 14-20 to 14-24).

Giardia lamblia (flagellate) (see page 65 and Fig. 12-35).

CECUM AND COLON

NEMATODES

Oesophagostomum radiatum (cattle), *Oe. columbianum* (sheep and goats), *Oe. venulosum* (sheep and goats), *Chabertia ovina* (sheep and goats) (18 to 22 mm., Strongyloidea) (see page 112 and Figs. 6-23 to 6-25). The fourth stage larvae of *Oe. radiatum* in cattle and *Oe. columbianum* in sheep may be found in abscesses in the gut wall (see Fig. 6-25).

Trichuris discolor (52 mm., cattle), *Trichuris ovis* (70 mm., sheep and goats) (Trichuroidea) (see page 136 and Figs. 6-61 and 12-23).

Skrjabinema ovis, *S. caprae* (8 to 10 mm., Oxyurida) (see page 122).

PROTOZOANS

Eimeria spp. (coccidia) (see page 67 and Figs. 12-28, 12-29, and 14-20 to 14-24).

Entamoeba bovis (ameba).

Buxtonella sulcata (ciliate).

LIVER

NEMATODES

Ascaris suum (Ascaridida). This swine ascarid sometimes matures in the bile ducts of sheep and cattle.

Stephanurus dentatus (Strongyloidea) (see page 115 and Fig. 6-28). Immature *S. dentatus* worms migrate through the bovine liver and cause severe trauma.

CESTODES

Thysanosoma actinoides, Wyominia tetonis (Anoplocephalidae) (see page 93).

CESTODE LARVAE

Echinococcus granulosus, E. multilocularis hydatids (Taeniidae) (see page 91 and Figs. 5-18, 5-19, 14-45, 14–51, and 14-52).

Taenia hydatigena cysticerci (Taeniidae) (see page 90, Table 5-1, and Fig. 5-15).

TREMATODES

Fasciola hepatica, F. gigantica, Fascioloides magna (Fasciolidae) (see page 77 and Figs. 4-1 to 4-7, 4-10, and 12-27A). *Fasciola hepatica* (30 mm.) is endemic in western and gulf states of U.S.A., Hawaii, Puerto Rico, British Columbia, and eastern provinces of Canada. *Fasciola gigantica* (75 mm.) is endemic in Hawaii and Africa. *Fascioloides magna* (100 mm.) is widely scattered over North America.

Dicrocoelium dendriticum (Europe, Asia, Africa, South America, and central New York State), *Eurytrema pancreaticum* (Asia and Brazil) (Dicrocoeliidae) (see page 82 and Figs. 4-17 and 12-27C).

PERITONEUM AND PERITONEAL CAVITY

NEMATODE

Setaria labiatopapillosa (Filarioidea) (see page 132 and Fig. 6-56).

CESTODE LARVA

Taenia hydatigena larva (Taeniidae) (see page 90, Table 5-1, and Figure 5-15).

PENTASTOMID NYMPH

Linguatula serrata (see page 140 and Fig. 6-71).

Respiratory System

NASAL CAVITY AND PARANASAL SINUSES

INSECT LARVA

Oestrus ovis larva in sheep and goats (Oestridae) (see page 20 and Fig. 1-21).

TRACHEA AND BRONCHI

NEMATODES

Dictyocaulus viviparus (80 mm.; cattle), *D. filaria* (100 mm.; sheep and goats) (Trichostrongyloidea) (see page 110 and Figs. 6-11, 6-22, and 12-26).

Protostrongylus rufescens (50 mm.; sheep) (Metastrongyloidea) (see page 117 and Figs. 6-32 and 12-26).

Mammomonogamus laryngeus (Syngamidae) (see page 116 and Fig. 6-29). Male and female worms are fused *in copula;* endemic in Puerto Rico.

LUNG PARENCHYMA

NEMATODES

Muellerius capillaris (Metastrongyloidea) (see page 117 and Figs. 6-33 and 12-26).

Oesophagostomum columbianum larvae (erratic migration) (see page 112 and Fig. 6-25).

CESTODE LARVA

Echinococcus granulosus (Taeniidae) (see page 91 and Figs. 5-18, 5-19, and 14-51).

Vascular System

HEART

CESTODE LARVAE

Taenia ovis, Taeniarhynchus saginatus (Taeniidae) (see page 90 and Table 5-1).

ARTERIES

NEMATODES

Elaeophora schneideri (sheep; Filarioidea) (see page 133).

Elaeophora poeli (cattle; Filarioidea).

Onchocerca armillata (cattle; Filarioidea).

Veins

TREMATODES

Schistosoma mathiei in sheep, *S. mansoni* in South American cattle (Schistosomatidae) (see page 78 and Fig. 4-11).

Lymph Nodes

PENTASTOMID

Linguatula serrata (see page 140 and Fig. 6-71).

Blood

NEMATODE MICROFILARIA

Setaria labiatopapillosa.

PROTOZOANS

Babesia bigemina, B. bovis, B. divergens, B. argentina, Theileria parva, T. annulata, T. mutans (piroplasms) (see page 70 and Fig. 3-8).

Trypanosoma theileri (cattle), *T. melophagium* (sheep) (hemoflagellates) (see page 62 and Fig. 3-1). Rarely seen in blood films; readily demonstrable by blood culture.

ORGANISMS OF UNCERTAIN CLASSIFICATION

Anaplasma marginale, Eperythrozoon wenyoni.

Skeletal Muscles and Connective Tissues

CESTODE LARVAE

Taeniarhynchus saginatus (Taeniidae) (Table 5-1). Cysticerci found most frequently in the muscles of mastication, tongue, heart, and muscular portion of the diaphragm of cattle; scolex with four suckers but no hooks.

Taenia ovis (Taeniidae) (Table 5-1). Pea-sized vesicles are found in the heart and esophagus and beneath the epicardium and diaphragmatic pleura of sheep and goats.

Taenia hydatigena (Taeniidae) (see page 90, Table 5-1, and Fig. 5-15). Sometimes found in skeletal muscles but more commonly in liver or on peritoneal membranes.

INSECT LARVAE

Hypoderma bovis, H. lineatum (Hypodermatidae) (see page 20 and Fig. 1-21).

NEMATODES

Onchocerca gutterosa, O. lienalis, O. bovis (Filarioidea) (see page 132). Adult *Onchocerca* worms are found in deep connective tissues, microfilariae in the dermis.

PROTOZOANS

Sarcocysts in Muscles

Sarcocystis spp. (coccidia) (see page 68, Table 3-1, and Fig. 14-26).

Urogenital System

PROTOZOAN

Tritrichomonas foetus (flagellate) (see page 64 and Fig. 3-2).

Nervous System

Brain, Spinal Cord, and Meninges

NEMATODE

Parelaphostrongylus tenuis (Metastrongyloidea) (see page 117 and Figs. 14-74 and 14-75).

CESTODE LARVA

Multiceps multiceps (Taeniidae) in brain of sheep and goats (see page 90 and Figs. 5-16 and 14-48).

INSECT LARVA

Hypoderma bovis (Hypodermatidae) (see page 20).

Eye

NEMATODES

Thelazia californiensis (sheep), *T. gulosa* (cattle), *T. skrjabini* (cattle) (Spirurida) (see page 129 and Fig. 6-51).

Skin and Hair

INSECTS

Musca autumnalis, Stomoxys calcitrans, Haematobia irritans (Muscidae) (see page 12 and Figs. 1-13, 1-14, and 1-16).

Glossina spp. (Africa) (see page 15 and Fig. 1-17).

Melophagus ovinus (Hippoboscidae) (see page 16 and Fig. 1-18).

Hypoderma bovis, H. lineatum (Hypodermatidae) (see page 20).

Tabanidae (see page 10 and Figs. 1-9 and 1-10).

Dipteran Larvae

Hypoderma bovis, H. lineatum (30 mm., Hypodermatidae) (see page 20 and Fig. 1-21).

Calliphoridae, Sarcophagidae (see page 17 and Figs. 1-11 and 1-20).

Anoplurans

Haematopinus eurysternus, H. quadripertussus, H. tuberculatus, Linognathus vituli, Solenopotes capillatus (cattle), *Linognathus ovillus, L. pedalis, L. oviformes* (sheep), *Linognathus oviformes, L. stenopsis* (goat) (see page 25 and Figs. 1-29 to 1-31).

Mallophagans

Damalinia bovis (cattle), *D. ovis* (sheep). *Damalinia caprae, D. limbatus, D. (Holokartikos) crassipes* (goats) (see page 29 and Fig. 1-34).

Siphonapterans

Echidnophaga gallinacea (see page 33 and Fig. 1-42).

ARACHNIDS

Metastigmata: Ixodidae

Ambylomma americanum, A. cajennense, A. imitator, A. inornatum, A. maculatum, A. oblongoguttatum (see page 43 and Fig. 2-1).

Boophilus annulatus, B. microplus (see page 43 and Fig. 2-13).

Dermacentor andersoni, D. albipictus, D. occidentalis, D. variabilis, D. (Otocentor) nitens (see page 43 and Figs. 2-14 to 2-16).

Haemaphysalis leporispalustris (see page 43 and Fig. 2-10).

Ixodes cookei, I. pacificus, I. scapularis (see page 43 and Figs. 2-2, 2-8, and 2-9).

Metastigmata: Argasidae

Otobius megnini ("spinose ear tick") (see page 40 and Fig. 2-5).

Ornithodorus coriaceus, O. turicata (see page 40 and Fig. 2-4).

Astigmata

Sarcoptes scabiei (see page 51 and Fig. 2-23).

Chorioptes bovis (see page 55 and Figs. 2-28 and 2-29).

Psoroptes communis, P. cuniculi (see page 53 and Fig. 2-27).

Prostigmata

Demodex bovis, D. ovis, D. caprae (see page 58 and Fig. 2-33).

Psorobia ovis (see page 59).

Trombiculidae (see page 60 and Fig. 2-36).

Mesostigmata

Raillietia auris (cattle), *R. caprae* (goats). Ear mites (see page 49 and Fig. 2-20).

PROTOZOAN

Besnoitia besnoiti (coccidian) (see page 69).

NEMATODES

Adult Filariids

Stephanofilaria stilesi (6 mm., Filarioidea). Very small adult filariids in skin of ventral abdomen.

Parafilaria bovicola (Filarioidea). Causes "summer bleeding" in cattle.

Microfilariae

Onchocerca gutterosa, O. lienalis, O. bovis (Filarioidea). Microfilariae found in dermis of cattle.

Elaeophora schneideri (Filarioidea) (see page 133).

Rhabditis strongyloides (Rhabditida) (see page 99 and Figs. 6-6, 14-57, and 14-58).

PARASITES OF HORSES

Alimentary System

MOUTH

INSECT LARVAE

Gasterophilus intestinalis, G. nasalis, G. hemorrhoidalis (see page 21).

PROTOZOAN

Trichomonas equibuccalis (mucosoflagellate). Found around gum margins of cheek teeth (see page 64).

STOMACH

NEMATODES

Draschia megastoma, Habronema muscae, H. microstoma (Spirurida) (see page 130 and Fig. 6-53).

Trichostrongylus axei (Trichostrongyloidea) (see page 105 and Figs. 6-11 and 6-15). May cause hypertrophic gastritis with wartlike mucosal proliferations.

INSECT LARVAE

Gasterophilus spp. (see page 21 and Figs. 1-21 and 1-23).

SMALL INTESTINE

NEMATODES

Parascaris equorum (Ascaridoidea) (see page 124 and Fig. 12-32).

Strongyloides westeri (Rhabditida) (see page 100 and Figs. 6-8, 12-32, and 14-59).

CESTODES

Anoplocephala magna, Paranoplocephala mamillana (see page 94 and Figs. 5-1, 5-22, and 12-31).

PROTOZOAN

Eimeria leuckarti (coccidian) (see page 67 and Figs. 12-30 and 14-29).

LARGE INTESTINE

NEMATODES

Oxyuris equi (150 mm.), *Probstmayria vivipara* (3 mm.) (Oxyurida) (see page 121 and Figs. 6-37 to 6-39 and 12-32).

Family Strongylidae

The horse is host to 56 species belonging to the family Strongylidae and as many as 20 different species are often found in the same horse.

Subfamily Strongylinae. Strongylus vulgaris, S. edentatus, S. equinus, Triodontophorus serratus, T. brevicauda, T. tenuicollis, T. nipponicus, Oesophagodontus robustus, Craterostomum acuticaudatum (see page 111 and Figs. 6-9, 13-7, and 13-10, bottom row).

Subfamily Cyathostominae. Genera: *Cyathostomum, Cylicocyclus, Cylicostephanus, Cylico-*

dontophorus, Poteriostomum, Gyalocephalus (see page 111 and Figs. 13-8 to 13-18).

Each species can be identified by careful study of the stomal region alone. With fresh specimens, detail sufficient for identification can be seen without recourse to clearing agents; simply mount the specimen under a coverslip in a drop of water. With this simple preparation, it is usually possible to roll the specimen so that both dorsal and lateral aspects may be studied. Even preserved specimens may be studied in this manner but tend to be considerably less transparent than fresh specimens. In order to facilitate comparisons, I have grouped together illustrations of the species that bear the greatest resemblance to one another. The nomenclature of J. Ralph Lichtenfels' excellent monograph *Helminths fo Domestic Equids* (Proc. Helminth. Soc. Wash., 42, 1975) is the system that has been applied in the following pictorial key.

CESTODE

Anoplocephala perfoliata (see page 94 and Figs. 5-4, 5-22, and 12-31). Found mainly in the cecum, this tapeworm tends also to cluster in the ileum near the ileocecal valve, where it is associated with ulceration and chronic inflammation of the ileal wall.

LIVER

NEMATODE LARVAE

Parascaris equorum (Ascaridoidea).

Strongylus edentatus, S. equinus (see page 111 and Figs. 14-64 through 14-68).

CESTODE LARVA

Echinococcus granulosus (Taeniidae) (see page 91 and Figs. 5-18, 5-19, and 14-51).

PANCREAS

NEMATODE

Strongylus equinus (see page 111 and Fig. 14-68).

PERITONEUM AND PERITONEAL CAVITY

NEMATODES

Setaria equina (150 mm.; Filarioidea) (see page 132 and Figs. 6-57 and 12-41).

Text continued on page 290

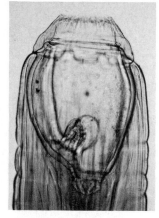

Strongylus vulgaris

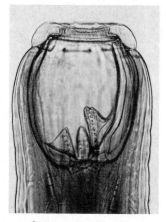

Strongylus equinus

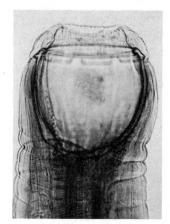

Strongylus edentatus

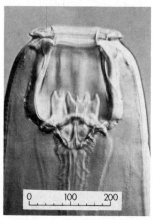

Triodontophorus brevicauda

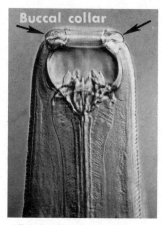

Triodontophorus serratus

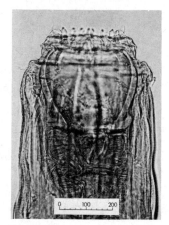

Oesophagodontus robustus

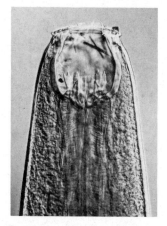

Triodontophorus nipponicus

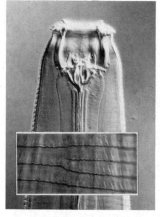

Triodontophorus tenuicollis

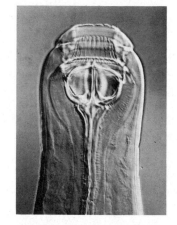

Gyalocephalus capitatus

Figure 13–7. Members of the subfamily Strongylinae (large strongyles) and *Gyalocephalus capitatus* (subfamily Cyathostominae). *Strongylus vulgaris* and *Oesophagodontus robustus* (x72); *Strongylus equinus* (x40); *Strongylus edentatus* (x33); *Triodontophorus* spp. and *Gyalocephalus capitatus* (x112). *Strongylus* spp. cleared and mounted by the glycol methacrylate method of Pijanowski *et al.* (1972): Cornell Vet., *62*, 333–336.

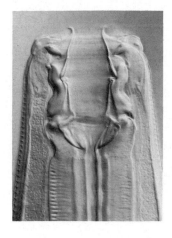
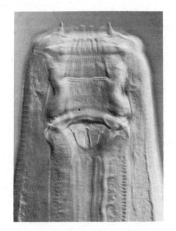
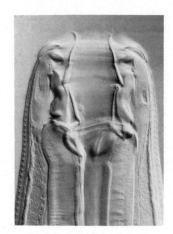

Cyathostomum coronatum

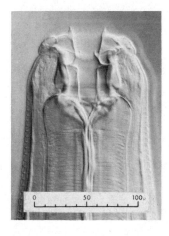
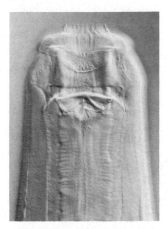
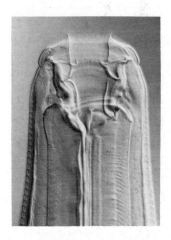

Cyathostomum catinatum

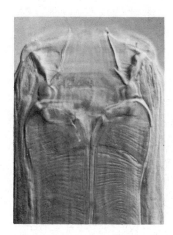
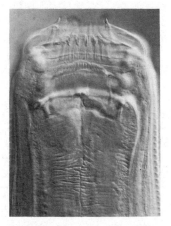
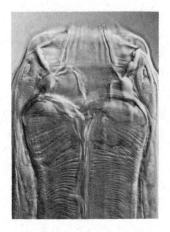

Cyathostomum tetracanthum

Figure 13–8. Members of the subfamily Cyathostominae. Dorsoventral (left), dorsal surface (center), and lateral (right) views of the heads of *Cyathostomum coronatum* (top row), *C. catinatum* (middle row), and *C. tetracanthum* (bottom row). (All x283.)

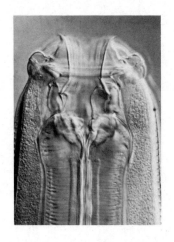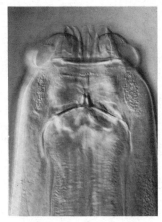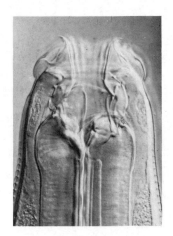

Cyathostomum labiatum

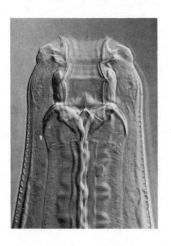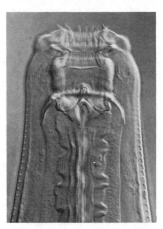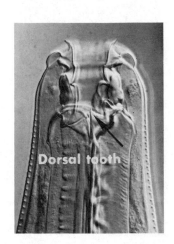

Cyathostomum labratum

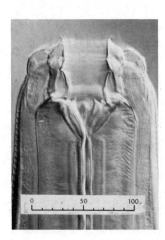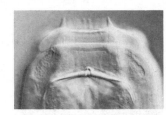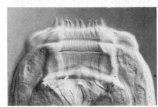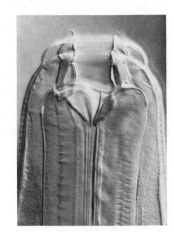

Cylicostephanus goldi

Figure 13–9. Members of the subfamily Cyathostominae. Dorsoventral (left), dorsal surface (center), and lateral (right) of the heads of *Cyathostomum labiatum* (top row), *C. labratum* (middle row), and *Cylicostephanus goldi* (bottom row). (All x283.)

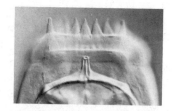
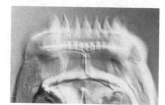
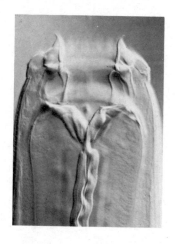
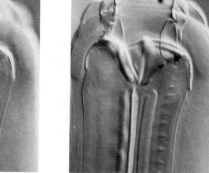

Cylicostephanus asymetricus

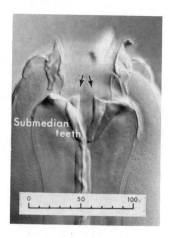
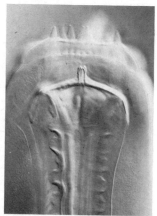

Cylicostephanus bidentatus

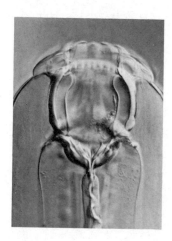
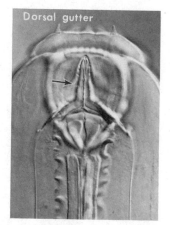
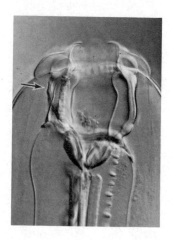

Craterostomum acuticaudatum

Figure 13–10. Members of the subfamily Cyathostominae and *Craterostomum acuticaudatum* (subfamily Strongylinae). Dorsoventral (left), dorsal surface (center), and lateral (right) views of the heads of *Cylicostephanus asymetricus* (top row), *C. bidentatus* (middle row), and *Craterostomum acuticaudatum* (bottom row). (All x283.)

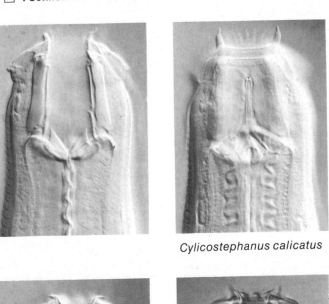

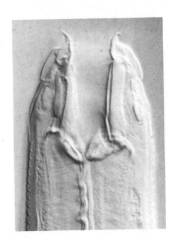

Cylicostephanus calicatus

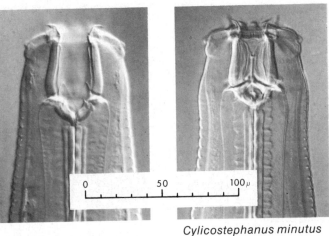

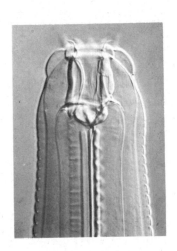

Cylicostephanus minutus

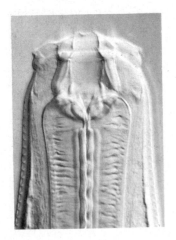

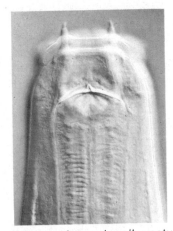

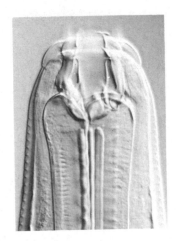

Cylicostephanus longibursatus

Figure 13–11. Members of the subfamily Cyathostominae. Dorsoventral (left), dorsal surface (center), and lateral (right) views of the heads of *Cylicostephanus calicatus* (top row), *C. minutus* (middle row), and *C. longibursatus* (bottom row). (All x425.)

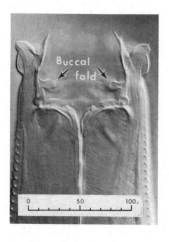
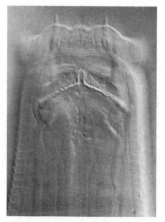
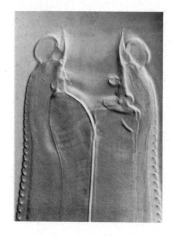

Cylicocyclus nassatus

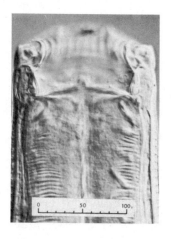
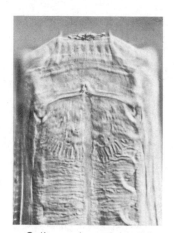
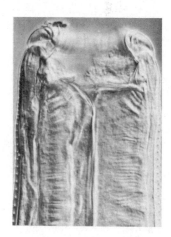

Cylicocyclus ashworthi

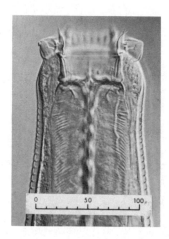
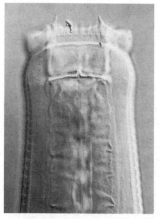
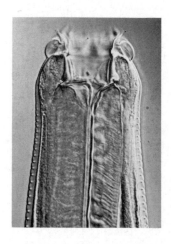

Cylicocyclus leptostomus

Figure 13–12. Members of the subfamily Cyathostominae. Dorsoventral (left), dorsal surface (center), and lateral (right) views of the heads of *Cylicocyclus nassatus* (top row), *C. ashworthi* (middle row), and *C. leptostomus* (bottom row). (*C. nassatus* and *C. leptostomus* x283, *C. ashworthi* x242.)

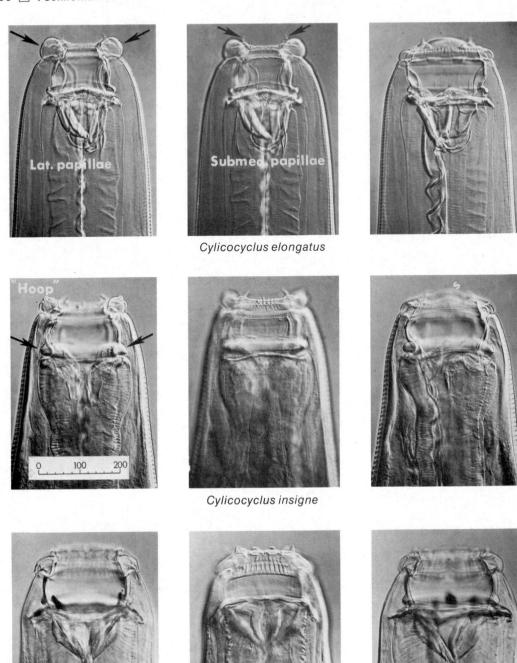

Cylicocyclus elongatus

Cylicocyclus insigne

Cylicocyclus ultrajectinus

Figure 13–13. Members of the subfamily Cyathostominae. Dorsoventral (left), dorsal surface (center), and lateral (right) views of the heads of *Cylicocyclus elongatus* (top row), *C. insigne* (middle row), and *C. ultrajectinus* (bottom row). (All x112.)

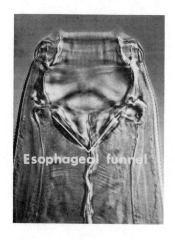 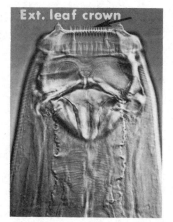 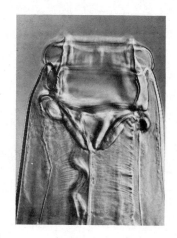

Poteriostomum imparidentatum

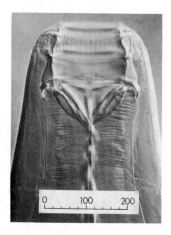 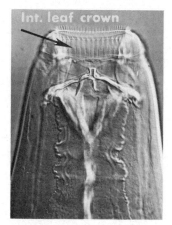 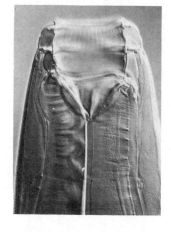

Poteriostomum ratzii

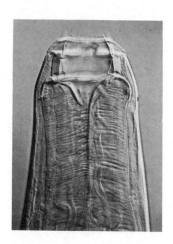 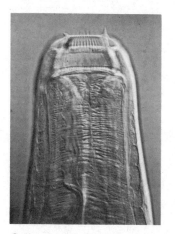 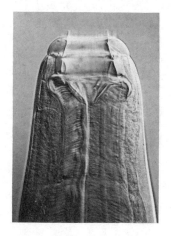

Cylicodontophorus mettami

Figure 13–14. Members of the subfamily Cyathostominae. Dorsoventral (left), dorsal surface (center), and lateral (right) views of the heads of *Poteriostomum imparidentatum* (top row), *Poteriostomum ratzii* (middle row), and *Cylicodontophorus mettami* (bottom row). (All x112.)

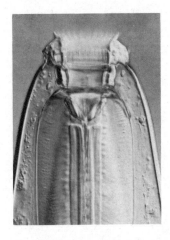
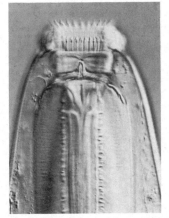
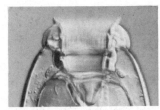
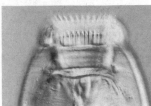

Cylicodontophorus bicoronatus

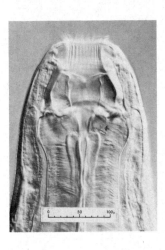
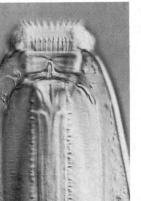
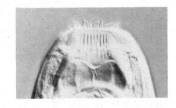
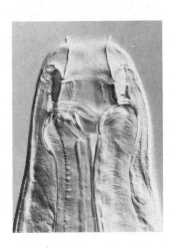
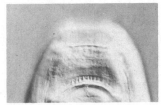

Cylicodontophorus euproctus

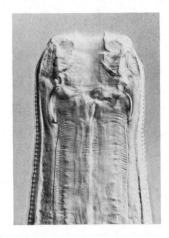
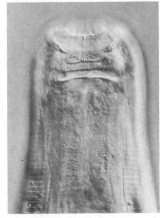
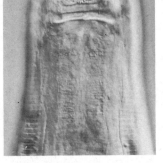
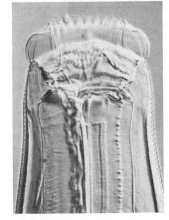

Cyathostomum pateratum

Figure 13–15. Members of the subfamily Cyathostominae. Dorsoventral (left), dorsal surface (center), and lateral (right) views of the heads of *Cylicodontophorus bicoronatus* (top row), *C. euproctus* (middle row), and *Cyathostomum pateratum* (bottom row). (All x170.)

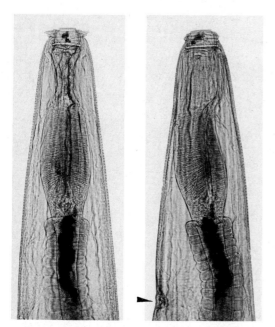

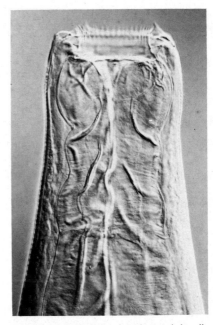

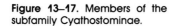

Figure 13–16. *Cylicocyclus auriculatus* (subfamily Cyathostominae) (x50). Note prominent lateral head papillae. Arrow indicates position of excretory pore.

Figure 13–18. *Cylicocyclus brevicapsulatus*, the only homely member of the subfamily Cyathostominae (x168).

Figure 13–17. Members of the subfamily Cyathostominae.

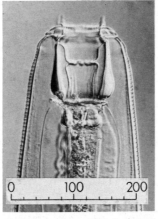

Cylicostephanus poculatus

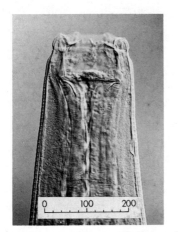

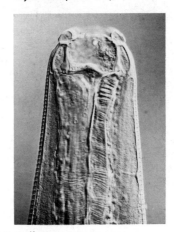

Cylicocyclus radiatus

Strongylus edentatus (44 mm. Strongylinae) (see page 111 and Figs. 14-64 to 14-67).

Respiratory System

PARANASAL SINUSES

INSECT LARVA

Rhinoestrus purpureus (Oestridae; exotic).

BRONCHI AND BRONCHIOLES

NEMATODE

Dictyocaulus arnfieldi (65 mm.; Trichostrongyloidea) (see page 110 and Figs. 6-11 and 6-22).

LUNG PARENCHYMA

PROTOZOAN OR FUNGUS?

Pneumocystis carinii (uncertain classification) (see page 311 and Fig. 14-34). Causes acute pneumonia in immunosuppressed hosts.

Vascular System

ARTERIES

NEMATODES

Strongylus vulgaris (see page 111 and Fig. 13-19).
Elaeophora böhmi (Filarioidea) (see page 264 and Fig. 12-41). Found in intimal nodules of the wall of the aorta and other vessels. Exotic.

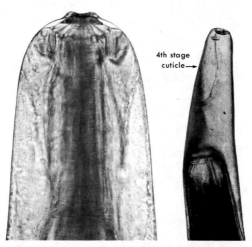

4th stage cuticle→

Figure 13–19. *Strongylus vulgaris* fourth stage (left, x108) and immature fifth stage (right, x38) from a mural thrombus of the cranial mesenteric artery of a horse.

BLOOD

NEMATODE MICROFILARIA

Setaria equina (Filarioidea) (see page 264 and Fig. 12-41).

PROTOZOAN

Babesia caballi (piroplasm) (see page 70).

SKELETAL MUSCLES AND CONNECTIVE TISSUES

PROTOZOAN CYSTS

Sarcocystis bertrami, S. fayeri (coccidians) (see page 68, Table 3-1, and Figs. 14-25 and 14-26).

INSECT LARVAE

Hypoderma bovis, H. lineatum (see page 20 and Fig. 1-21). In dorsal subcutaneous tissues of horse erratically.

NEMATODE MICROFILARIAE

Onchocerca cervicalis, O. reticulata (Filarioidea) (see page 264 and Fig. 12-41). Microfilariae in dermis.

Urogenital System

KIDNEYS

PROTOZOAN

Klossiella equi (coccidian) (see page 310 and Fig. 14-32).

TESTES

NEMATODE

Strongylus edentatus (see page 111 and Figs. 14-64 to 14-67). Immature fifth stage in vaginal tunics.

Nervous System

BRAIN AND SPINAL CORD

NEMATODES

Strongylus vulgaris (see page 111 and Figs. 13-7 and 13-19). Fourth or fifth stages migrating erratically; even one worm can cause fatal neurological disease.
Setaria spp. (Filarioidea) (see page 132 and

Figs. 6-56, 6-57, and 12-41). Erratic migration with neurological disease.

Micronema deletrix (Rhabditida) (see page 99).

Draschia megastoma (Spirurida) (Mayhew *et al.*, 1983).

INSECTS

Hypoderma bovis, H. lineatum (Diptera) (see page 20). Erratic migration in abnormal host; one larva can cause fatal neurologic disease.

PROTOZOAN

Equine protozoan myelitis organism (EPM).

EYE

NEMATODES

Thelazia lacrymalis (Spirurida) (see page 129 and Fig. 6-51). Found in conjunctival sac and lacrimal ducts.

Draschia megastoma and *Habronema* spp. larvae may cause habronemic conjunctivitis (see page 130).

Onchocerca spp. microfilariae (see page 264 and Fig. 12-41).

Skin and Hair

INSECTS

Musca autumnalis, Stomoxys calcitrans (Diptera: Muscidae) (see page 12 and Fig. 1-13).

Hippobosca equina, Lipoptena cervi (Diptera: Hippoboscidae) (see page 16 and Fig. 1-18).

Gasterophilus intestinalis, G. nasalis, G. hemorrhoidalis (Diptera) (see page 21).

Tabanus spp., *Chrysops* spp. (Diptera: Tabanidae) (see page 10 and Figs. 1-9 and 1-10).

Haematopinus asini (Anoplura) (see page 26 and Fig. 9-1).

Damalinia equi (Mallophaga: Ischnocera) (see page 29).

Echidnophaga gallinacea (Siphonaptera) (see page 33 and Fig. 1-42).

Triatoma sanguisuga (Hemiptera: Triatominae) (see page 35 and Fig. 1-48).

INSECT LARVAE

Hypoderma bovis, H. lineatum (Diptera) (see page 20 and Fig. 1-21). In subcutis of the saddle area.

ARACHNIDS

Metastigmata: Ixodidae

Amblyomma, Anocentor, Boophilus, Dermacentor, Haemaphysalis, Hyalomma, Ixodes, Rhipicephalus (see pages 43 to 45 and Figs. 2-6 to 2-16).

Astigmata

Sarcoptes scabiei (Sarcoptidae) (see page 51 and Fig. 2-23).

Psoroptes communis, P. cuniculi, Chorioptes bovis (Psoroptidae) (see pages 53 to 55 and Figs. 2-27, 2-28, and 2-29).

Prostigmata

Trombiculidae (see page 60 and Fig. 2-36).

Demodex equi (see page 58 and Fig. 2-33).

NEMATODE MICROFILARIAE AND LARVAE

Parafilaria multipapillosa (Filarioidea) (see page 263 and Fig. 12-41). Microfilariae in serosanguineus discharge from ulcerated nodules.

Onchocerca cervicalis, O. reticulata (Filarioidea) (see page 264 and Fig. 12-41). Microfilariae of *Onchocerca* are almost universally present in the dermis of horses, especially the dermis of the ventrum.

Rhabditis strongyloides (Rhabditida) (see page 99 and Fig. 6-6).

Draschia megastoma, Habronema muscae, H. microstoma (Spirurida) (see page 130). Larvae of these species excite exuberant granulomatous reactions in skin wounds, areas of skin subject to frequent wetting, and ocular conjunctiva.

PARASITES OF SWINE

Alimentary System

ESOPHAGUS

NEMATODE

Gongylonema pulchrum (150 mm.; Spirurida) (see page 129 and Fig. 13-26).

STOMACH

NEMATODES

Physocephalus sexalatus (Fig. 6-52), *Ascarops strongylina, Gnathostoma hispidum* (Fig. 6-48), and *Simondsia paradoxum* (Spirurida).

Hyostrongylus rubidus (9 mm.) and *Ollulanus tricuspis* (1 mm.) (Trichostrongyloidea) (see page 109 and Figs. 6-11 and 6-19).

Capillaria putorii (Trichuroidea) (see page 136 and Fig. 12-20).

INSECT LARVAE

Gasterophilus intestinalis, G. hemorrhoidalis (Diptera) (see page 21 and Fig. 1-21).

Small Intestine

NEMATODES

Ascaris suum (410 mm.; Ascaridoidea) (see page 124 and Figs. 6-40 and 12-34).

Globocephalus urosubulatus (6 mm.; Ancylostomatoidea) (see page 113 and Fig. 6-27).

Strongyloides ransomi (5 mm.; Rhabditida) (see page 100 and Fig. 6-8).

Trichinella spiralis (4 mm.; Trichuroidea) (see page 134 and Fig. 6-59).

ACANTHOCEPHALAN

Macracanthorhynchus hirudinaceus (470 mm.) (see page 138 and Fig. 6-66).

PROTOZOANS

Eimeria debliecki and about 10 other species of *Eimeria, Isospora suis* (coccidians).

Giardia lamblia (mucosoflagellate) (see page 65 and Fig. 12-35).

Cecum and Colon

NEMATODES

Oesophagostomum dentatum, Oe. brevicaudum, Oe. georgianum, Oe. quadrispinulatum (Strongyloidea) (see page 112 and Fig. 6-23).

Trichuris suis (Trichuroidea) (see Figs. 6-63 and 12-34).

PROTOZOANS

Entamoeba histolytica, E. coli, E. suis, Endolimax nana, Iodamoeba buetschlii (amebas) (see page 65).

Chilomastix mesnili, Tetratrichomonas buttreyi, Trichomitus rotunda, T. suis (mucosoflagellates) (see page 64).

Balantidium coli (ciliate) (see page 65 and Fig. 12-19).

Liver, Pancreas, and Peritoneal Cavity

NEMATODE LARVAE

Ascaris suum (Ascaridoidea) (see page 124 and Fig. 6-42). Migrating larvae cause "milk spot" lesions on the liver surface.

Stephanurus dentatus (Strongyloidea) migrating larvae in liver and pancreas (see page 115 and Fig. 6-28).

TREMATODES

Fasciola hepatica, F. gigantica (see page 76 and Figs. 4-1 and 4-10).

CESTODE LARVAE

Echinococcus granulosus (Taeniidae) (see Figs. 5-18, 5-19, and 14-51).

Taenia hydatigena (Taeniidae) (see page 91 and Fig. 5-15).

Respiratory System

Bronchi and Bronchioles

NEMATODES

Metastrongylus apri, M. salmi, M. pudendotectus (Strongylida) (see page 116 and Fig. 6-30).

Lung Parenchyma

NEMATODE LARVA

Ascaris suum (see page 124 and Fig. 6-42).

CESTODE LARVA

Echinococcus granulosus (Taeniidae) (see page 91 and Figs. 5-18, 5-19, and 14-51).

TREMATODE

Paragonimus kellicotti (Troglotrematidae) (see page 80 and Figs. 4-12 and 12-17B).

Skeletal Muscles and Connective Tissues

⸫ NEMATODE LARVA

Trichinella spiralis (Trichuroidea) (see page 134 and Figs. 12-42 and 14-87).

CESTODE LARVAE

Taenia solium (Taeniidae) (see page 90, Table 5-1, and Figs. 14-46 and 14-47).

Spirometra mansonoides (Diphyllobothriidae) (see page 95 and Figs. 5-27 and 14-55).

TREMATODE LARVA

Alaria (mesocercaria, Diplostomatidae) (see page 81).

PROTOZOAN CYSTS

Sarcocystis miescheriana, S. porcifelis, S. suihominis (coccidians) (see page 68, Table 3-1 and Figs. 14-25 and 14-26).

Urogenital System

NEMATODE

Stephanurus dentatus (45 mm.; Strongylida) (see page 115 and Fig. 6-28). Stout, white worms in the kidneys, ureters, urinary bladder, perirenal fat, pork chops, spinal canal, and elsewhere as a result of erratic migrations.

Skin and Hair

INSECTS

Musca, Stomoxys (Diptera) (see page 12 and Figs. 1-13 and 1-14).
Haematopinus suis (Anoplura) (see page 26).
Pulex irritans, Echidnophaga gallinacea, Tunga penetrans (Siphonaptera) (see page 33 and Figs. 1-42 and 1-44).

ARACHNIDS

Metastigmata (ticks) (see pages 43 to 45 and Figs. 2-6 to 2-17).
Sarcoptes scabiei (Astigmata) (see page 51 and Fig. 2-23).
Demodex phylloides (Prostigmata) (see page 58).

COMMON PARASITES OF LABORATORY ANIMALS

Many parasites lose all opportunity to complete their life histories the day their host becomes a member of a laboratory animal colony. Although they may limit the usefulness of their immediate hosts as experimental subjects, such parasites present no continuing problem of control. Heartworm infection, for example, renders a dog unfit for experi-

ments involving the circulatory or respiratory system but, in the absence of mosquitoes, must remain confined to the host it arrived in. On the other hand, a surprising variety of arthropod, protozoan, and helminth parasites do succeed in maintaining impressive populations even in reasonably hygienic laboratory animal colonies. Hair-clasping mites, mucosoflagellates, coccidians, *Hymenolepis* tapeworms, and pinworms are particularly common. The following incomplete outline includes only the common parasites of laboratory rabbits, rats, mice, guinea pigs, monkeys, and apes.

PARASITES OF RABBITS

Alimentary System

STOMACH

NEMATODES

Obeliscoides cuniculi, Graphidium strigosum (18 to 20 mm.; Trichostrongyloidea) (see Fig. 13-20). Spicules of *O. cuniculi* 0.54 mm.; of *G. strigosum* 2.4 mm.

INTESTINE

NEMATODES

Trichostrongylus retortaeformis, Nematodirus leporis (Trichostrongyloidea) (see Figs. 6-11 and 6-15).

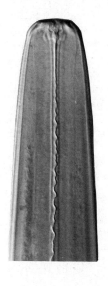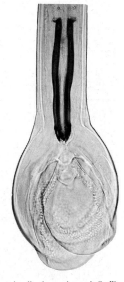

Figure 13–20. *Obeliscoides cuniculi*, stomal end (left) and bursa and spicules of male (right) (x120).

Strongyloides papillosus (6mm.; Rhabditida) (see page 100).
Passalurus ambiguus (11 mm.; Oxyurida) (see Fig. 6-36).
Trichuris leporis (Trichuroidea) (see page 136).

CESTODE

Cittotaenia ctenoides (Anoplocephalidae) (see Fig. 12-35).

PROTOZOANS

Eimeria spp. (coccidian) (see page 67 and Fig. 12-35). Ten species of *Eimeria* parasitize the intestinal epithelium and cause diarrhea and emaciation.
Entamoeba cuniculi (ameba). Nonpathogenic.

LIVER AND PERITONEAL CAVITY

PROTOZOAN

Eimeria stiedae causes biliary coccidiosis.

CESTODE LARVA

Taenia pisiformis (Taeniidae) (see page 90; Fig. 13-21).

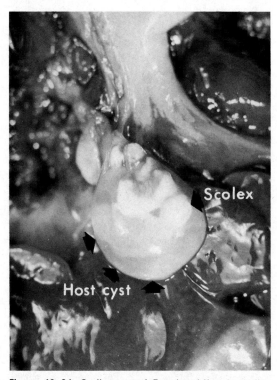

Figure 13–21. Cysticercus of *Taenia pisiformis* on the surface of the liver of a domestic rabbit (about x3).

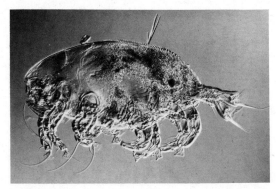

Figure 13–22. *Leporacarus gibbus,* a hair-clasping mite of rabbits (x100). (Specimen courtesy of Dr. Stephen Weisbroth.)

Skin and Hair

ARACHNIDS

Psoroptes cuniculi (Astigmata) (see page 55 and Fig. 2-27).
Sarcoptes, Chorioptes (Astigmata) (see Figs. 2-23, 2-28, and 2-29).
Leporacarus gibbus (see Fig. 13-22).
Cheyletiella parasitovorax (Prostigmata) (see page 59 and Fig. 2-34).

PARASITES OF RATS

Alimentary System

STOMACH AND INTESTINES

NEMATODES

Nippostrongylus brasiliensis (6 mm.; Trichostrongyloidea) (see Fig. 13-23).
Strongyloides ratti (Rhabditida) (see page 100 and Fig. 6-8).
Gongylonema neoplasticum (Spirurida) (see page 129).
Syphacia muris, Aspiculuris ratti (Oxyurida) (see Fig. 13-24).
Heterakis spumosa (16 mm., Ascaridida).
Trichinella spiralis (Trichuroidea) (see page 134 and Fig. 6-59).
Trichuris muris (Trichuroidea) (see page 136).

CESTODE

Hymenolepis diminuta (Hymenolopidae) (see page 94 and Fig. 12-35). Scolex without hooks.

PROTOZOANS

Eimeria nieschultzi and other species (coccidians) (see page 67 and Fig. 12-35).

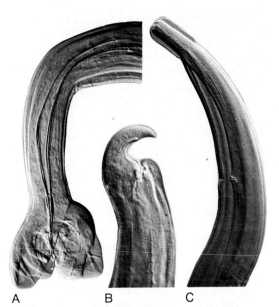

Figure 13–23. *Nippostrongylus brasiliensis.* A. Bursa and spicules of male (x125). B. Caudal end of female (x150). C. Esophageal region (x150).

Giardia (mucosoflagellate) (see page 65 and Fig. 12-35).

LIVER

NEMATODE

Capillaria hepatica (Trichuroidea) (see page 136 and Fig. 14-89).

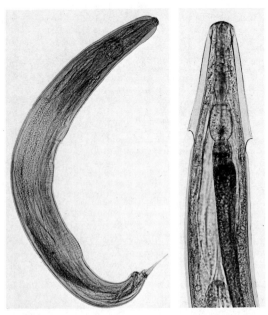

Figure 13–24. Pinworms of mice: *Syphacia obvelata* male (left) and *Aspiculuris tetraptera* anterior end (right) (x80).

CESTODE LARVA

Hydatigera taeniaeformis (Taeniidae) (see page 90 and Fig. 14-50).

PROTOZOAN

Hepatozoon muris (plasmodium). Schizogony takes place in the hepatic cells; gamonts are found in the monocytes of the circulating blood. The vector is a mesostigmatid mite, *Echinolaelaps echidninus.*

Urogenital System

NEMATODES

Capillaria spp., *Trichosomoides crassicauda* (Trichuroidea) (see page 137 and Fig. 6-64).

Skin and Hair

INSECTS

Polyplax spinulosa (Anoplura) (see page 29 and Fig. 13-25).

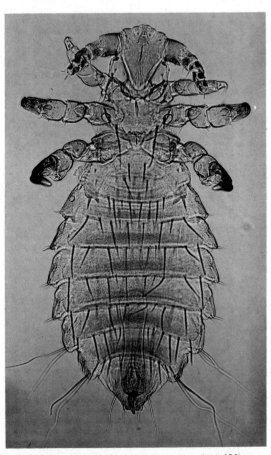

Figure 13–25. *Polyplax spinulosa* male (x108).

Xenopsylla cheopis (Siphonaptera) (see page 33 and Fig. 1-43).

ARACHNIDS

Ornithonyssus bacoti (Mesostigmata) (see page 47).

Radfordia ensifera (Prostigmata) (see page 60).

Notoedres muris (Astigmata) (see page 52 and Figs. 2-24 and 2-25).

PARASITES OF MICE

Alimentary System

STOMACH AND INTESTINES

PROTOZOANS

Cryptosporidium muris (stomach) and *C. parvum* (small intestine).

NEMATODES

Heligmosomoides polygyrus (syn. *Nematospiroides dubius;* Trichostrongyloidea). Reddish, tightly coiled.

Nippostrongylus brasiliensis (6 mm.; Trichostrongyloidea) (Fig. 13-23).

Syphacia obvelata, Aspiculuris tetraptera (Oxyurida) (see Fig. 13-24).

Heterakis spumosa (Ascaridida).

Trichuris muris (Trichuroidea) (see page 136).

CESTODES

Hymenolepis nana, H. diminuta (Hymenolepididae) (see page 94 and Fig. 12-35). The scolex of *H. nana* is armed with hooks, that of *H. diminuta* is unarmed.

Urogenital System

KIDNEYS

PROTOZOAN

Klossiella muris (coccidian) (see page 310).

Skin and Hair

INSECTS

Polyplax serrata (Anoplura) (see page 29 and Fig. 1-32).

ARACHNIDS

Myobia musculi, Radfordia affinis (Prostigmata) (see page 60 and Fig. 2-35). Myobiids do not migrate away from a dead host; the carcass must be scanned carefully with a stereoscopic microscope to find them.

Myocoptes musculinus (Astigmata) (see page 56 and Fig. 2-32).

Ornithonyssus bacoti, Allodermanyssus sanguineus (Mesostigmata) (see pages 47 to 49).

PARASITES OF GUINEA PIGS

Alimentary System

NEMATODE

Paraspidodera uncinata (Oxyurida).

CESTODE

Hymenolepis nana (see page 94 and Fig. 12-35).

PROTOZOANS

Eimeria caviae (coccidian).

Balantidium sp. (ciliate) (see page 65 and Fig. 12-19).

Cryptosporidium wrairi.

Skin and Hair

INSECTS

Gliricola porcelli, Gyropus ovalis, Trimenopon hispidum (Mallophaga) (see page 30 and Fig. 1-39).

ARACHNIDS

Chirodiscoides caviae (Astigmata) (see page 56 and Fig. 2-31).

PARASITES OF MONKEYS AND APES

The kinds of parasites to be found depends on the species and geographical origin of the monkey and upon the duration and environmental conditions of its captivity. Certain parasites (e.g., *Strongyloides* and *Oesophagostomum*) flourish in captive monkeys. Others, especially those whose natural intermediate hosts are no longer available, tend to fade away. In mixed colonies, parasites that are not discriminating in their selection of hosts may spread to species of monkeys that, for geographical or ecological reasons, they rarely or never infect in the wild. Such cross-infections are more likely to cause disease because of the lack of mutual adaptation of host and parasite. The following therefore represents a composite listing of the more common parasites of monkeys and apes without particular regard to natural host species preferences or geographical origins.

Alimentary System

NEMATODES

Cephalobus parasiticus (Rhabditida). These harmless parasites of the stomach and intestines of *Macaca iris mordax* (and probably others) resemble the free-living generation of *Strongyloides*. Their rhabditiform larvae may be confused with those of *Strongyloides* on fecal examination. They do not, however, develop into filariform larvae, so the dilemma may be resolved by culturing the fecal specimen.

Strongyloides fuelleborni, S. stercoralis (Rhabditida) (see page 100 and Fig. 6-8). Simian strongyloidosis is a human health hazard.

Nochtia nochti (Trichostrongyloidea). Bright red worms lying within or protruding from gastric papillomata in the prepyloric region of the stomach. Cross sections of *N. nochti* in histological preparations display 16 distinct longitudinal cuticular ridges and channeled lateral alae.

Trichostrongylus, Molineus, Nematodirus (Trichostrongyloidea) (see page 105 and Fig. 6-11).

Oesophagostomum (Conoweberia) apiostomum, Oe. stephanostomum, Ternidens deminutus (Strongyloidea) (see page 112; Fig. 13-26). Stout-bodied "nodular worms" with leaf crowns and transverse ventral cervical groove.

Necator, Ancylostoma, Globocephalus (Ancylostomatoidea) (see page 113 and Figs. 6-10 and 6-27).

Ascaris lumbricoides (Ascaridoidea) (see page 124 and Fig. 6-40).

Trichuris spp. (Trichuroidea) (see page 136).

Enterobius spp. (Oxyurida) (see page 121; Fig. 13-26). Pinworms are quite host-specific; a species of pinworm infects a genus of monkeys. *Enterobius vermicularis* occurs in chimpanzees. *Enterobius* spp. are usually considered nonpathogenic, but sometimes they invade the wall of the intestine and produce serious or even fatal disease.

Streptopharagus, Gongylonema, Protospirura, Physocephalus, Rictularia, Physaloptera (Spirurida) (see pages 127 to 129 and Figs. 6-49, 6-50, 6-52 and 13-26). *Protospirura muricola*, a parasite of rodents that uses the cockroach *Leucophaea maderae* as intermediate host, has been observed to cause perforation of the stomach in captive monkeys (Foster and Johnson, 1939).

CESTODES

Bertiella studeri (Anoplocephalidae). Large, four suckers, no hooks.

Hymenolepis nana (Hymenolepidae) (see page 94 and Fig. 12-35). Very small, four suckers, hooks.

ACANTHOCEPHALANS

Prosthenorchis, Moniliformis (see page 139 and Fig. 12-36).

TREMATODE

Gastrodiscoides hominus (Paramphistomatidae).

PROTOZOANS

Balantidium coli (ciliate) (see page 65 and Fig. 12-19). Acute enteritis (Teare and Loomis, 1982).

Entamoeba spp.

Giardia lamblia (flagellate) (see page 65 and Fig. 12-35).

Liver and Pancreas

PROTOZOAN

Hepatocystis kochi schizonts (see page 72).

NEMATODES

Capillaria hepatica (Trichuroidea) (see page 136 and Fig. 14-89). Worms and eggs in hepatic parenchyma.

Trichospirura leptostoma. A 10 to 20 mm. worm with a long capillary pharynx; associated with varying degrees of fibrosing pancreatitis. Found in pancreatic duct of American primates.

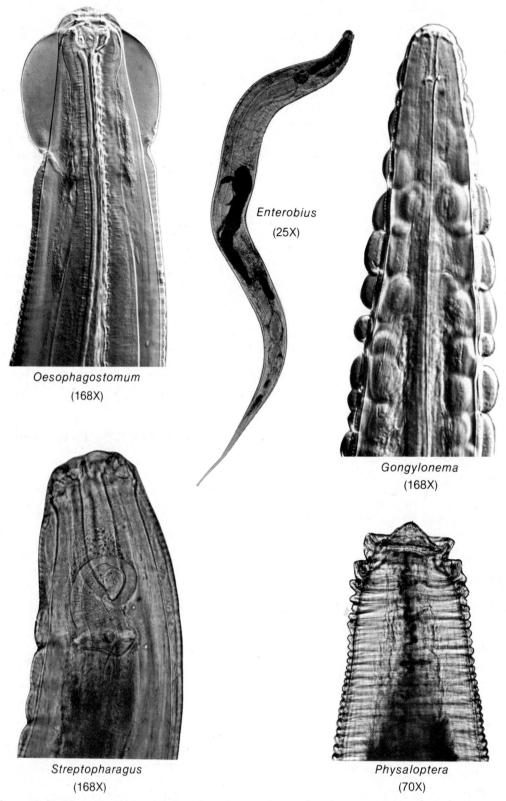

Figure 13–26. Some nematode parasites of monkeys and apes. (Specimens courtesy of Dr. M. M. Rabstein.)

Respiratory System

NOSE AND THROAT

NEMATODE

Anatrichosoma (Trichuroidea) (see page 137 and Fig. 12-36).

ANNELIDS

The leeches that attack the pharyngeal mucosa of monkeys are large, black annelids with a large cup-shaped caudal sucker. The presence of this bloodsucking parasite is suggested by chronic epistaxis in a recently captured monkey. When the host drinks infested water, the young leeches enter the mouth, nose, pharynx, or larynx and attach to the mucous membrane. They remain in these locations for several weeks unless removed.

ARACHNID

Rhinophaga spp.

LUNGS

NEMATODES

Filaroides (Metastrongyloidea).
Metathelazia (Spirurida).

CESTODE LARVA

Echinococcus granulosus (Taeniidae) (see page 90 and Figs. 5-18, 5-19, and 14-51).

ARACHNID

Pneumonyssus simicola (Mesostigmata) (see page 49).

SEROUS CAVITIES

NEMATODE

Dipetalonema spp. (Filarioidea) (see page 132 and Figs. 6-58, 14-85, and 14-86).

CESTODE LARVAE

Taenia hydatigena (Taeniidae) (see page 90 and Fig. 5-15).
Mesocestoides (Mesocestidae) (see page 95 and Figs. 14-53 and 14-54).
Spirometra mansonoides (Diphyllobothriidae) plerocercoid larva (see page 95 and Figs. 5-27 and 14-55).

PENTASTOMID NYMPHS

Porocephalus, Armillifer, Linguatula (see pages 140 and 305).

ACANTHOCEPHALANS

Prosthenorchis spp. and others (see page 139). Acanthocephalan nymphs may be found encysted on the peritoneal membranes of all sorts of vertebrates, even those that are the normal definitive hosts for the parasite in question.

BLOOD

NEMATODE MICROFILARIAE

Dirofilaria, Dipetalonema, Tetrapetalonema, Loa, Brugia (Filarioidea). Differentiation of the many kinds of microfilariae found in monkeys from all parts of the tropics is a task for the specialist. Many species remain to be described.

PROTOZOANS

Hemosporidians.

Muscles and Connective Tissues

NEMATODES

Onchocerca, Dirofilaria, Dipetalonema, Tetrapetalonema, Loa, Brugia (Filarioidea) (see page 130 and Figs. 6-54 and 6-58). *Onchocerca* microfilariae are found in the dermis.

CESTODE LARVAE

Taenia (cysticercus) (see page 90).
Mesocestoides (tetrathyridium) (see page 95 and Figs. 14-53 and 14-54).
Spirometra (plerocercoid) (see page 95 and Figs. 5-27 and 14-55).

Skin and Hair

INSECTS

Pedicinus, Pthirus (Anoplura) (see page 25 and Fig. 1-27).

NEMATODES

Anatrichosoma cutaneum (Trichuroidea) (see page 137 and Fig. 12-36). Very slender (25 by

0.2 mm.) worms give rise to subcutaneous nodules, edema about the joints, and elongated, serpiginous blisters of the palms and soles. Adult females burrow in the epidermis of the palms and soles.

Onchocerca microfilariae.

Dracunculus (Spirurida) (see page 127 and Figs. 6-46 and 6-47).

REFERENCES

The host lists of this chapter are based on the checklists of Becklund (1964) and of Benbrook (1963) and are supplemented from literature reports and personal observations.

Becklund, W. W. (1964): Revised check list of internal and external parasites of domestic animals in the United States and possessions and in Canada. Am. J. Vet. Res., *25*, 1380-1416.

Benbrook, E. A. (1963): Outline of Parasites Reported for Domesticated Animals in North America. Sixth Ed. Iowa State University Press. Ames, Iowa.

Foster, A. O., and Johnson, C. M. (1939): A preliminary note on the identity, life cycle, and pathogenicity of an important nematode parasite of captive monkeys. Am. J. Trop. Med., *19*, 265-277.

Georgi, J. R. (1979): Differential characters of *Filaroides milksi* Whitlock, 1956 and *Filaroides hirthi* Georgi and Anderson, 1975. Proc. Helminth. Soc. Wash., *46*, 142-145.

Lichtenfels, J. R. (1975): Helminths of Domestic Equids. Proc. Helminth. Soc. Wash. (Special Issue) *42*, 92 pp.

Mayhew, I. G., Lichtenfels, J. R., Greiner, E. C., MacKay, R. J., and Enloe, C. W. (1983): Migration of a spirurid nematode through the brain of a horse. J. Am. Vet. Med. Assoc., *180*, 1306-1311.

Teare, J. A., and Loomis, M. R. (1982): Epizootic of balantidiasis in lowland gorillas. J. Am. Vet. Med. Assoc. *181*, (11), 1345-1347.

14

HISTOPATHOLOGICAL DIAGNOSIS

Marion E. Georgi and Jay R. Georgi

If it is difficult to identify whole parasites, it is far more difficult to identify pieces of them in histological sections. Therefore, it is necessary to exploit every source of available information, including knowledge of the kinds of parasites most likely to be found in the particular host and tissue under study, and the life histories and intrahost migration patterns of all suspects. The host-organ listing of parasites in the preceding chapter should be consulted as a checklist of possibilities. Page references are listed in parentheses to assist the reader in finding pertinent information on the structure, life history, and migration patterns of each parasite considered below. The histological characteristics of various groups of parasites add yet another set of diagnostic criteria, and the exposition of this subject is the principal business of this chapter. Special stains and electron microscopy are valuable investigative tools and, when available, marvellous diagnostic aids. However, the following exposition is restricted, for the most part, to diagnostic features that can be perceived with the compound light microscope and routine H + E staining. Definitive identification of parasites in histological sections often comes down to retrieving the tissue block or wet tissues and teasing this material apart to find a critical fragment (e.g., the head or tail of a worm).

A distinguished monograph dealing with the present subject is *Identification of Parasitic Metazoa In Tissue Sections* by MayBelle Chitwood and J. Ralph Lichtenfels, first published in Experimental Parasitology, *32*, 407-519, 1972, and later reprinted by the U.S. Department of Agriculture. Another outstanding source of information is *Pathology of Tropical and Extraordinary Diseases*, Volumes One and Two, by C. H. Binford and D. H. Connor, Armed Forces Institute of Pathology, 1976, Washington, D.C..

ARTHROPODS

Arthropods typically have paired, jointed legs, and segmented chitinous exoskeletons.

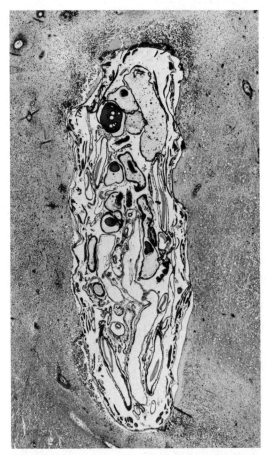

Figure 14–1. *Cuterebra* in a cat's brain (x22). The internal organs lie in a body cavity rather than in a parenchymatous matrix.

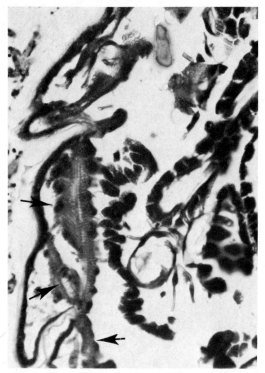

Figure 14–2. Dipteran larva in a calf's brain (x250). The body is segmented and striated muscles (arrows) attach at various points to the exoskeleton.

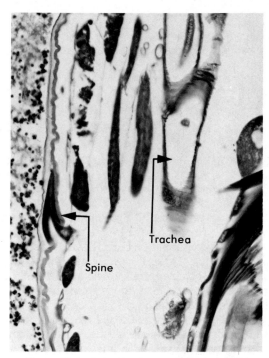

Figure 14–3. *Cuterebra* in a cat's brain (x220).

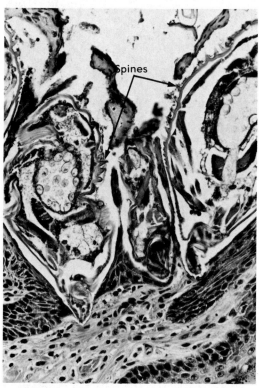

Figure 14–4. *Sarcoptes* in a dog's skin (x230).

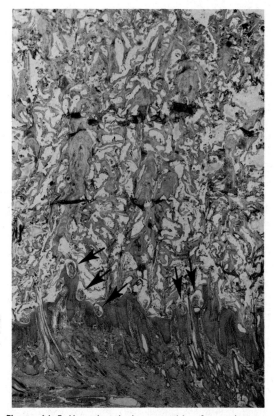

Figure 14–5. Hyperkeratosis caused by *Sarcoptes scabiei* in the fox (x22). The mites (arrows) are found in the deeper layers of the greatly thickened epidermis.

They have striated muscles that attach at different points on the inside of this exoskeleton. Some have tracheal respiratory systems.

INSECTS

Dipterans (see pages 17 to 24). Fly maggots in tissue sections display a body cavity (see Fig. 1-11; Fig. 14-1), segmentation, striated muscles attached at various points to the chitinous exoskeleton (Fig. 14-2), and tracheae formed of rings of cuticle; some species have prominent spines (Fig. 14-3). *Cuterebra* larvae are obligate endoparasites of rodents and lagomorphs. These larvae frequently invade dogs and cats, where they are usually found in the cervical subcutaneous tissues but have been reported to migrate through the central nervous system with disastrous result (see page 22 and Fig. 1-12; Figs. 14-1 and 14-3). First stage *Hypoderma* larvae migrate extensively in cattle; erratic migration through the brain of horses has been reported (see page 21). The spiracular plate is very important in identification of larval dipterans and may need to be retrieved from the wet tissues or paraffin block (see Figs. 1-20 and 1-21).

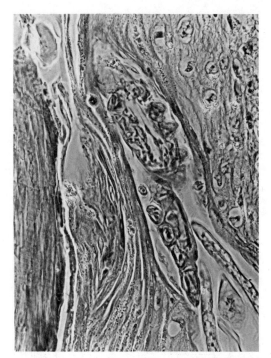

Figure 14–7. *Demodex canis* in a dog's hair follicle (x430).

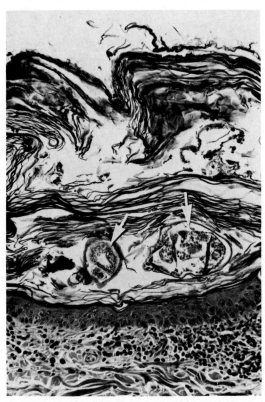

Figure 14–6. *Cheyletiella yasguri* in the skin of a dog (x150). These mites (arrows) lie in the stratum corneum.

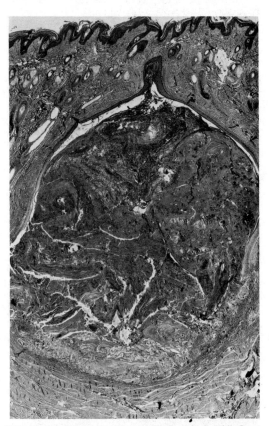

Figure 14–8. Demodectic mange in a bull (x16). Demodectic mange in cattle takes the form of nodular accumulations of myriads of mites and cellular debris in proportions depending on the age of the lesion.

ARACHNIDS

Mites. Mites parasitic in tissues have legs, and their striated muscles are attached at different points on the exoskeleton, but they lack tracheae. *Sarcoptes, Notoedres, Trixacarus,* and the like have spines on their dorsum (see page 51 and Figs. 2-23 and 2-24) and feed at the stratum germinativum and dermis (Fig. 14-4). In some hosts such as the red fox *Vulpes fulva,* sarcoptic mange is characterized by extraordinary hyperkeratosis (Fig. 14-5). Hyperkeratosis is also typical of manges caused by *Chorioptes* and *Cheylietiella,* but the mites lie more superficially in the stratum corneum (Fig. 14-6).

Demodex spp. are cigar-shaped mites found in the hair follicles or associated sebaceous glands (see page 58 and Fig. 2-33; Fig. 14-7). In severe demodectic mange in dogs, *D. canis* may be found in the lymph nodes. Demodectic mange in cattle and swine tends to be nodular (see page 58 and Fig. 14-8).

Mites of the respiratory tract (e.g., *Pneumonyssus, Sternostoma*) have more delicate exoskeletons than their ectoparasitic relatives

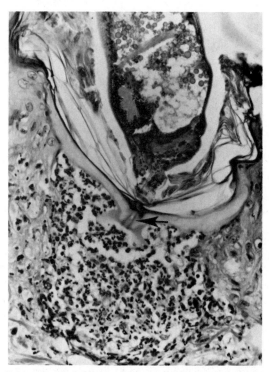

Figure 14–10. *Walchia americana* in a cat's skin (x225). The *stylostome* or feeding tube extends to an area of dermis infiltrated with inflammatory cells.

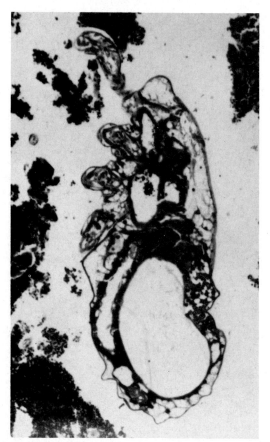

Figure 14–9. *Pneumonyssoides caninum* in a dog's nasal sinus (x92).

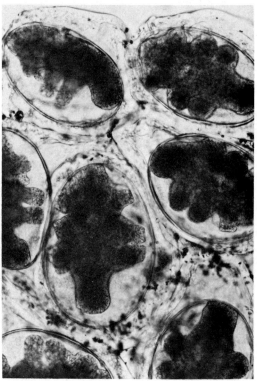

Figure 14–11. Pentastomid eggs with developing embryos (x160).

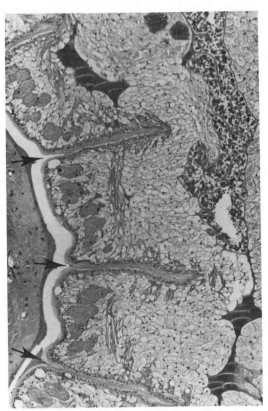

Figure 14-12. Pentostomid in a lymph node of a South American otter (x94). The cuticle is marked by deep annulations (arrows).

(see page 49). *Pneumonyssoides caninum* (Fig. 14-9) of the canine nasal passages may be compared with *Sarcoptes scabiei* (Fig. 14-4).

Trombiculid larvae (chiggers) feed through a stylostome or feeding tube extending into the dermis (see page 60; Fig. 14-10).

PENTASTOMIDS

Pentastomid adults are wormlike parasites of the respiratory passages of predacious reptiles, birds, and mammals that become infected when they ingest encysted pentastomid nymphs in the tissues of their prey (see page 140 and Fig. 6-71). The intermediate host becomes infected by ingesting the egg, which contains a larva with four or six appendages, depending on the species in question (Fig. 14-11). Pentastomids have annulated bodies (Fig. 14-12) with striated muscles (Fig. 14-13); these muscles are not arranged for moving appendages, which are lacking in all but the embryonic and larval stages. The cuticle is perforated by pores that appear as pits in surface view (Fig. 14-14) and as short cylinders of sclerotized material connected to vacuoles in histological sections (Fig. 14-15). Most characteristic, however, are the acidophilic glands, which stain bright pink with striking blue nuclei in H + E sections (Figs. 14-12, 14-13, and 14-15).

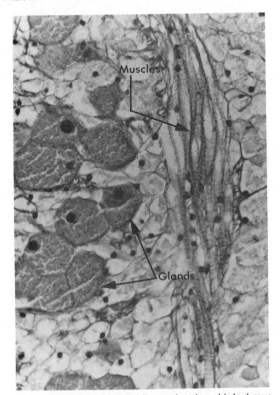

Figure 14-13. Pentastomid tissue showing striated muscle and acidophilic glands (x460).

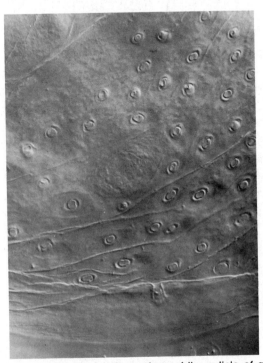

Figure 14-14. Pores in the surface of the cuticle of a pentastomid (x440).

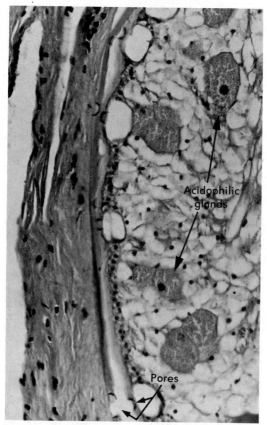

Figure 14–15. Pores in a histological section of a pentastomid (x290). A molt is in progress and pores can be seen in both cuticles.

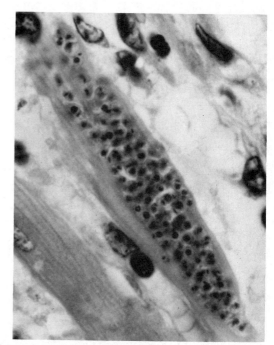

Figure 14–16. *Trypanosoma cruzi* amastigotes in cardiac muscle (x1300). Both nucleus and kinetoplast can be seen in individual organisms.

PROTOZOANS

FLAGELLATES

At the light microscope level, it is often very difficult to distinguish even distantly related intracellular protozoans purely on the basis of structure. It is one matter to start out with a known experimental infection and recognize the salient features of a particular organism but it is quite another to be able to identify the same organism in material submitted for diagnosis. For example *Trypanosoma cruzi* amastigotes should be easy to distinguish from *Toxoplasma gondii* bradyzoites because the former have a kinetoplast and the latter do not. However, the kinetoplast may be visible in only a small proportion of the amastigotes and might be overlooked. It is usually necessary to take into account the history, clinical signs, and pathological changes in reaching a diagnosis. Electron microscopy provides more definitive evidence but is expensive and frequently not feasible.

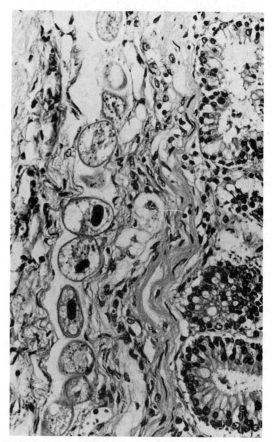

Figure 14–17. *Balantidium coli* in the submucosa of the large intestine of a pig (x280).

Trypanosoma. *Trypanosoma cruzi* amastigotes are generally found in muscle cells of the esophagus, colon, and heart, where they may be responsible for megaesophagus, megacolon, and myocarditis, respectively. These very small parasites have a nucleus and a kinetoplast and do not store PAS-positive material (see page 62; Fig. 14-16).

CILIATES

Balantidium coli trophozoites may secondarily invade the wall of the large intestine of swine suffering from various forms of enteritis. They are characterized by a macronucleus and cilia (see page 65 and Fig. 12-19; Fig. 14-17). Rumen ciliates may be found in the lung as a result of terminal inhalation of rumen contents (Fig. 14-18), in which case there is no evidence of inflammatory reaction. Rumen ciliates may also be found in hepatic vessels in cases of very severe enteritis (Fig. 14-19). In horses with severe enteritis, the extravagantly shaped ciliates normally present in the large intestine may

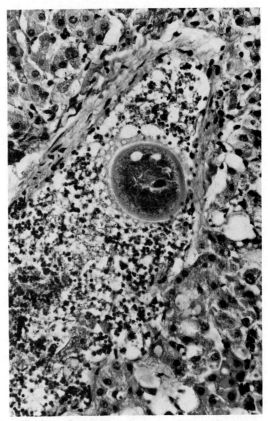

Figure 14–19. Ciliate in vein in the liver of a bull with severe enteritis (x250).

secondarily penetrate the submucosa. These ciliates have large, often polymorphic macronuclei and some have tufts of long cilia.

COCCIDIANS

The life history and development of the major genera of coccidians are described on pages 67 to 69 and diagrammed in Figures 3-3 to 3-7. A description of the histological appearance of the various stages follows but host specificity, site specificity, and details of development characteristic of the genera and species of coccidia must also be taken into consideration in arriving at a diagnosis.

Asexual Stages

Trophozoites. When a sporozoite enters a cell, it rounds up as a *trophozoite* in a membrane-lined *parasitophorous vacuole* (Fig. 14-20).

Schizonts. Schizonts develop from trophozoites by endopolygony. Depending on the species, schizonts may be found in enterocytes (Figs. 14-21 and 14-22), biliary epithelial

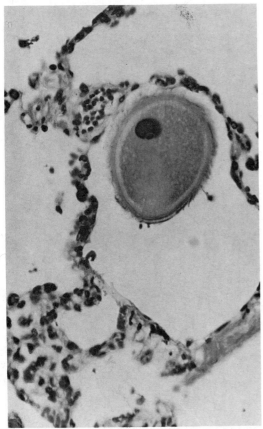

Figure 14–18. Rumen ciliate in the lung of a cow (x360). Agonal inhalation of ruminal contents accounts for the atypical location of this ciliate.

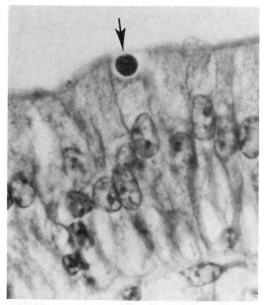

Figure 14–20. *Eimeria* trophozoite (arrow) in an intestinal epithelial cell of a chicken (x1300).

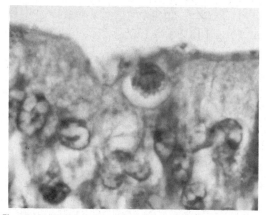

Figure 14–21. *Eimeria* schizont in an intestinal epithelial cell of a chicken (x1400).

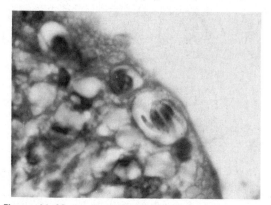

Figure 14–22. Another *Eimeria* schizont in an intestinal epithelial cell of a chicken (x1400).

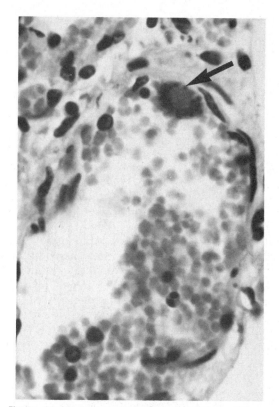

Figure 14–23. *Sarcocystis cruzi* schizont (arrow) in endothelium of a small artery of a calf with a fatal, naturally acquired infection (x812). (Specimen provided by Dr. Paul Frelier.)

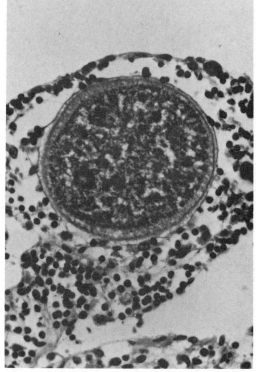

Figure 14–24. *Eimeria bovis* developing megaschizont in central lacteal of an intestinal villus (x425).

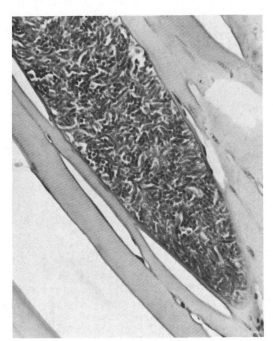

Figure 14–25. Sarcocyst of *Sarcocystis muris* in skeletal muscle of a mouse (x1300). (Specimen provided by Dr. Marguerite Frongillo.)

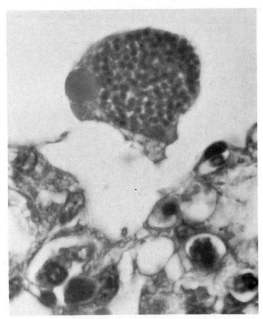

Figure 14–27. *Toxoplasma gondii* in the lung of a fatally infected cat (x1200). A macrophage has engulfed many *T. gondii* tachyzoites and two erythrocytes.

cells (e.g., *Eimeria stiedae* /rabbit), endothelial cells (Figs. 14-23 and 14-24), renal epithelial cells, or even uterine epithelial cells. Ordinary schizonts contain from less than ten to hundreds of merozoites. Megaschizonts (Fig. 14-24) may contain over 100,000.

Sarcocysts. Sarcocysts are found in skeletal and cardiac muscle fibers (Figs. 14-25 and 14-26); these vary in size from a few μm in diameter to macroscopically visible objects, stain intensely with hematoxylin, and are packed full of bradyzoites that are larger than those of *Toxoplasma* and rounded at both ends. Septa subdivide the interior of the

sarcocyst but may escape notice because they stain poorly or not at all with H + E.

Toxoplasma Cysts. Tachyzoites accumulate as "groups" in intracellular vacuoles (Fig. 14-27), bradyzoites become tightly packed in intracellular "cysts" (Fig. 14-28); the latter,

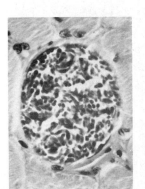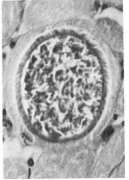

Figure 14–26. Sarcocysts of *Sarcocystis cruzi* (left) and *Sarcocystis bovifelis* (right) in skeletal muscle of the calf in Figure 14–23 (x300). The cyst wall of *S. bovifelis* is thicker and appears striated.

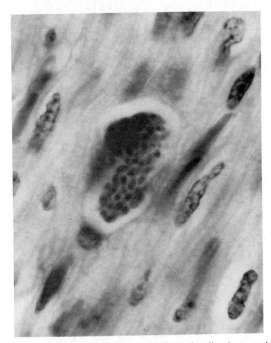

Figure 14–28. *Toxoplasma gondii* bradyzoites in a cyst in cardiac muscle of a puppy (x1200).

when found in striated muscle fibers, might be confused with either sarcocysts or accumulations of *T. cruzi* amastigotes.

Sexual Stages

A merozoite produced by the final schizogonic generation enters a fresh host cell and develops into either a male or a female *gamont*. The female gamont enlarges, stores food materials, and induces a hypertrophy of both the cytoplasm and the nucleus of its host cell. When mature, the gamont is called a *macrogamete*. The male gamont also induces hypertrophy of the cytoplasm and the nucleus of its host cell (Fig. 14-29 and 14-30) as it undergoes repeated nuclear division and becomes multinucleate. Each nucleus is finally incorporated into a flagellated *microgamete*. When a macrogamete is penetrated and fertilized by a microgamete, it becomes a *zygote*. Presently, wall-forming bodies, already present in the macrogamete, become clearly visible as large, spherical, eosinophilic granules in the cytoplasm of the zygote; these later coalesce to form the oocyst wall (Figs. 14-30 and 14-31).

Klossiella. A parasite of the equine kidney,

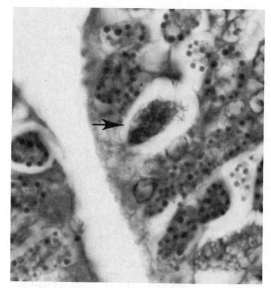

Figure 14–30. Male gamont (arrow) of *Eimeria* in an intestinal epithelial cell of a chicken (x1400). The surrounding female gamonts contain wall-forming bodies.

Klossiella equi is usually an accidental histopathological finding. Schizogony occurs in the glomerular endothelium and in the proximal convoluted tubules. The distinctive sporonts (Fig. 14-32) in the renal tubular epithe-

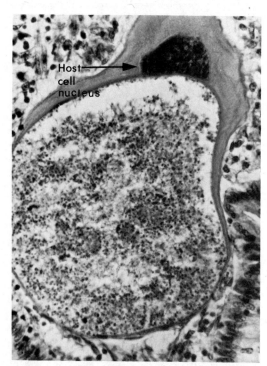

Figure 14–29. Male gamont of *Eimeria leuckarti* in the submucosa of the small intestine of a horse (x350). The cytoplasm and nucleus of the host cell (arrow) are greatly hypertrophied and enormous numbers of flagellated microgametes have developed.

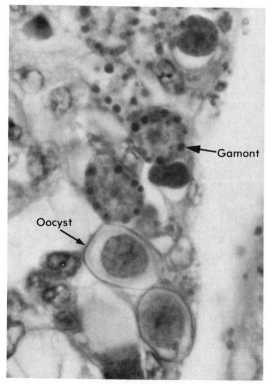

Figure 14–31. Female gamonts and oocysts of *Eimeria* in an intestinal epithelial cell of a chicken (x1400). The female gamonts contain wall-forming bodies.

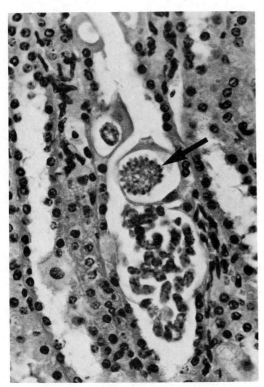

Figure 14–32. Sporont of *Klossiella equi* (arrow) in the renal tubular epithelium of a horse (x425).

lium produce as many as 40 sporoblasts, which develop into sporocysts, each of which may contain 8 to 15 sporozoites.

Cryptosporidium. The minute (5 μm) organisms appear as basophilic spheres on the luminal surface of epithelial cells of the

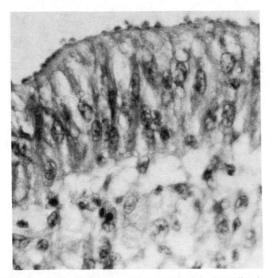

Figure 14–33. *Cryptosporidium* projecting from the luminal surface of intestinal epithelial cells of a chicken (x765).

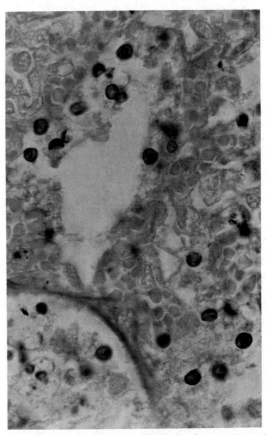

Figure 14–34. *Pneumocystis carinii* in horse lung; Gomori methenamine silver stain (x1000). (Specimen provided by Dr. J. M. King.)

intestinal and respiratory tracts of vertebrates (Fig. 14-33). Diarrhea has been associated with *Cryptosporidium* infection in man, calves, lambs, and pigs.

Pneumocystis. The taxonomic position of *Pneumocystis* is unclear; it may be a protozoan or perhaps a fungus. *Pneumocystis* causes interstitial pneumonia, especially in horses with immune deficiencies. These organisms stain brownish black with Gomori's methenamine silver stain (Fig. 14-34).

TREMATODES

The general anatomy of trematodes is briefly outlined on page 76 (see Fig. 4-9). The internal organs of these dorsoventrally flattened worms are embedded in a parenchymatous matrix; there is no body cavity (Fig. 14-35). Trematodes differ from cestodes in having a gut (Fig. 14-36) and in lacking the calcareous corpuscles found scattered about the parenchyma of cestodes; some trematodes have tegumental spines. Circular and longitudinal nonstriated muscles are

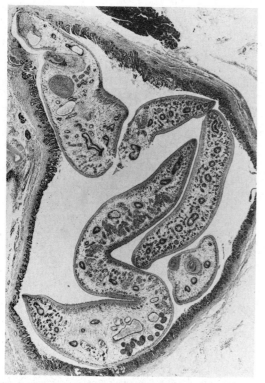

Figure 14–35. *Fasciola hepatica* in a bile duct of a rat (x13). (Specimen provided by Dr. Helen Han Hsu.)

poorly developed and found immediately under the tegument, whereas in cestodes there are two distinct zones of muscle fibers (Figs. 14-43 and 14-44). Although both trematodes and cestodes have suckers, in trematodes the oral sucker surrounds a stoma that is connected to a gut (Fig. 14-37), whereas a gut is lacking in cestodes; the ventral sucker of trematodes is also not connected to a gut. Sections through the uterus contain eggs, which, by their size and state of embryonic development, may provide clues to the identity of the specimen (Fig. 14-38; see also Chapter 13). The distribution of vitelline glands (Fig. 14-39) in the trematode body is a much used taxonomic character. For example, these glands lie both dorsal and ventral to the gut in *Fasciola* but they all lie ventral to the gut in *Fascioloides*. The body form of some trematodes is distinctive. For example, diplostomatids are divided into a flattened forebody and cylindrical hindbody (see Fig. 4-15; Fig. 14-40) and in the dioecious schistosomatids, the slender female is enclosed in the gynecophoric groove of her stouter male partner (see Fig. 4-11; Fig. 14-41). Schistostomatid eggs tend to excite granulomatous inflammatory reactions in tissues (Fig. 14-42). Anatomical details not available in Chapter 4 may be found in Schell (1970). Refer to Chapter 13 for information on site specificity.

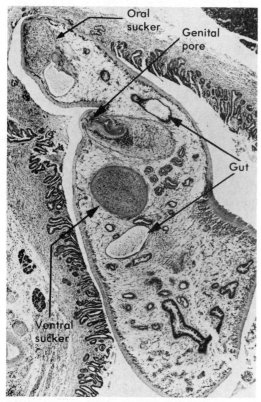

Figure 14–36. *Fasciola hepatica* in a bile duct of a rat (x27). (Specimen provided by Dr. Helen Han Hsu.)

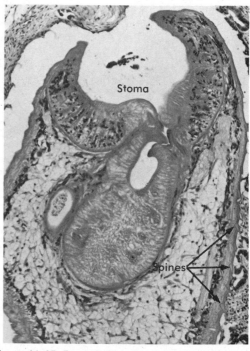

Figure 14–37. *Fasciola hepatica* in a bile duct of a rat (x90). (Specimen provided by Dr. Helen Han Hsu.)

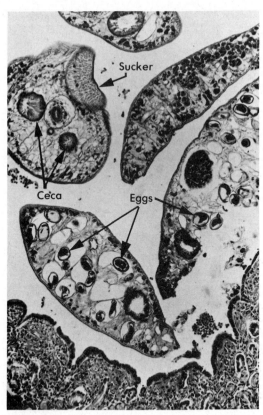

Figure 14-38. Trematodes in the pancreatic duct of a cat (x100).

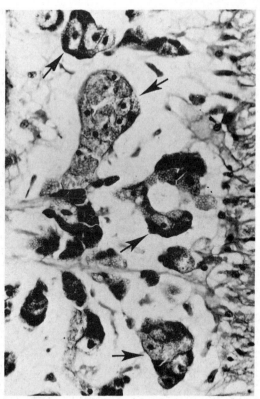

Figure 14-39. *Fasciola hepatica* in a bile duct of a rat. Vitelline glands (arrows) filled with secretion granules (x250). (Specimen provided by Dr. Helen Han Hsu.)

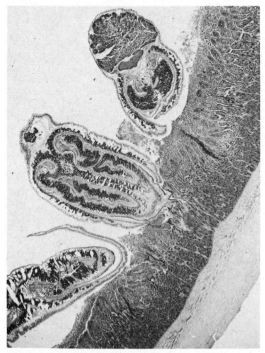

Figure 14-40. *Alaria* in the small intestine of a dog (x10). *Alaria*, typical of the family Diplostomatidae, is divided into fore- and hindbody.

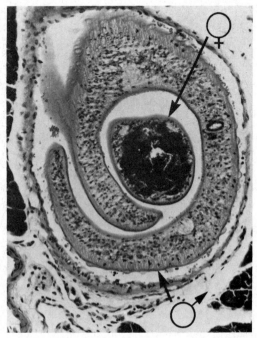

Figure 14-41. *Schistosoma mansoni* in a mesenteric vein of a mouse (x130). (Specimen provided by Dr. Helen Han Hsu.)

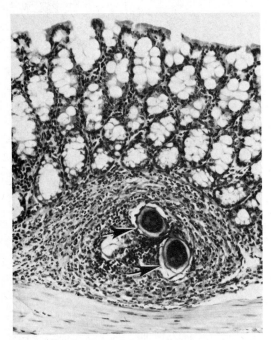

Figure 14–42. Granuloma containing eggs (arrows) of *Schistosoma mansoni* (x120). (Specimen provided by Dr. Helen Han Hsu.)

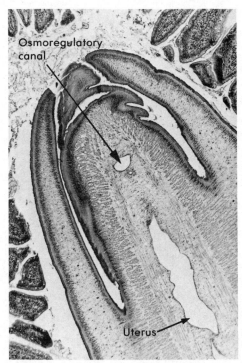

Figure 14–43. *Hydatigera taeniaeformis* in the small intestine of a cat; section through two adjoining segments (x50).

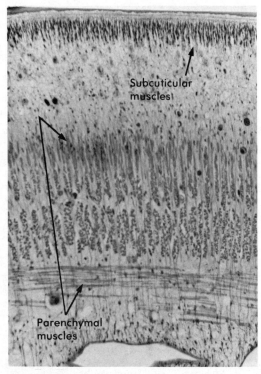

Figure 14–44. *Hydatigera taeniaeformis* of Figure 14–43 at higher power showing the subcuticular and parenchymal muscle layers (x140).

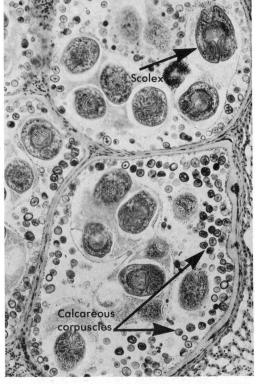

Figure 14–45. *Echinococcus multilocularis* alveolar hydatid (x108).

CESTODES

Like trematodes, the internal organs of
cestodes are embedded in a parenchymatous
matrix, there being no body cavity (see page
84). There are two principal zones of nonstriated muscle fibers, *subcuticular* and *parenchymal* (Figs. 14-43 and 14-44). The parenchymal zone divides the parenchyma into a
cortex lying outside a longitudinal layer of
fibers and a *medulla* lying within a transverse
layer of muscle fibers; the medulla contains
the osmoregulatory ducts and reproductive
organs if these are present. Calcareous corpuscles are typical of cestode tissues and,
especially in metacestodes, may provide the
only evidence that the specimen is a tapeworm (Fig. 14-45). Because adult cestodes are
parasites of the lumen of the intestine and
bile ducts, metacestodes (i.e., larvae) are the
forms most frequently encountered in histological sections.

Taeniid metacestodes are the most common and important representatives of Cestoda found in tissues of domestic animals.
For information on site specificity, refer to
Chapter 13, a general discussion of the structure of the cysticercus, coenurus, strobilocercus, hydatid cyst; alveolar hydatid is presented in Chapter 5 and Figures 5-15 through
5-19. If the section includes only bladder
wall, there will be little more than calcareous

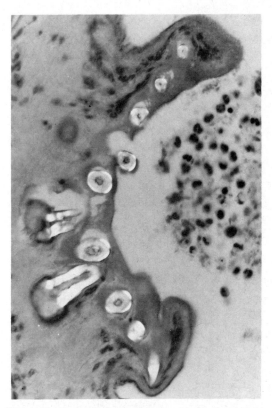

Figure 14–47. Cysticercus of Figure 14–46, showing bi-
refringence of hooks in polarized light (x425).

corpuscles to identify it as cestode tissue. A
section through the scolex that includes
hooks identifies the specimen as a taeniid
(Figs. 14-46 and 14-47). *Taeniarhynchus saginatus*, the "beef tapeworm" of man, forms an
exception in having no hooks at all.

Tentative identification of particular species of taeniid metacestodes may be based on
their host and site specificity (see Chapter
13). For example, a cysticercus attached to
the peritoneal membranes of a cottontail rabbit has a very small probability of being
anything other than *Taenia pisiformis*. Further
evidence may be provided by hook length
measurements if both long and short hooks
happen to lie in the plane of section or if
they can be isolated from the wet tissues.
Verster (1969) may be consulted for hook
length data. If there is more than one scolex
connected to the same bladder wall, the metacestode is probably a coenurus of the genus
Multiceps (Fig. 14-48). *Taenia crassiceps* presents a source of confusion in this regard by
forming many cysticerci by budding. These
all lie within the same host cyst but are not
attached to a common bladder wall (Fig. 14-
49). Strobilocerci of *Hydatigera taeniaeformis*
are cysticerci that have precociously begun

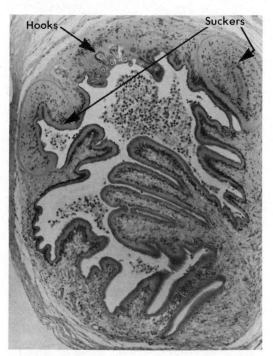

Figure 14–46. Cysticercus of *Taenia solium* (x96).

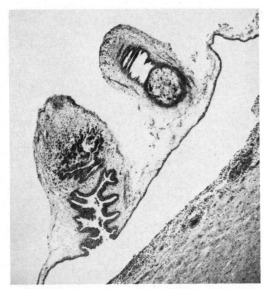

Figure 14–48. Coenurus in the brain of a cat showing two scolices on a thin bladder wall (x45).

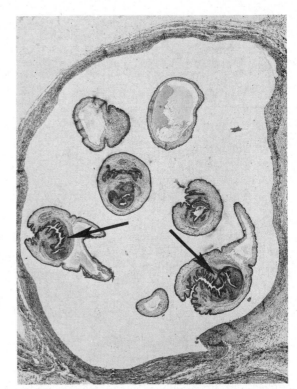

Figure 14–49. Cysticerci of *Taenia crassiceps* in a subcutaneous cyst of a gray squirrel (x16). Note inversion of scolices (arrows). This is an unusual cysticercus in that it proliferates by budding and may be found widely disseminated in various tissues of rodents.

to elongate and segment as metacestodes; these are found in the livers of rodents (Fig. 14-50).

Hydatid cysts manifest *expansive growth* and have thick, laminated membranes separating the germinative layer, which bears sessile scolices or brood capsules, from the surrounding host connective tissue capsule (Fig. 14-51). In sterile hydatid cysts, the laminated membrane is the only diagnostic character available. Alveolar hydatids have much thinner laminated membranes; their manner of growth is *invasive* instead of expansive (Fig. 14-52).

Tetrathyridia of *Mesocestoides* (see page 95) differ from taeniid larvae in lacking a bladder. Tetrathyridia have four suckers and no hooks; the calcareous corpuscles are large but not as dense as those of other metacestodes (Figs. 14-53 and 14-54).

Plerocercoids of *Spirometra* (see page 96 and Fig. 5-27), also called "spargana" in medical literature, have no bladder, no suckers, and no hooks. There is little besides calcareous corpuscles in a parenchymatous matrix to identify the plerocercoid as a metacestode larva; the invaginated scolex may fortuitously lie in the plane of section (Fig. 14-55).

NEMATODES

The general structure of nematodes is discussed in Chapter 6, and nematode eggs are illustrated in Chapter 12. For information on host and site specificity, refer to Chapter 13.

Nematodes are round in cross section,

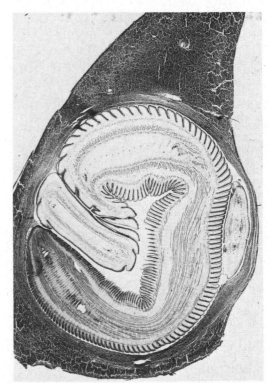

Figure 14–50. Strobilocercus of *Hydatigera taeniaeformis* encysted in the liver a muskrat (*Ondatra zibethica*) (x12).

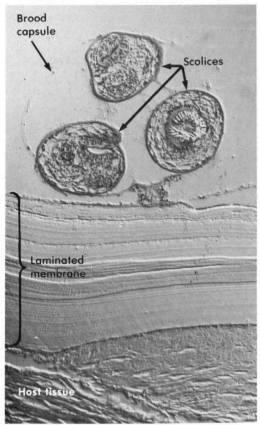

Figure 14–51. *Echinococcus granulosus* hydatid cyst (x202).

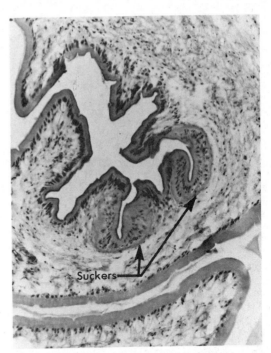

Figure 14–53. *Mesocestoides* tetrathyridium from the peritoneal cavity of a baboon (*Papio* sp.); region of scolex showing two suckers (x200).

have a body cavity containing tubular organs including a digestive tract and a male or female reproductive tract. The body wall consists of three contiguous layers: an outer cuticle, an intermediate hypodermal layer, and an inner layer of muscle cells. The hypodermis is often expanded as longitudinal *lateral chords* that divide the muscle layer into dorsal and ventral fields (Fig. 14-56). Dorsal

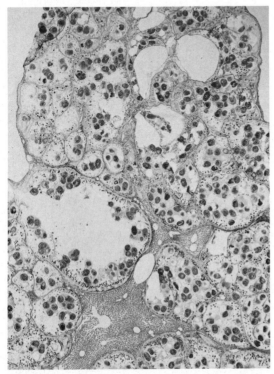

Figure 14–52. *Echinococcus multilocularis* alveolar hydatid (x24).

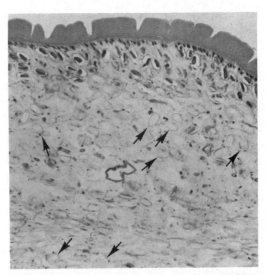

Figure 14–54. *Mesocestoides* tetrathyridium of Figure 14–53 parenchyma with large, "empty" calcareous corpuscles (arrows) (x250).

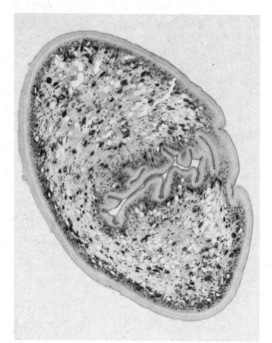

Figure 14-55. *Spirometra mansonoides* plerocercoid from the subcutaneous tissues of a mouse (x108).

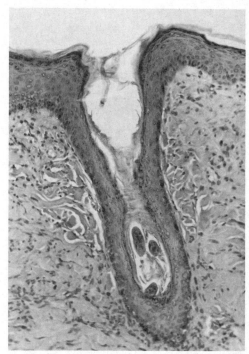

Figure 14-57. *Rhabditis (Pelodera) strongyloides* in a hair follicle of a dog (x130).

and ventral chords are also present in certain regions of the body of some nematodes, and the adenophoreans (e.g., *Dioctophyme, Eustrongylides, Trichuris*) have several, asymmetrically distributed, longitudinal chords. Except in the region of the chords, the

hypodermis is thinner than the somatic muscle layer. This is in contrast to the situation in acanthocephalans, in which the hypodermis is thicker than the muscle layer (Fig. 14-92).

RHABDITIDA

Rhabditis (Pelodera) strongyloides. These larvae are found in the hair follicles of dogs, swine, and cattle (Fig. 14-57); they have double lateral alae (see page 99; Fig. 14-58).

Strongyloides. *Strongyloides* larvae (see Fig. 12-8) also have double lateral alae. The adult parasitic female worms are found deep in the mucous membrane of the small intestine (see page 100 and Fig. 6-8; Fig. 14-59).

STRONGYLIDA

Trichostrongyloidea

With the exception of *Trichostrongylus*, the cuticle of trichostrongyloid nematodes has longitudinal ridges (Fig. 14-60). Fourth stage larvae are found in the mucosae of the stomach and intestines of ruminants and a wide range of other hosts. *Trichostrongylus axei* fourth stage larvae and juvenile adults are found between the basement membrane and epithelial cells of the abomasal mucosa (Fig. 14-61). *Ostertagia* fourth stage larvae and ju-

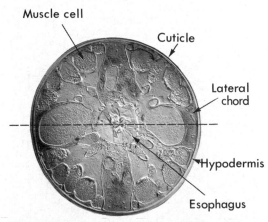

Figure 14-56. Cross section through the esophageal region of *Strongylus vulgaris* showing the division of somatic musculature into dorsal and ventral fields by the lateral cords. In this particular body region of *S. vulgaris*, the dorsal and ventral cords are exceptionally well developed and these anatomically separate their respective muscle fields into halves. However, functional separation, expressed in terms of coordinated muscular activity, remains predominantly dorsoventral (x62).

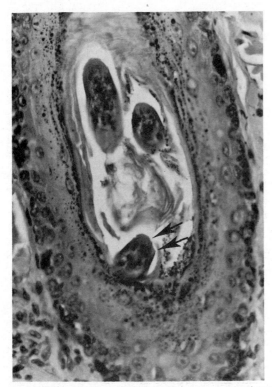

Figure 14–58. Same as Figure 14–57, enlarged to show double lateral alae (arrows) (x400).

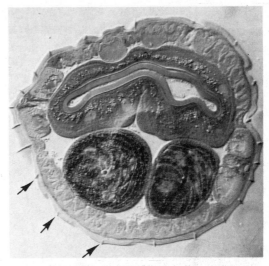

Figure 14–60. Cross section through *Haemonchus contortus* (x140). The entire circumference of the cuticle is marked by longitudinal ridges (arrows).

venile adults are found in dilated gastric glands of the abomasum (see page 106; Figs. 14-62 and 14-63).

Strongyloidea

Strongylus vulgaris, S. edentatus, and *S. equinus* migrate extensively and occasionally erratically in the horse. See Chapter 13 for

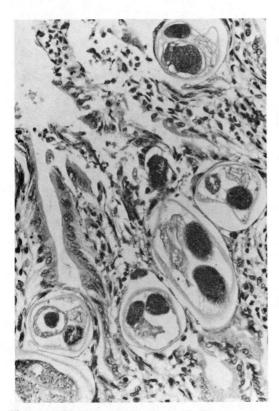

Figure 14–59. *Strongyloides westeri* in the mucosa the small intestine of a horse (x250).

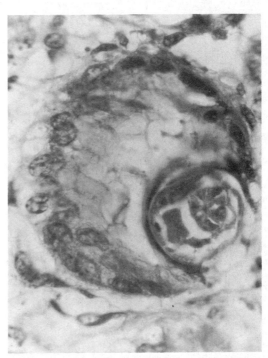

Figure 14–61. *Trichostrongylus axei* in the abomasal mucosa of a heifer (x1000).

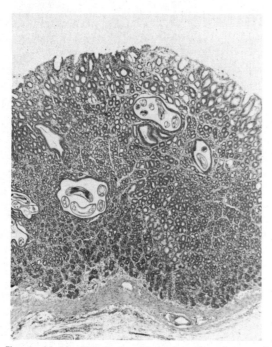

Figure 14–62. *Ostertagia ostertagi* in the abomasal mucosa of a heifer (x25). (Specimen provided by Dr. Lois Roth.)

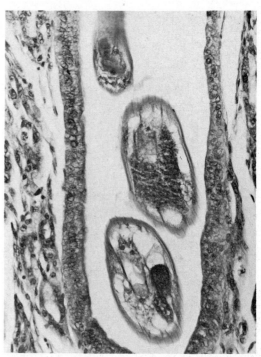

Figure 14–63. *Ostertagia ostertagi* in the abomasal mucosa (x370). Higher magnification of Figure 14–62. shows longitudinal cuticular ridges typical of the superfamily Trichostrongyloidea.

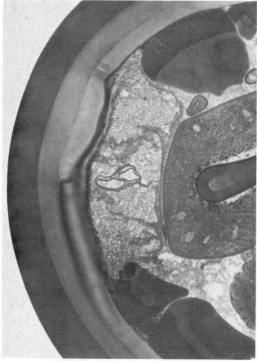

Figure 14–64. Cross section of *Strongylus edentatus* showing the thick, multilayered cuticle of this species (x220).

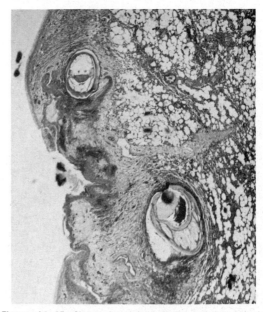

Figure 14–65. *Strongylus edentatus* immature male in the lung of a horse (x15). Two sections of worm are visible. The upper is a cross section near the caudal end of the worm (see also Fig. 14–66), and the lower is an oblique section through the buccal capsule (see also Fig. 14–67).

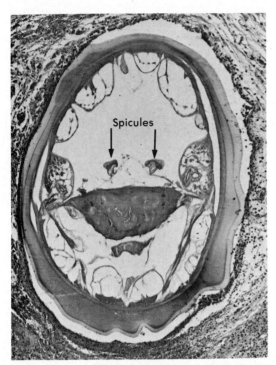

Figure 14–66. Higher magnification of Figure 14–65, showing a section through the caudal end of the worm (x100). Note the thick, multilayered cuticle, spicules, and prominent lateral cords. The cytoplasm of the somatic muscle cells was lost in histological processing (see also Fig. 14–64).

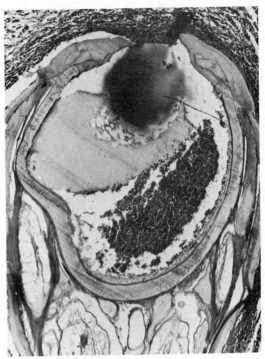

Figure 14–67. Higher magnification of Figure 14–65, showing the buccal capsule (x100).

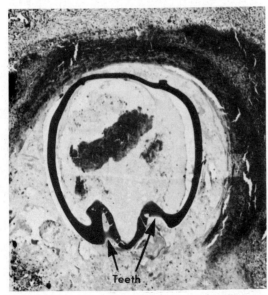

Figure 14–68. *Strongylus equinus* defunct immature adult worm in the pancreas of a horse (x100). The teeth in the base of the buccal capsule distinguish this species from *S. edentatus.*

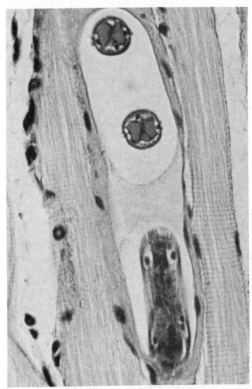

Figure 14–69. *Ancylostoma caninum* third stage larvae within skeletal muscle fibers (x650). From Lee, K. T., Little, M. D., and Beaver, P. C. (1975): Intracellular (muscle-fiber) habitat of *Ancylostoma caninum* in some mammalian hosts. J. Parasitol., *61*, 589–598. Note the double lateral alae.

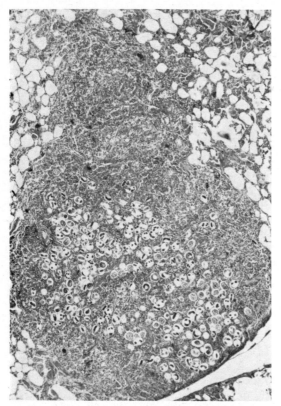

Figure 14–70. Eggs and larvae of *Aelurostrongylus abstrusus* in a nodule in the lung of a cat (x32).

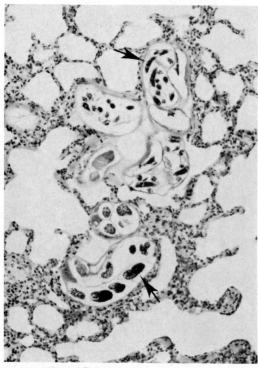

Figure 14–71. *Filaroides hirthi* in normal canine lung tissue (x108). The dark objects are eggs and larvae (arrows) in the uterus of female worms.

normal and erratic organ distribution of these species in the horse. *Strongylus edentatus* tends to migrate retroperitoneally and is characterized by a very thick, multilayered cuticle (Figs. 14-64, 14-65, 14-66, and 14-67). *Strongylus equinus* immature adults are frequently found in the pancreas; sections through the buccal capsule reveal the presence of teeth at their base (Fig. 14-68).

Ancylostomatoidea

Hookworms. Hookworm larvae have double lateral alae (see page 113; Fig. 14-69).

Metastrongyloidea

Aelurostrongylus abstrusus is the most common nematode parasite of the lungs of the domestic cat. Adults, eggs in varying stages of development, and larvae are found in

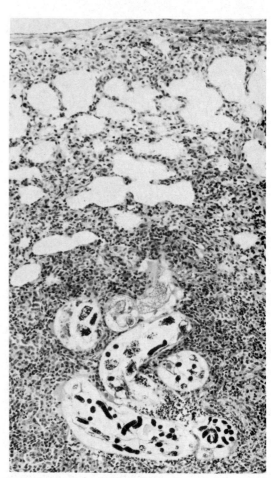

Figure 14–72. *Filaroides hirthi* worm surrounded by a cellular inflammatory reaction (x108).

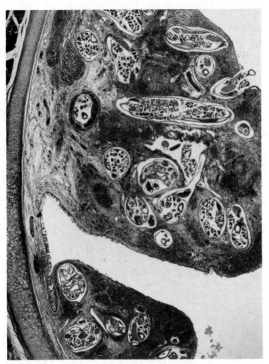

Figure 14–73. *Filaroides osleri* in fibrous nodules in the trachea of a dog (x2).

nests in the lung parenchyma (Fig. 14-70). *Angiostrongylus vasorum* adults may be found in the right heart and pulmonary vessels, while the eggs and larvae are found in the lung parenchyma. *Filaroides hirthi* adults are found in the lung parenchyma of the dog surrounded either by normal lung tissue (Fig. 14-71) or by a cellular inflammatory reaction (Fig. 14-72). Eggs contain first stage larvae when laid and tend not to accumulate in the lung tissue. Autoinfection by *Filaroides hirthi* may lead to a state of hyperinfection in which lung tissue is almost completely replaced by adult worms and larvae may be found widely scattered in lymph nodes, pancreas, gut wall, liver, and brain. *Filaroides osleri* adults are found in fibrous nodules projecting into the lumen of the trachea and principal bronchi (see Fig. 6-35; Fig. 14-73).

Muellerius capillaris of sheep and goats, like *A. abstrusus*, is found in nodules in the parenchyma; these contain adult worms, eggs in varying stages of development, and larvae. If the tails of larvae can be located in the section, *Muellerius* can be distinguished from *Protostrongylus* (see Fig. 12-26). *Protostrongylus* adults may be found either in parenchymal nodules or in the airways. *Dictyocaulus* adults are found in the airways. *Parelaphostrongylus tenuis* adults are found in the meninges and nervous tissue of the spinal cord and brain of sheep and goats (Figs. 14-74 and 14-75). Their eggs and larvae, indistinguishable from those of *Muellerius*, are found widely scattered in the lung parenchyma rather than concentrated in nests.

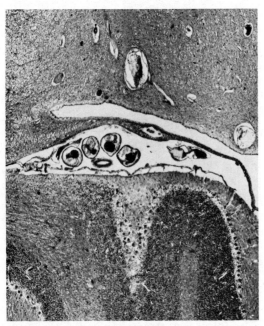

Figure 14–74. *Parelaphostrongylus tenuis* in the meninges of a goat (x25).

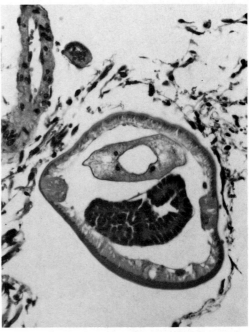

Figure 14–75. *Parelaphostrongylus tenuis* (x290).

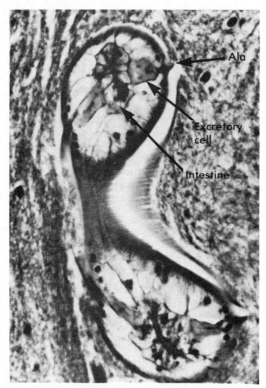

Figure 14–76. *Baylisascaris procyonis* in the brain of a Chukar partridge showing relationship of the intestine and excretory cells to the single lateral alae (x530). Specimen provided by Dr. Malcolm Peckham.

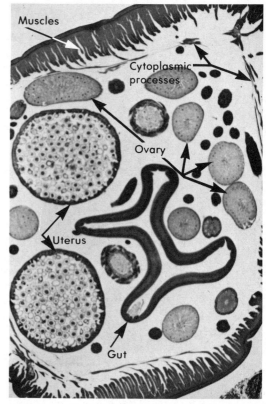

Figure 14–77. Cross section of *Parascaris equorum* (x25).

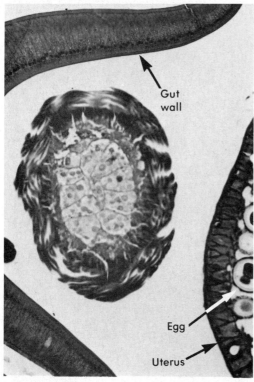

Figure 14–78. Enlargement of Fig. 14–77, showing the columnar intestinal cells with one nucleus near the base of each cell (x140).

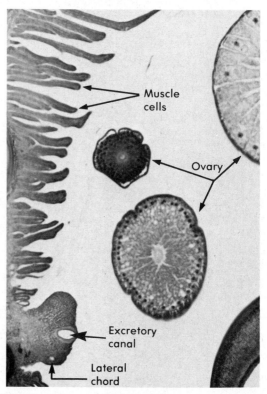

Figure 14–79. Enlargement of Fig. 14–77, showing other details (x120).

ASCARIDIDA

Ascarid larvae have single lateral alae. An excretory cell in each lateral chord lies directly apposed to the intestine, forming a bridge to the lateral ala of each side (Fig. 14-76). *Toxocara* larvae migrating or arrested in somatic tissues tend not to exceed 26 μm in diameter (Nichols, 1956a, 1956b) but *Baylisascaris* larvae continue to grow as they migrate and may reach 55 to 69 μm (Kazacos, 1983). See page 126.

Ascarid adults, as typified by *Parascaris equorum*, have many tall somatic muscle cells; cytoplasmic processes connect dorsal field muscles with the dorsal nerve, and ventral field muscles with the ventral nerve (Fig. 14-77). The intestinal cells are columnar, with one nucleus near the base of each cell; microvillae are present, and typical thick-walled ascarid eggs may be seen in cross sections of the uterus (Figs. 14-78 and 14-79).

SPIRURIDA

Spirocerca lupi (Fig. 14-80) provides an example of the superfamily Spiruroidea. The

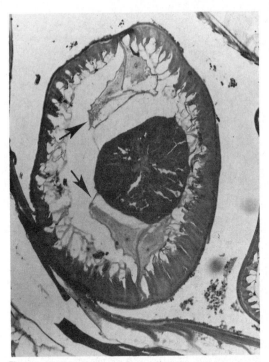

Figure 14–81. Cross section of *Spirocerca lupi* in the region of the glandular esophagus showing the lateral chords (arrows) projecting into the pseudocoelom (x95).

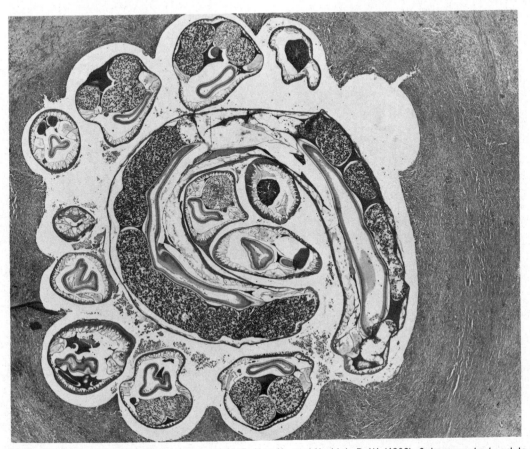

Figure 14–80. *Spirocerca lupi* (x22; from Georgi, M. E., Han H., and Hartrick, D. W. (1980): *Spirocerca lupi* nodule in the rectum of a dog. Cornell Vet., *70*, 43-49.).

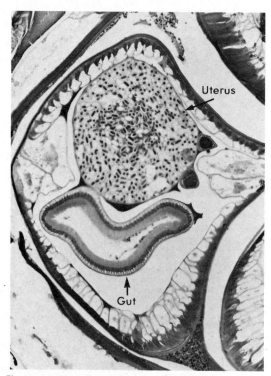

Figure 14–82. Cross section of *Spirocerca lupi* showing the three-layered intestine and uterus filled with tiny eggs (x95).

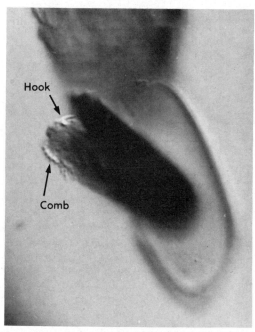

Figure 14–83. *Spirocerca lupi* egg with broken shell from which the larva projects (x1800).

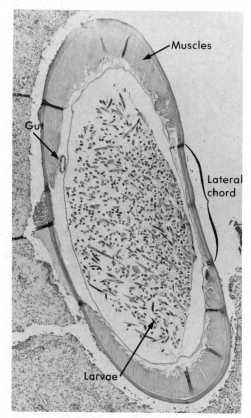

Figure 14–84. Cross section of *Dracunculus insignis* in a subcutaneous granuloma in a dog (x39). (Specimen provided by Dr. S. Neuenschwander.)

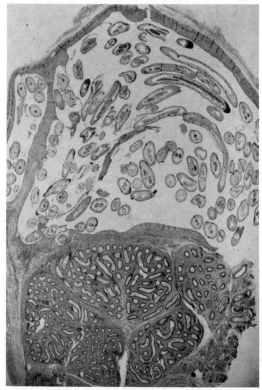

Figure 14–85. *Dipetalonema gracilis* in the vaginal tunics of a monkey (x10). Many cross sections are visible above the host testicular tissue.

adults are typically found in nodules in the wall of the esophagus. On cross section, they are characterized by large lateral chords that project into the body cavity, deeply stained glandular esophagus (Fig. 14-81), a three-layered intestine, and uterus filled with small eggs containing deeply staining larvae (Fig. 14-82). The larvae have hooks and combs associated with the stoma; these structures require oil immersion microscopy to be seen properly (Fig. 14-83).

Dracunculus insignis of the order Camallanina is characterized by flat lateral chords separating semilunar dorsal and ventral muscle fields, a very reduced intestine, and a large uterus filled with larvae (see page 127; Fig. 14-84).

The structure of *Dipetalonema gracilis* (Fig. 14-85) is reasonably typical of the superfamily Filarioidea. The lateral chords do not project into the body cavity in the manner, for example, of *Spirocerca lupi* and have a cuticular thickening at their base; the dorsal and ventral muscle fields are semilunar, rather like those of *Dracunculus;* the lumen of the glandular esophagus is not triradiate; and the muscular vagina may be found in the same sections as the esophagus (Fig. 14-86). Microfilariae in the uterus present the most convincing evidence that the worm in question is a member of the Filarioidea.

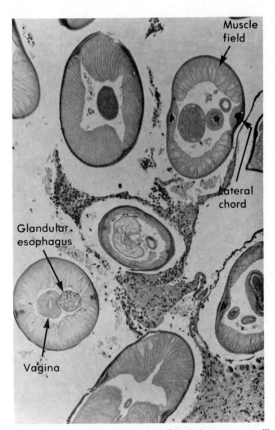

Figure 14–86. Cross sections of *Dipetalonema gracilis* (x108). Specimen provided by Dr. R. S. Hirth.

ENOPLIDA

Superfamily Trichuroidea

Trichuroids display a high order of site specificity and, with the conspicuous exception of *Trichinella spiralis,* a high order of host specificity as well. The host-organ listings of Chapter 13 should prove helpful in dealing with this group of parasites.

Trichinella spiralis larvae are found in a "nurse cell" (Fig. 14-87) in striated muscle; these larvae have a stichosome esophagus (see page 133 and Fig. 6-59). Adult *T. spiralis* are found in the mucosa of the small intestine (Fig. 14-88). In section, *T. spiralis* somewhat resembles *Strongyloides* except that they have a stichosome esophagus and the uterus contains prelarvae instead of segmenting eggs. *Capillaria* spp. infecting the intestinal mucosa are somewhat larger than *Trichinella* and have eggs with bipolar plugs in their uteri.

Capillaria has bilateral *bacillary bands* that run the length of the body, but these are not conspicuous and may be difficult to recognize compared with the single bacillary band of *Trichuris* (see further on). The presence of

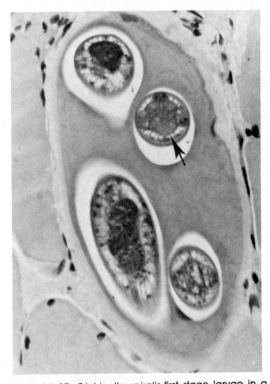

Figure 14–87. *Trichinella spiralis* first stage larvae in a skeletal muscle fiber showing a cross section of the stichosome esophagus (arrow) (x425).

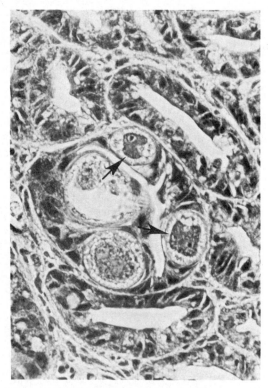

Figure 14–88. *Trichinella spiralis* adult in the mucosa of the small intestine of a rat (x480). Two cross sections of stichosome esophagus (arrows) are visible.

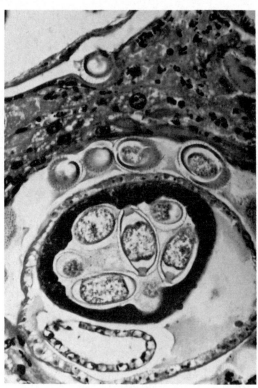

Figure 14–89. *Capillaria hepatica* in the liver of a rat (x360). Eggs with bipolar plugs are visible in the uterus.

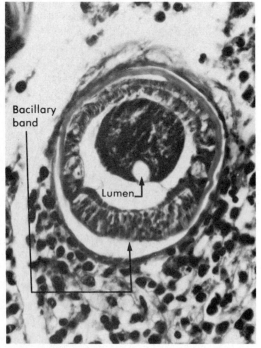

Figure 14–90. Cross section of the esophageal region of *Trichuris discolor* in the cecum of a heifer (x500).

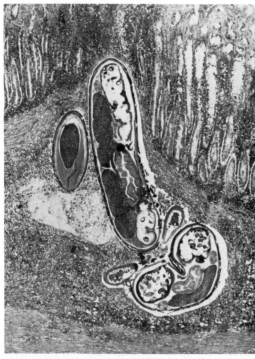

Figure 14–91. *Trichuris vulpis* in the submucosa of the large intestine of a dog (x33).

single-celled eggs with bipolar plugs in the uterus is the best criterion for identifying *Capillaria* in tissue sections (Fig. 14-89). *Trichuris* has similar eggs but is found only in the large intestine, about the only site eschewed by *Capillaria*. *Anatrichosoma* in the nasal mucosa of primates and *Trichosomoides* in the bladder of rats have larvated eggs with bipolar plugs (see Figs. 6-64 and 12-36).

Trichuris has one bacillary band in the esophageal region; this is always located opposite the capillary lumen of the stichosome esophagus (Fig. 14-90). The stout "handle" portion of the adult normally lies free in the lumen of the large intestine, while the thin "whiplash" esophageal portion is threaded through the mucous membrane. Immature *Trichuris* lie entirely within the mucosa and are of uniform diameter. In an unusual case of *Trichuris vulpis* infection marked by persistent diarrhea, entire worms lie in the submucosa (Fig. 14-91).

ACANTHOCEPHALANS

Acanthocephalans are round in cross section, have a body cavity, but lack a digestive tract. The hypodermis is much thicker than the longitudinal somatic muscle layer lying internal to it. The hypodermis contains

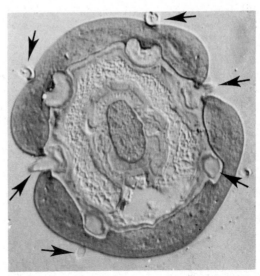

Figure 14–93. Cross section through the proboscis of *Neoechinorhynchus* showing hooks (arrows) (x320).

spaces called *lacunae;* eggs are found floating free in the body cavity of females (Fig. 14-92). The proboscis, armed with many hooks, is the structure most likely to be encountered in sections of intestine (Fig. 14-93).

Acanthocephalan cystacanths are typically found in the arthropod intermediate hosts but occasionally also encysted in the tissues

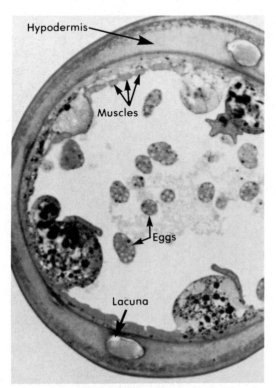

Figure 14–92. Cross section of a female acanthocephalan, *Neoechinorhynchus* (x240).

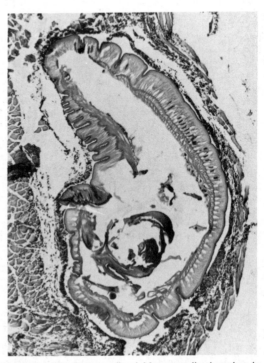

Figure 14–94. Cystacanth of *Macracanthorhynchus ingens* in skeletal muscle of a golden hamster (*Mesocricetus auratus*) (x66). (Specimen provided by Dr. G. R. Fahnestock.)

of paratenic hosts (Fig. 14-94). The thick hypodermis lying external to the muscle layer provides the principal clue to the identity of the cystacanth.

REFERENCES

Binford, C. H., and Connor, D. H. (Editors) (1976): Pathology of Tropical and Extraordinary Diseases. Vols. I and II. A.F.I.P. Washington, D. C.

Chitwood, M. B., and Lichtenfels, J. R. (1972): Identification of Parasitic Metazoa in Tissue Sections. Exp. Parasitol., 32, 407-519.

Kazacos, K. R. (1983): Raccoon roundworms (Baylisascaris procyonis)—A cause of Animal and Human Disease. Station Bulletin No. 422. Agr. Expt. Sta., Purdue University.

Nichols, R. L. (1956a): The etiology of visceral larva migrans. I. Diagnostic morphology of infective second-stage Toxocara larvae. J. Parasit., 42, 349-362.

Nichols, R. L. (1956b): The etiology of visceral larva migrans. II. Comparative larval morphology of Ascaris lumbricoides, Necator americanus, Strongyloides stercoralis, and Ancylostoma caninum. J. Parasitol., 42, 363-399.

S. C. Schell (1970): How to Know the Trematodes, Wm. C. Brown Company, Dubuque, Iowa.

INDEX

Note: Page numbers in *italics* represent illustrations; a t following a number indicates a table. Entries in all capitals are trade names.